CHILD HEALTH IN THE TROPICS

Sixth Nutricia – Cow & Gate Symposium

CHILD HEALTH
IN THE TROPICS

Leuven, 18–21 October 1983

EDITORS:

R.E. EECKELS, O. RANSOME-KUTI, C.C. KROONENBERG

1985 **MARTINUS NIJHOFF PUBLISHERS**
a member of the KLUWER ACADEMIC PUBLISHERS GROUP
BOSTON / DORDRECHT / LANCASTER

Distributors

for the United States and Canada: Kluwer Academic Publishers, 190 Old Derby Street, Hingham, MA 02043, USA
for the UK and Ireland: Kluwer Academic Publishers, MTP Press Limited, Falcon House, Queen Square, Lancaster LA1 1RN, UK
for all other countries: Kluwer Academic Publishers Group, Distribution Center, P.O. Box 322, 3300 AH Dordrecht, The Netherlands

Library of Congress Cataloging in Publication Data

```
Nutricia-Cow & Gate Symposium (6th : 1983 : Louvain,
  Belgium)
  Child health in the tropics.

  Includes index.
  1. Child health services--Tropics--Congresses.
2. Children--Tropics--Nutrition--Congresses. 3. Diarrhea
in children--Tropics--Congresses. 4. Infants (Newborn)--
Tropics--Congresses. I. Eeckels, R. E. II. Ransome-
Kuti, O. III. Kroonenberg, C. C. IV. Title. [DNLM:
1. Child Nutrition--congresses. 2. Diarrhea--congresses.
3. Perinatology--congresses. 4. Primary Health Care--
congresses. 5. Tropical Medicine--congresses.
W3 NU777 6th 1983c / WC 680 N976 1983c]
RJ103.T76N88   1983      362.1'9892'00913     85-8895
```

ISBN-13: 978-94-010-8719-3   e-ISBN-13: 978-94-009-5012-2
DOI: 10.1007/978-94-009-5012-2

Copyright

Preface

It is almost twenty years ago since under Nutricia's auspices the first Nutricia Symposium took place. Professor Jonxis was mainly responsible for the organization of the earlier symposia, whilst Professor Visser organized the fifth Nutricia Symposium in 1978.

This book is the commitment to paper of the lectures given during the sixth Nutricia/Cow & Gate Symposium held in Louvain in 1983. Both Professor Eeckels and Professor Ransome-Kuti succeeded in collecting a panel of experts on 'Child Health in the Tropics'.

We hope, in fact we are sure, that you will consider the contents of this book a daily stimulation in your medical profession.

October 1984

Contents

SESSION I
FEEDING, FEEDING PRACTICES AND GROWTH
Chairman: Chap-Yung Yeung

SESSION II
DIARRHOEAL DISEASES
Chairman: O. Ransome-Kuti

SESSION III
NUTRITION
Chairman: J.H.P. Jonxis

SESSION IV
THE NEWBORN INFANT
Chairman: O.P. Ghai

SESSION V
TRAINING AND TEACHING – PRIMARY HEALTH CARE SYSTEMS
Chairman: R.G. Hendrickse

List of authors

A. Alisjahbana, Department of Child Health, Medical School, University Padjadjaran, Bandung, Indonesia
Co-author: A. Usman

A. Bamisaiye, Institute of Child Health and Primary Care, College of Medicine, University of Lagos, P.M.B. 1001, Surulere, Lagos, Nigeria

J.M. Bengoa, Vittoria, Spain

E.R. Boersma, St. Elisabeth Hospital, Willemstad, Curaçao, Netherlands Antilles
Co-authors: Th.M. Hoorntje, N.H. Hutter, P.J. Offringa, J.H.P. Jonxis, R.A. Soer

D. Brasseur, Department of Pediatrics, Free University of Brussels, Belgium
Co-authors: Ph. Goyens, H.L. Vis

R.E. Brown, St. Joseph's Hospital and Medical Centre, Department of Community Medicine, 703 Main Street, Paterson, New Jersey 07503, U.S.A.

S.R. Daga, Institute of Child Health and Department of Preventive & Social Medicine, Grant Medical College & J.J. Hospital, Bombay, 400 008 India
Co-author: A.S. Daga

J.M. Feris, Children's Hospital 'Dr. Robert Reid Cabral', Santo Domingo, Dominican Republic
Co-author: R. Mendoza

R.G. Hendrickse, Department of Tropical Pediatrics, School of Tropical Medicine, Pembroke Place, Liverpool L3 5QA, U.K.

Z. Isani, National Institute of Child Health, Jinnah Postgraduate Medical Centre, Karachi, Pakistan

P.G. Janssens, Former Director, Institute of Tropical Medicine, Nationale Straat 155, 2000 Antwerp, Belgium

S.R. Khan, King Edward Medical College, Lahore, Pakistan

W. Klaver, International Course in Food Science and Nutrition, Lawickse Allee 11, 6701 AN Wageningen, The Netherlands

J.A. Kusin, Royal Tropical Institute, Amsterdam, The Netherlands
Co-author: S. Kardjati

S. Martodipuro, Research and Development Center for Health Service, Ministry of Health, 17 Indrapura Surabaya, Indonesia

Y.N. Mathur, National Institute of Nutrition, Indian Council of Medical Research, Hyderabad-500 007, India
Co-author: D.H. Rao

A. Molla, International Centre for Diarrhoeal Disease Research, Bangladesh, GPO Box 128, Dhaka-2, Bangladesh

Co-authors: A.M. Molla, M. Khatun

A.M. Molla, International Centre for Diarrhoeal Disease Research, Bangladesh, GPO Box 128, Dhaka-2 Bangladesh
Co-authors: S.A. Sarker, A. Molla, M. Khatoon, W.B. Greenough III

D. Morley, Institute of Child Health, University of London, Tropical Child Health Unit, 30 Guildford Street, London WC1N 1EH, U.K.

T.C. Okeahialam, Department of Pediatrics, University of Nigeria Teaching Hospital, P.M.B. 1129, Enugu, Nigeria

S.A. Olowe, Department of Pediatrics, College of Medicine, University of Lagos, P.M.B. 12003, Lagos, Nigeria

A. Omololu, University of Ibadan, Department of Human Nutrition, Ibadan, Nigeria

A. Pradilla, World Health Organisation, 1211 Geneva 27, Switzerland

M.G.M. Rowland, Medical Research Council Laboratories, P.O. Box 273, Bangul, Gambia
Co-authors: S.G.J. Goh, S. Tulloch, D.T. Dunn, R.J. Hayes

R. Sakr, Pediatric Department and the Biochemistry Department, Cairo University, al Falaki Square, Bab El Louk, Cairo, Egypt
Co-authors: D. Fleita, S. Samuel, A. Abdelwahab

L. Sinisterra, Human Ecology Research Foundation, Apartado Aereo 7308, Cali, Colombia

J.P. Stanfield, University of Newcastle upon Tyne, Department of Child Health, Newcastle upon Tyne NE1 4LP, U.K.

Suharyono, Department of Child Health, Medical School, University of Indonesia/Dr. Cipto Mangunkusumo General Hospital, Jakarta, Indonesia

N. Tafari, Department of Pediatrics and Child Health, Perinatal Care Unit, P.O. Box 1768, Addis Ababa, Ethiopia

V. Tanphaichitr, Division of Nutrition and Biochemical Medicine, Department of Medicine and Research Centre, Faculty of Medicine, Ramathibodi Hospital and Institute of Nutrition, Mahidol University, Rama 6 Road, Bangkok 10400, Thailand

V.S. Tanphaichitr, Division of Hematology and Endocrinology, Department of Pediatrics, Faculty of Medicine Siriraj Hospital, Mahidol University, Bangkok, 10700, Thailand
Co-authors: C. Tuchinda, V. Suvatte, S. Tuchinda

Chap-Yung Yeung, Department of Pediatrics, University of Hong Kong, Queen Mary Hospital, Hong Kong

List of participants

W.Y. Aalbersberg, Ede, The Netherlands
B.S.F. Adjou-Moumouni, Cotonou, Republic of Benin
A. Alisjahbana, Bandung, Indonesia
A. Bamisaiye, Lagos, Nigeria
E.R. Boersma, Willemstad, Curaçao, Netherlands Antilles
C. Bourgeois, Brussels, Belgium
D. Brasseur, Brussels, Belgium
R.E. Brown, Paterson, New Jersey, U.S.A.
C.A. Canosa, Valencia, Spain
C. Chintu, Lusaka, Zambia
S.R. Daga, Bombay, India
A.M.F.L.P. da Graca, Maputo, Mozambique
G.A. de Jonge, Amsterdam, The Netherlands
R. de Meijer, Leuven, Belgium
N.A. de Soto, Santo Domingo, Dominican Republic
R. Eeckels, Leuven, Belgium
E. Eggermont, Leuven, Belgium
H. Ejoh, Onitsha-Anabra State, Nigeria
J.M. Feris, Santo Domingo, Dominican Republic
J. Fernandes, Groningen, The Netherlands
O.P. Ghai, New Delhi, India
Ph. Goyens, Brussels, Belgium
R. Gyselings, Mons, Belgium
K. Haque, Riad, Saudi Arabia
R.G. Hendrickse, Liverpool, U.K.
R.J.J. Hermus, Zeist, The Netherlands
Z. Isani, Karachi, Pakistan
P.G. Janssens, Antwerp, Belgium
J.H.P. Jonxis, Groningen, The Netherlands
S. Kardjati, Amsterdam, The Netherlands
H. Khalifa, Casablanca, Maroc
S.R. Khan, Lahore, Pakistan
W. Klaver, Wageningen, The Netherlands
J.A. Kusin, Amsterdam, The Netherlands
A.A.O. Laditan, Ibadan, Nigeria
B. Madukwe, Lagos, Nigeria
S. Martodipuro, Surabaya, Indonesia

Y.N. Mathur, Hyderabad, India
A. Molla, Dhaka, Bangladesh
A.M. Molla, Dhaka, Bangladesh
C. Morley, London, U.K.
T.C. Okeahialam, Enugu, Nigeria
S.A. Olowe. Lagos, Nigeria
A. Omololu, Ibadan, Nigeria
M. Parent, Liège, Belgium
A. Pradilla, Geneva, Switzerland
L.H.J. Ramaekers, Maastricht, The Netherlands
O. Ransome-Kuti, Lagos, Nigeria
M.G.M. Rowland, Banjul, The Gambia
R. Sakr, Cairo, Egypt
E.D.A.M. Schretlen, Nijmegen, The Netherlands
J. Senecal, Rennes, France
J. Senterre, Liège, Belgium
L. Sinisterra, Cali, Colombia
J.P. Stanfield, Newcastle upon Tyne, U.K.
Suharyono, Salemba-Jakarta, Indonesia
A.H. Sutanto, Medan, Indonesia
N. Tafari, Addis Ababa, Ethiopia
V. Tanphaichitr, Bangkok, Thailand
V.S. Tanphaichitr, Bangkok, Thailand
Tu Giay, Hanoi, Vietnam
K. Vallante, Leuven, Belgium
J.L. van den Brande, Utrecht, The Netherlands
H.H. van Gelderen, Leiden, The Netherlands
H. van Loon, Antwerp, Belgium
V.W.A. Vermeulen, Curaçao, Netherlands Antilles
H.K.A. Visser, Rotterdam, The Netherlands
J. Vuylsteke, Antwerp, Belgium
H.W.A. Voorhoeve, Rijswijk, The Netherlands
O.C. Ward, Crumlin-Dublin, Eire
C.A. Winkel, Colombia
J.L. Yntema, Curaçao, Netherlands Antilles
Chap-Yung Yeung, Hong Kong

Participants Nutricia/Cow & Gate

C. Bosmans
G. de Graaf
C.C. Kroonenberg
J. Norton-Booth

O.D. Suurenbroek
J. Wells
B. van Woelderen

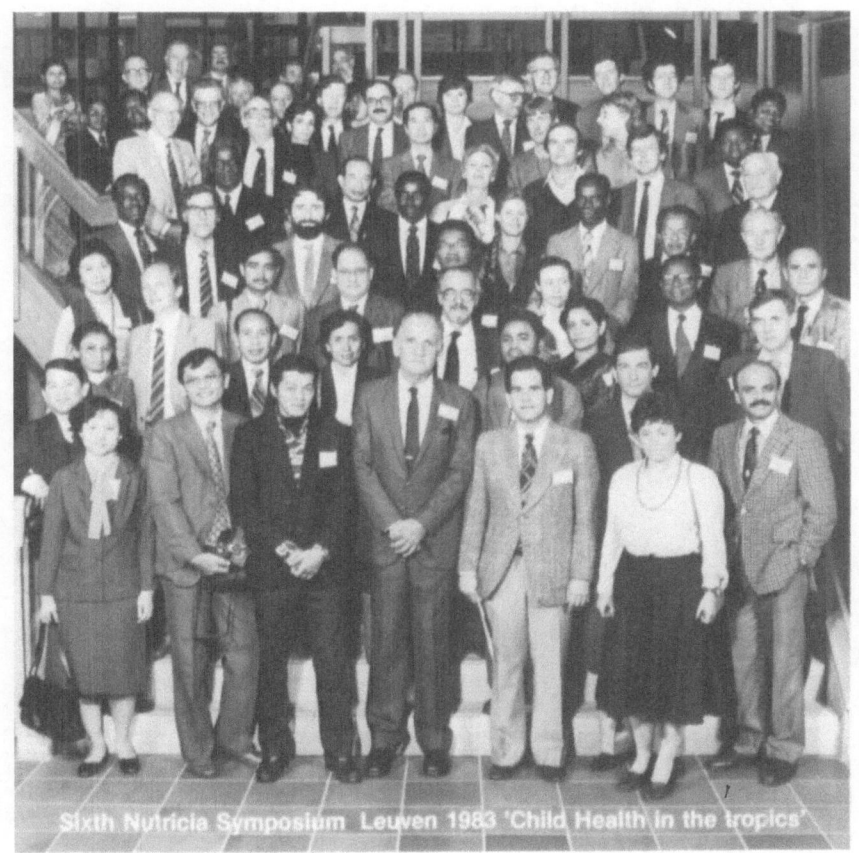

Sixth Nutricia Symposium Leuven 1983 'Child Health in the tropics'

Feeding, feeding practices and growth

Chairman: Chap-Yung Yeung

The practice of breastfeeding

A. OMOLOLU

Introduction

The practice of breastfeeding, it is agreed, is as old as human beings and, yet, over the past thirty years as scientific interest in the practice has revived, we have not endeavoured to study the practice in an environment where it is still the norm. On the other hand, theoretical questions like 'How long can breast milk alone support a child?' have been our concern; instead of 'How do the people who have been and still practise breastfeeding deal with supplementation?'. The practice of breastfeeding must have worked over the centuries in these communities – why is it now breaking down? What can now be done to make it work?

Over the past ten years, the Department of Human Nutrition, University of Ibadan, has had the opportunity of carrying out studies both in the rural as well as urban populations of the country. With the support of the World Health Organisation, the Nestlé Nutrition Research Council and the University of Ibadan, cross-sectional, longitudinal and in-depth studies have been carried out into the present practices of breastfeeding, the intakes of breastmilk by babies as well as the factors – traditional, social, economic, foetal and maternal – that could and do affect the practice of breastfeeding.

This paper will discuss the present practice of breastfeeding in the rural areas, show why it works, the strains and stresses that affect it as well as the modifications that now take place amongst the urban populations.

Present practice amongst the rural and urban poor

Breastfeeding is still practised by these groups because it is the only way of feeding the baby that they know, that they have seen work and that they can afford. Even in the rural areas, mothers have heard of and seen babies being artificially fed. Over 50% of the rural mothers believe that artificial feeding is better than breastfeeding; but they know that it is expensive and that they cannot afford it. In the urban areas, most feeding mothers hope and look forward to the time when they will be able to afford to feed their babies artificially. To the illiterate mothers in both rural and urban areas, artificial feeding is a mystique whose dangers and details they do not know. For example, these mothers cannot believe that artificial feeding can cause the death of babies, for it is their own babies who are breastfed that die, not the babies of the well-to-do who are artificially fed! They breastfeed their babies, therefore, because it is the only way they know. To them, there is no practical alternative; anyway, breastfeeding is widely practised.

As soon as the baby is born and separated from the mother, the first feed that is given is water – in sips. Small amounts are given, either by spoon or by force-feeding. Water feeding is continued until the child cries vigorously and makes 'the motions of sucking' and the mother is rested and strong enough to breastfeed. In a recent study, the average time interval between birth and the first breastfeed was 10 hours, ranging between a few minutes and 25 hours. Thus, breastfeeding is not rushed. Both the mother and baby are fit and ready before it is carried out, and, invariably, the first act of breastfeeding is enjoyed by both. This is a lesson for us.

After this first enjoyable act of breastfeeding, the frequency depends on the mother and baby. Primips usually breastfeed the baby whenever it cries. When the mother gets tired and complains, she is then advised to give water feeds alternately. Multiparas usually know this and, whenever the baby cries, decide whether to give the breast or water. Thus, there is never a question of giving the breast every four hours – mothers decide whether to give the breast or water.

During the first 14 days of life, if a baby cries for food frequently – every 2 hours instead of 3 to 4 hours – mothers were observed to give relatively large amounts of water by force-feeding (up to 40 ml or more at a time). This amount of water enlarged the stomach, made the abdomen full and tense and normally caused some discomfort for the baby for about 30 minutes. This water feeding was repeated two or three times in the day. Usually, when next offered the breast, the baby would take a larger amount and be satisfied for a longer period. Thus, the mother had a longer rest between feeds.

It was also noticed that as the baby got older, night feeding was stopped by the use of water feeds. Babies, who were adequately fed on the breast during the day and who cried during the night were offered only water during the night. Sometimes, they were force-fed water whenever they cried for food during the night. Within a week or so, these babies stopped crying for food at night, but they were usually given the breast at about 10 pm and again between 5 am and 6 am. In this way, the mother was assured of a good night's rest by the time the baby was 2 months old at the latest.

Support for breastfeeding

One important practice that ensures the proper initiation of breastfeeding is found in most tribes and communities, not only in Nigeria but all over Africa. This practice stipulates that a woman after child-birth does not go out of her home for 40 days. The main preoccupation and duty of the husband during the wife's pregnancy is to make adequate preparations for this 40-day confinement. He has to provide enough food or staples, fire wood and other necessities for the wife; also a companion from his family, usually his mother, a sister, etc. or someone from the wife's family. During these 40 days, the mother does no housework. She is bathed, massaged and fed – all she has to do is to look after and feed the baby. She thus gets the rest she needs after child-birth, eats enough to make up for her losses during pregnancy and parturition and also builds up a reserve for lactation. She comes out after the 40 days' confinement in new clothes and accessories to show the new baby to the world.

Thus, traditional societies ensure adequate rest and food for the mother after delivery. She is excluded from any housework, massaged and pampered by a women companion and relieved of any responsibilities to husband or home. For 40 days she has a holiday with her baby. What can modern society offer the breastfeeding mother? A maternity leave which leaves her full of housework, care of her other children and husband? Christening parties and visitors?

By the end of the 40 day-confinement, the mother's family or husband would have designated a young girl – 8, 10, 12 or 14 years old – who would live with and help her look after the baby. If she is a multipara, she may already have an older girl who will play this part. It is the responsibility of the husband to provide for this helper.

After the confinement, the mother takes on her household duties but is not usually allowed to go to the fields or do work outside the house until the baby is 3 months old. During this time, the mother is expected to have the baby with her all the time – on her back, in her hands or on her lap. If she has to go out, the baby goes with her and she is expected to breastfeed whenever the baby cries for food. No one looks twice at a breastfeeding mother – except to give support.

During the confinement, mother trains the baby so that what we call 'on demand' feeding is usually a 3 or 4 hourly feeding. Thus, the mother has a very good idea of when the baby will cry for food and thus plan her activities. She also knows that if she is away from the child at this time, the 'let down reflex' will release the milk.

Number of feeds

The concept that most of us have is that the African baby is always on the breast and that on many occasions the breast is offered as a pacifier. This image is not true.

In one sample of 45 infants aged 1 month and from a rural setting, the highest number of breast feeds given during 24 hours was 8 – and the average number of feeds amongst the group was 6. In another group of 25 infants aged 3 months who were fully breastfed, the highest and mean numbers of breastfeedings per day were 6. In both cases, the interval between feeds works out at 3 hours. In the case of the 1 month olds, 8 feeds in 24 hours; and in the 3 months olds, 6 feeds in 18 hours as there are no night feeds. The breast is never used as a pacifier except on rare occasions when mother is at an important meeting or discussion which she cannot leave and the child cries incessantly. On such rare occasions, the mother tries every other means of pacifying the child – playing, making faces, change of nappies, cooling – before resorting to the breast as a pacifier.

Supplementation

Though water is regularly given to babies, it is not looked upon as a food. The first supplement given in rural areas is a gruel made of maize and water, millet, sorghum or rice and water. The gruel is cooked thick. At the time of feeding, the gruel is made thin with hot water; as the child gets older, less water is added. The gruel is given by force-feeding, spoon or cup, and alternate feeds of the gruel are given with the breast.

There is no set age or weight for introducing the gruel. Most mothers, when asked why they decided to give the gruel when they did, replied 'I just decided' or 'the child was old enough'. Only a few mothers said that the child was hungry or cried and that was when the gruel was introduced. By force-feeding, large amounts of the gruel may be fed – much more than the child would take voluntarily. Thus, the gruel is usually given by force-feeding when the mother is going to be away and does not want the baby to cry or when she wants to have a rest.

Though a gruel may be introduced into the feeding pattern as early as 3 months, it was found that it was only by 6 months that more than 50% of mothers used the gruel. The gruel was given *not* to stop breastfeeding but to augment it. Breast-feeding usually continued till the baby was 12 months or more.

The addition of other foods to the baby's diet depends upon the baby. If he is forward and grabs adult food during meals, he is allowed to eat and play with the morsel. Soon, he will be offered the food whenever it is eaten. In this way, the forward child, in a family that eats together, has better chances of getting to know and have adult food than the shy or sickly child, who is corseted by the mother, in a family that eats at different times.

End of breastfeeding

The mother is the only person who decides when breastfeeding should stop. This is because if the child gets sick or dies, it is the mother who has the blame. Traditionally, she is not expected to get pregnant whilst breastfeeding. The husband, on the other hand, tries to induce her to start marital relationships as early as possible. If she agrees and becomes pregnant, she must then stop breastfeeding and wean the child. This is why it seems to some observers that weaning is abrupt in Africa. The stoppage of breastfeeding is decided by another pregnancy. If the mother did not plan to wean the child but falls for the inducement of her husband, she may find herself in this predicament. The older the woman gets, the more she learns and thus takes her time in starting marital relationships. This is why older women and mothers that have lost a previous baby tend to breastfeed longest. They are afraid to take the chance.

Discussion

With the above discussion as a background, one can look at the problems of breastfeeding from the point of view of the modern woman.

The working mother, who has to travel away from home for fixed hours everyday, is becoming a common phenomenon all over the world. In most countries of Africa, the government departments and some commercial houses allow a 'maternity leave'. This is at most three months – 6 weeks before and 6 weeks after delivery. This means that the mothers who wishes to breastfeed her baby has only 6 weeks in which to institute and then stop breastfeeding! It takes 40 days to institute breastfeeding satisfactorily; yet the mother now has to stop in two weeks! This is not good enough. Most mother who satisfactorily start breastfeeding before returning to work complain of the 'let-down reflex' which soaks their dresses for weeks after their return to work. The answer to this problem is for doctors and nutritionists to insist on mothers having at least two months of their maternity leave after delivery.

The provision of crèches for breastfeeding mothers and their babies only works where mother live close to their working places. In most developing countries, most working mothers live far from their working places and travel long distances in overcrowded public transport to get to work. These mothers find it impractical to bring their small babies to their working places.

In most traditional societies – and most societies in both developed and developing countries are still traditional when it comes to the roles of men and women, fathers and mothers – men are not expected to be involved in household duties and child care. There is a great need for education. Education at home, in schools, at work and in all aspects of life – that, with the unitary family, cooperation and support between the father and mother in all types of household duties and chores make for a better family life.

Growth and weaning in urban Gambian infants

M.G.M. ROWLAND, S.G.J. GOH, S. TULLOCH, D.T. DUNN
and R.J. HAYES

Introduction

It is well known that the early childhood years in developing countries are a critical period in terms of survival [1]. We are aware that malnutrition in the preschool child often has its origins in infancy [2]; the beginning of the onslaught of infectious diseases to which young children are subjected is similarly timed. The relationship between these two aspects of impaired health is well documented [3]. One of the best known examples of this nutrition-infection interaction is the inter-relationship between diarrhoeal disease and growth impairment. So striking is the association of this synergistic phenomenon with early feeding patterns that the term 'weanling diarrhoea' was coined more than 20 years ago [4].

A clear example of this problem is seen in The Gambia where there is widespread and severe growth faltering in rural children starting around three months of age and an increasing burden of diarrhoea occurring in the second half of infancy; both events occur around the time of the onset of the weaning period [5]. There is a marked deficit in energy intake at the time of deviation from normal growth standards [6] and a highly significant negative correlation between diarrhoea and growth has been demonstrated at this age [7]. Also described is the potential importance of contaminated weaning foods in the epidemiology of the early childhood diarrhoeas [8]. Despite the importance attached to the 'weaning dilemma' [5] – i.e. the balance to the struck between the merits of early dietary supplementation and the dangers of gastrointestinal infection carried with it – there has been remarkably little effort to try and define the precise impact of the initiation of weaning on health and growth. A good attempt was made by Watkinson who claimed that children receiving the highest breast milk intakes had later weaning dates, a delayed onset of diarrhoea-induced weight loss and significantly greater weight than their less privileged counterparts by the age of one year [9].

An important controversy centres on this scenario; it is the question of whether mothers, particularly in the third world, introduce weaning foods inappropriately early, sabotaging their lactation, prematurely exposing their infants to the risk of gastrointestinal infection and thus contributing significantly and unnecessarily to the epidemiology of early childhood malnutrition in their own offspring.

Materials and methods

In 1981 a cohort study was started in an urban community in The Gambia in the town of Bakau some ten kilometres from the capital Banjul. This community numbers approximately 10,000 people inhabiting an area of 0.5 km², being around the sixth largest and densest urban population in the country.

Living conditions are typical of the underprivileged third world. Roads in the town are unsurfaced and often lined by open drains. Houses are mostly terraced and of mud-brick, or less often of cement, with corrugated metal roofs. About 85% of the dwelling clusters or compounds have some sanitational facilities, usually in the form of pit latrines [10]. There is a fairly comprehensive public standpipe system delivering potable chlorinated water. Primary health care is provided by the Government Health Centre about one kilometre distant and more medical facilities are available at the neighbouring Medical Research Council Laboratories in Fajara. The vast majority of mothers in Bakau obtain antenatal care at the health centre and are subsequently delivered there or report with their baby for a check up within twenty four hours of delivery.

In this study 126 infants were recruited within two weeks of birth at a rate of approximately ten per month. Eighty per cent were studied for one year or more, default mainly arising from migration. Morbidity was monitored by weekly questionnaires administered in the homes by visiting field workers who also documented feeding details. Routine anthropometry (weight and length) was carried out at monthly call clinics and complementary morbidity data were obtained at these and other clinics. Routine childhood immunizations were carried out according to the current policies of the Gambian Government Maternal and Child Health Programme and all illnesses were actively treated with appropriate medication. Breast milk intakes were regularly monitored in a 75% sample of the cohort until weaning was established and again at one year of age. The aim was to determine the relationships between breast feeding and weaning practices and infant growth and morbidity with special emphasis on diarrhoeal diseases. Analysis of the data is not yet complete but some of the results are described below.

Results

Selected maternal characteristics

The foregoing description of the township has shown that this was not a privileged urban area nor were the cohort subjects in any sense an urban elite. Of the cohort mothers approximately half were illiterate and only one in six had proceeded to secondary school or beyond. Twenty five per cent were teenagers and only one half were older than twenty three years. One quarter of the mothers were single and the same proportion were primiparous. In contrast to the rural situation, however, two thirds of the mothers were housewives with no other form of employment.

Feeding practices

All mothers breast fed their children from birth. The onset of weaning, defined as the regular addition of other foods to the infant's diet documented in three successive weeks, occurred between one and forty six weeks with a median of thirteen weeks. These data are illustrated in Figure 1. About one third of the children started weaning before their earliest Keneba counterparts [11]. Despite this, the urban nature of the community and the availability of a number of alternatives, traditional weaning foods only were given to 75% of children, the remainder being weaned using predominantly commerical infant formula or a mixture of traditional and processed foods. Perhaps predictably formula foods tended to be used when children started weaning earlier, the median age of introduction being six weeks (Figure 1). One reason for early weaning was the mother's return to paid employment, often around six weeks after the birth of the child. Some of these women introduced bottle feeds as early as one week of age in order to establish a pattern of supplementary feeding before starting work. Despite this, all women regularly breast fed into the second year of life except for one mother who completed weaning at 11 months. There is little doubt that within this community there were mothers who were regularly maintaining lactation for a year or more despite periods of around 8 hours per day of separation from their infants. Breast milk intake data is not yet complete but preliminary results suggest that volumes consumed were high compared with those documented in rural women in Keneba [12].

Growth

Birthweights obtained at the health centre at or shortly after birth were lower than normal standards with a mean weight of 3.2 (SD 0.4) kg for boys and 3.0

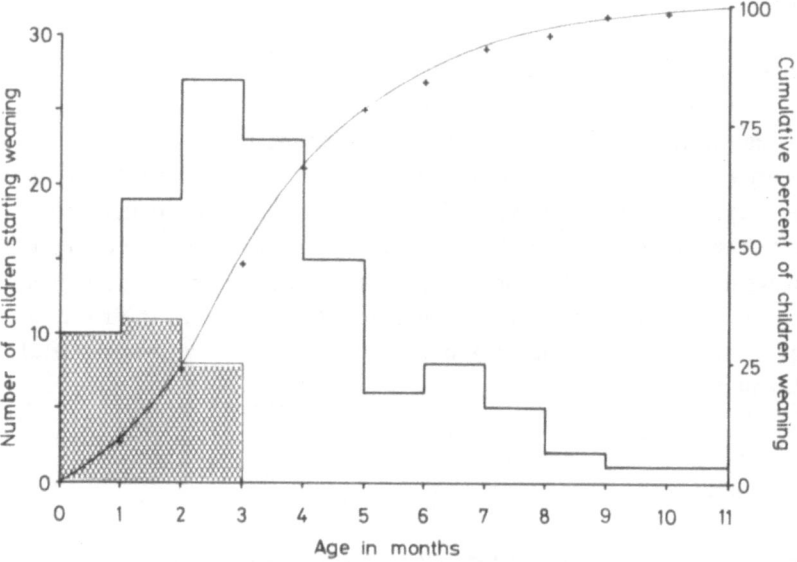

Figure 1. Age at onset of weaning in urban Gambian infants (n = 117). ■ indicates use of an infant formula food. Cumulative percentages calculated using life table methods (n = 126).

(SD 0.4) kg for girls. There was no evidence of seasonal variation, in contrast to earlier Keneba findings [13].

Nutritional status in the first half of infancy was strikingly good and by three months these urban children had overshot the accepted norm for weight. Growth in weight and length is illustrated in relation to the currently used American NCHS standards [14] in Figure 2. The possible reasons and implications underlying this pattern have been discussed elsewhere [12].

From three months of age growth velocity declined markedly and from six months mean weights fell below the international standards to levels which appear inadequate even in relation to the more conservative estimates that have recently been proposed for predominantly breast fed communities [15]. This change in growth performance occurred around the time when the majority of children were being introduced to weaning foods.

Impact of weaning on growth

What role does weaning play in this quite marked alteration in growth performance which follows such a promising start? The first exercise was to compare the growth of children who were weaning with those as yet unweaned and these data are illustrated in Figure 3. After three months of age, exclusively breast fed children were significantly heavier than those who had started the weaning

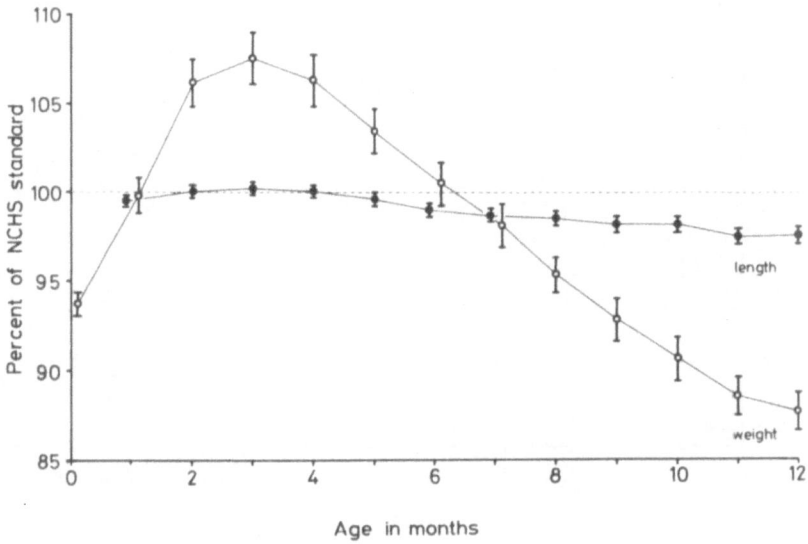

Figure 2. Growth in weight (—○—) and length (—●—) of urban Gambian infants expressed as Mean ± SE in relation to the NCHS [14] standards (n between 90 and 126).

process. Though compatible with the concept that the onset of weaning led to impaired growth performance, such results are in fact open to other interpretations. For example this picture could also arise as a result of the children who were smallest being weaned earliest.

To examine this possibility, birthweights were compared between infants starting to wean in the first month of life and those weaning later. Similarly, weights at one month of age were compared between children starting to wean in the second month of life and those weaning after two months of age. Corresponding analysis were carried out at monthly intervals and the results are illustrated in Figure 4. From three months of age onwards infants starting to wean during a given month tended to be lighter at the beginning of this month than those who remained exclusively breast fed. Using a rank test for each month and combining the results from three months onwards, this difference was just significant (p<0.05). There was no such trend below three months of age. These data are compatible with the hypothesis that at least from three months of age mothers tend to start weaning the smaller infants.

The nature of the growth pattern following weaning was next investigated to determine whether infants who had just been weaned appeared to be growing less well in the subsequent month than those who remained exclusively breast fed. In children starting weaning before three months of age there was a consistent trend towards slower growth and lower weight in the month following weaning compared with their non-weaning counterparts.

14

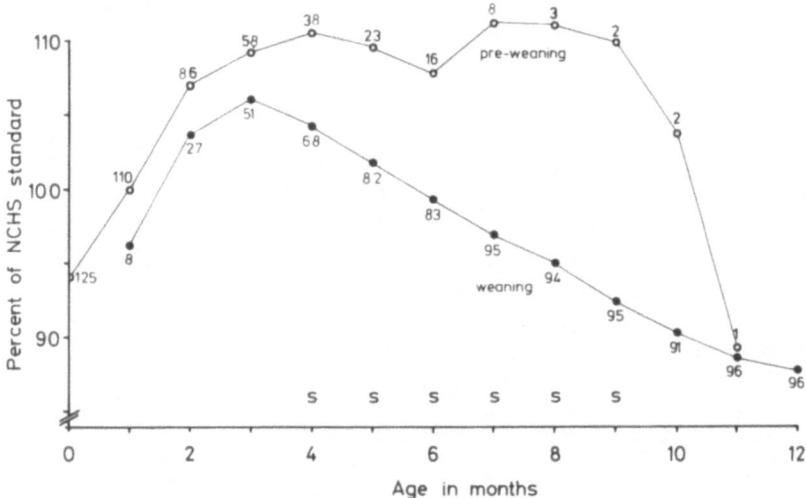

Figure 3. Mean weight-for-age of pre-weaning (—○—) and weaning (—●—) Gambian infants. S indicates a statistically significant difference (p<0.05).

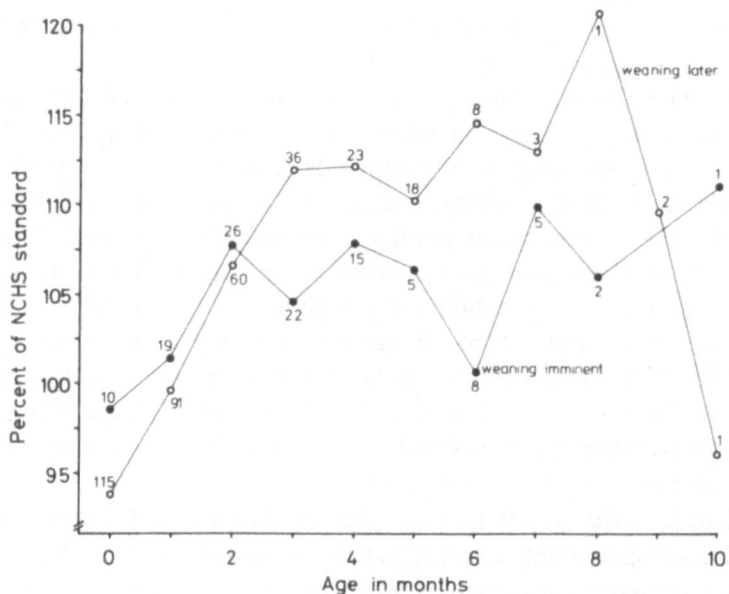

Figure 4. Mean weight-for-age of infants weaning in the subsequent month (—●—) compared with those weaning later (—○—).

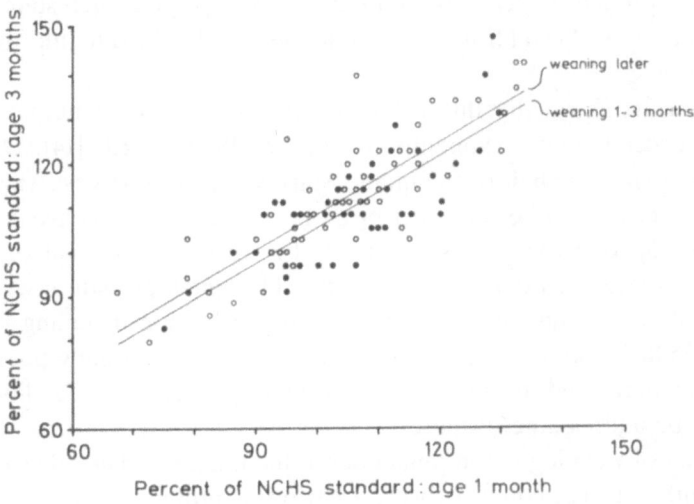

Figure 5. Relationship between weight-for-age of infants at ages 1 and 3 months, and fitted regression lines in those weaning between these ages (—●—) and in those weaning later (—○—) (n = 100).

This effect is illustrated in Figure 5 in which weight-for-age at one month is plotted against that at three months in two groups of infants, those starting to wean between one and three months and those weaning subsequently. Regression lines were fitted for these two groups, assuming equal slopes, and may be used to estimate the mean weight-for-age at three months for a given value at one month of age. It can be seen that this value is lower in those infants starting to wean between one and three months than in those who continue to be exclusively breast fed. This difference was close to statistical significance (p≈0.05).

No such effect on growth was apparent in children starting to wean at a later age; subjects were too few to permit this analysis beyond six months of age.

Discussion

The weaning period has long been recognised as a particularly hazardous phase in childhood [16]. Because of this some have advocated the strategy of delaying the onset of weaning in underprivileged communities even when there are nutritional grounds for starting to complement the diet of breast fed infants [17]. There has been considerable international interest and effort expended in identifying the point at which weaning is appropriate, with a view to avoiding an unnecessarily early introduction of other foods [18] though the futility of attempting to make generalizations on this subject has been recently emphasised [19]. It is assumed that weaning should not be started so early as to deliberately or inadvertently result in the premature cessation of breast feeding [18] but such statements are valueless in terms of establishing guidelines designed to lead to improved weaning practices.

Our data have shown that during the first three months of infancy mean growth in weight exceeds that documented in the NCHS standards [14]. During this period approximately half of the infants start weaning, a process which usually continues over a period of one year or more. There is no evidence in this early weaning group that the process is initiated in response to small size or poor growth and there is an overal tendency for subsequent growth in weight to be adversely affected. This could be due to a number of factors including a reduction of breast milk intake consequent upon weaning, a nutritionally poor weaning food supplement, and an increase in morbidity, particularly diarrhoea. These issues will be addressed elsewhere.

The onset of weaning in the remainder of the infants, which takes place after three months of age, coincides with a period of prolonged decline in growth performance in relation to the international standards, and tends to be carried out earlier in lower weight infants or those who are growing more slowly in the preceding month. The use of these two criteria, particularly the latter in the absence of an obvious non-dietary cause, would constitute normal clinical practice in judging whether an individual breast fed child should receive additional food. The lack of any deleterious effect on growth would support the concept that the decision by many of these mothers to start weaning was not inappropriate. Though relatively uneducated and inexperienced they may have been aided in their decision by the collective wisdom of their extended families. It may also be that after three months of age the timing of the onset of weaning at least in this community is not a critical issue.

If we are to suggest that at least after the age of three months there is no narrow critical age range for these individual infants to start weaning then one must ask how relevant these results are to communities elsewhere. Enough has been said here to show that we have not been studying an urban elite group. Environmental hygiene was in no sense adequate nor was diarrhoeal morbidity trivial [20]. However there are two important ways in which the mothers in Bakau differ from those in Keneba. The first relates to nutritional status. Bakau mothers appear to be some 10% heavier (and are also taller) than Keneba women on crude comparison of their mid-pregnancy weights. This almost certainly has some bearing on early lactation performance. Secondly, in the periods before and after the birth of their children even the minority of mothers who go out to work in Bakau have far less rigorous physical demands upon them than their rural subsistence farming counterparts [21]. The resultant advantage in physical wellbeing and the time available for normal child care, two factors which are rarely assessed, are surely of fundamental importance. There is mounting evidence to suggest that if we can only look after mothers from early enough in their reproductive life then they are well equipped to rear their children, through early infancy. The nature and significance of the fall off in growth widely documented in the second half of infancy and later has yet to be fully explained.

Summary

In a relatively underprivileged urban Gambian community the initiation of the weaning process before three months of age appeared to be unrelated to the prior size or growth performance of the individual breast fed infant. In this early weaning group there was a general trend for growth faltering to ensue. Where the onset of weaning was delayed until three months or later there was a trend for the smaller infants or those who were growth-faltering to be weaned earlier. In this group weaning had no apparent deleterious effect on growth.

A prolonged weaning period extending into the second year of life was observed in virtually all children and mothers were able to continue breast feeding even in those infants who started weaning earliest. However growth in weight and length of the group as a whole fell progressively below the international standards from around six months of age, for reasons which were not analysed in this paper.

Acknowledgements

The authors thank Dr Peter Smith for advice on the analysis of these data.

References

1. Dyson T: Levels, trends, differentials and causes of child mortality – a survey. World Health Stat Rep 30(4):282–311, 1977.
2. Whitehead RG, Coward WA, Lunn PG, Rutishauser IHE: A comparison of the pathogenesis of protein energy malnutrition in Uganda and The Gambia. Trans R Soc Trop Med Hyg 74:189–195, 1977.
3. Scrimshaw NS, Taylor CE, Gordon JE: Interactions of nutrition and infection. World Health Organization Monograph Series No 57. WHO Geneva, 1968, p 329.
4. Gordon JE, Chitkara ID, Wyon JB: Weanling diarrhoea. Am J Med Sci 245:345–377, 1963.
5. Rowland MGM, Barrell RAE, Whitehead RG: Bacterial contamination in traditional Gambian weaning foods. Lancet 1:136–138, 1978.
6. Tully M: Nursing with a research unit in Africa. Nurs Times 74:401–405, 1978.
7. Rowland MGM, Cole TJ, Whitehead, RG: A quantitative study into the role of infection in determining nutritional status in Gambian village children. Brit J Nutr 37:441–450, 1977.
8. Barrell RAE, Rowland MGM: Infant foods as a potential source of diarrhoeal illness in rural West Africa. Trans R Soc Trop Med Hyg 73:85–90, 1979.
9. Watkinson M: Delayed onset of weanling diarrhoea associated with high breast milk intake. Trans R Soc Hyg Trop Med 75:432–435, 1981.
10. Pickering H: Social and environmental factors associated with high rates of diarrhoea in young children. Unpublished doctoral dissertation, London University, in preparation.

11. Whitehead RG: Infant feeding practices and the development of malnutrition in rural Gambia. Food Nutr Bull 1(4):36–41, 1979.
12. Rowland MGM: Growth in young breast-fed Gambian infants and some nutritional implications. In: Falkner F, Kretchmer N (eds) Introduction of foods to infants: why, when and which? in press.
13. Prentice AM: Variations in maternal dietary intake, birthweight and breast milk output in the Gambia. In: Aebi H, Whitehead RG (eds) Maternal nutrition during pregnancy and lactation. Bern, Hans Huber Publishers 1980, pp 167–183.
14. Hamill PVV, Drizd TA, Johnson CL, Reed RB, Roche AF, Moore WM: Physical growth: National Center for Health Statistics percentiles. Am J Clin Nutr 32:607–696, 1979.
15. Chandra RK: Physical growth of exclusively breast fed infants. Nutr Res 2(3):275–276, 1982.
16. Welbourn HF: The danger period during weaning. J Trop Pediatr 1:34–46, 1955.
17. Editorial: A Swedish code of ethics for marketing of infants foods. Acta Paediatr Scand 66(2):129–132, 1977.
18. Scrimshaw NS, Underwood BA: Timely and appropriate complementary feeding of the breast-fed infant – an overview. Food Nutr Bull 2(2):19–22, 1980.
19. Whitehead RG, Paul AA: Infant growth and human milk requirements – a fresh approach. Lancet 2:161–163, 1981.
20. Lloyd-Evans N, Pickering H. Goh SGJ, Rowland MGM: Food and water hygiene and diarrhoea in young Gambian children – a limited case control study. Trans R Soc Trop Med Hyg, in press.
21. Paul AA, Müller EM: Seasonal variations in dietary intake in pregnant and lactating women in a rural Gambian village. In: Aebi H, Whitehead RG (eds) Maternal nutrition during pregnancy and lactation. Bern, Hans Huber Publishers, 1980, pp 105–116.

Some considerations on the formulation of weaning mixes

W. KLAVER

Summary

The following presentation proposes the cross-tabulation of so called 'double mixes' of foods as an 'abacus' for those working on the formulation of weaning foods and for those engaged in teaching basic concepts of the nutritive value of foods. These considerations were developed in the context of the training of nutrition workers.

Comparing the nutritive value of foods

In teaching basic concepts of nutrition science, food composition tables are used to provide a link between the nutrients that we distinguish and the foods that contain them. However, reading through the columns of a food composition table does not allow easy comparison of the nutritive value of the various foods. In particular, 'dry' foods suggest they contain high amounts of nutrients compared to 'wet' foods, while it may very well be that the dry food has to be cooked and so becomes similar in nutritive value to the wet food. In this way, starchy fruits, roots and tubers have been proclaimed particularly 'bulky' – which they are – but in fact cereals are often as bulky after cooking. It requires some calculations to verify that fresh beans (classified as a vegetable) contain as much nutritive value per unit as the dry beans; the latter only do not have all that water.

In sum, it is not an easy job to derive meaningful data from food composition tables. In the International Course in Food Science and Nutrition in Wageningen we train each year for 5 months 25 participants from developing countries. As a part of their refresher training in basic nutrition, they are offered a practical exercise based on the calculation of nutrient densities of foods for a given amount of energy. This provides the participants also with an opportunity to manipulate real foods in preparing an exhibition in which they rank foods according to their nutrient:energy density.

The formulation of food combinations

Formulating diets begins with the proximate components of foods, particularly their content of protein and fat, and the amount of metabolizable energy that these are supposed to provide. In terms of foods, this means dealing with staple foods, complementary (protein-rich) foods and energy-dense foods. The latter are particularly important for small children and their mothers. Micro-nutrients will be discussed as a next step only.

The former 'protein gap' in developing countries has been replaced by the 'energy gap'. However, adding oil or sugar to a food mixture dilutes its protein: energy density; so it seems wise to continue keeping an eye on the protein content of food mixtures.

Going into this usually requires that the whole theory of amino acid complementation be explained and that an additional book lands on the nutritionist's desk: the table of amino acids. Besides adding to the workload, it conferes a risk that protein quantity and protein quality are not given their proper place, i.e. when only the latter aspect is considered so that one searches essentially for the proportion of foods that give a maximum amino acid score. Such proportions exist where two foods are combined that have different limiting amino acids.

However, it should be borne in mind that protein quality is an attribute of a certain quantity of protein. The fact that foods of animal origin are rich in proteins in the first place, but have also a high protein quality – while the reverse is true for plant foods – makes confusion understandable. The criterion for food mix formulation should be protein quantity corrected for quality. Platt and Miller [1] proposed the net dietary-protein value that later became known as net dietary-protein calorie percent: NDp Cals% [2].

Double mixes

A tool exists that has the potential to save much of such calculation time to many nutritionists. That is the cross-tabulation of double mixes of a staple food and a protein-rich food. Such a table appeared in applied nutrition literature in 'The health aspects of food and nutrition' [3]. Food mixtures were tabulated that provided 360 kcal and an NDpCal of 8% (no oil added).

In the first edition (1971) of their Manual on feeding infants and young children, Cameron and Hofvander [4] included a double mix table with 10 g of oil added (except with the legumes) and an NDpCal of 7–8%. Both these tables used food composition data from Platt [5], amino acid composition data from Orr and Watt [6] and the FAO (1957) amino acid scoring pattern [7]. In the second edition (1976) of their manual, Cameron and Hofvander [4] included a table providing about 6% NDpCal. To the legumes, 5 g of oil was added. In the third edition (1983) of their manual [4] they present the same proportion figures as in 1976, be it that the legumes are included in the table with 10 g oil added. This time they write that each mix has the same protein value and provides the approximate equivalent of 5–6 g of reference protein.

Pellett and Mamarbachi [8] recalculated the table of double mix proportions using more recent amino acid content data [9] and the FAO/WHO (1973) amino acid scoring pattern [10]. They realized that the original equation for the calculation of NDpCals% [2] is mathematically cumbersome, as it is a complicated function of the protein energy percentage and the chemical score. Pellett and Mamarbachi proposed a modified equation which represents a one-to-one relationship with the protein energy percentage, multiplied by the chemical score. This product can be called 'net protein energy percentage'. Their double mixes were calculated for a (modified) NDpCal of 6.6%, which corresponds to a net protein energy level of 8.0%.

The table of Pellett and Mamarbachi [8] is limited in that the legumes (beans or peas) are left out and that they only give one level of oil added (10 g of oil per 350 kcal). Below a recalculated table is presented which includes legumes and groundnuts and which contains the proportions in grams of double mix quantities at three levels of added oil: 0, 5 and 10 g.

The principle of calculation is visualized in Figure 1. The ordinate on the left represents the crude and net protein energy percentages for 100% maize and the ordinate on the right represents the same for 100% soybean. Straight lines are drawn which represent the protein values of the range of intermediate mixtures of maize and soybeans for any given point on the abscissa.

The double mix proportion without oil added is sought at the level of 8% net protein energy. The latter is determined by the line corresponding to the limiting amino acid. The double mix proportions with 5 and 10 g oil added per 350 kcal are sought at the net protein energy levels of 9.2% and 10.7% to compensate for the diluting effect of the oil: the maize and bean mixture before addition of the oil has to provide 305 kcal in the first instance and 260 kcal in the second instance.

The results of these calculations performed on 13 staple foods and 8 complementary foods are presented in Table 1. The composition references of the individual foods are summarized in Table 2. Proximate food composition data are from Chatfield [11] and amino acid data from FAO [9]. The amino acid scores were derived using the FAO/WHO (1973) scoring pattern [10].

Using double mix proportions as an 'abacus'

The table of double mix proportions can be exploited further than has been reported up to now. In the first place, it allows to compare the protein value of various foods in terms of quantities of the foods, not quantities of protein. For instance, millet and oats require less complementary food than wheat, rice, sorghum and maize; sweet potato, bananas and plantains require more comple-

Table 1. Composition of mixtures of staple and supplement to give approximately 1.46 MJ (350 kcal) with a net protein energy percentage of 8.0 (which corresponds to an NDpEn% between 6.75 and 7.36 in these mixes). Supplement quantities were rounded to the nearest gram and staple quantities according to the exact proportion.

STAPLE	SUPPL. Oil	Oats	Wheat flour	Rice	Millet meal	Sorghum meal	Maize	Irish potato	Sweet potato	Yam	Taro/ Cocoyam	Banana	Plantain	Cassava flour	Double mix kcal range
Egg	+10	63_{13}	59_{31}	61_{25}	68_{19}	63_{28}	59_{29}	268_{24}	169_{41}	206_{26}	198_{32}	218_{34}	177_{39}	55_{48}	346–354
	+ 5	80_{7}	70_{28}	75_{22}	83_{14}	76_{25}	74_{27}	323_{20}	210_{38}	258_{22}	246_{27}	277_{30}	216_{35}	67_{46}	344–365
	+ 0	90_{0}	83_{26}	91_{19}	96_{9}	93_{23}	86_{24}	377_{18}	250_{35}	296_{18}	293_{24}	320_{27}	261_{32}	81_{45}	341–358
DSM	+10	62_{4}	61_{10}	64_{9}	69_{6}	64_{9}	66_{10}	255_{13}	179_{15}	208_{11}	214_{11}	233_{12}	184_{13}	59_{17}	340–359
	+ 5	72_{2}	71_{9}	76_{7}	93_{5}	77_{8}	78_{9}	316_{12}	215_{14}	244_{9}	253_{9}	289_{11}	222_{12}	74_{17}	330–378
	+ 0	90_{0}	90_{9}	90_{6}	100_{3}	88_{7}	89_{8}	378_{11}	250_{13}	309_{8}	304_{8}	349_{10}	283_{12}	84_{16}	327–364
DWM	+10	62_{7}	52_{15}	52_{14}	66_{10}	57_{14}	53_{14}	199_{20}	133_{22}	163_{17}	168_{17}	182_{18}	144_{20}	43_{24}	344–363
	+ 5	65_{3}	66_{14}	67_{11}	78_{7}	69_{12}	67_{13}	259_{18}	177_{21}	222_{15}	230_{15}	234_{16}	186_{18}	57_{24}	310–358
	+ 0	90_{0}	80_{13}	83_{9}	103_{5}	85_{11}	83_{12}	316_{16}	221_{20}	266_{12}	278_{12}	305_{15}	234_{17}	69_{23}	340–375
Fresh fish	+10	67_{6}	66_{15}	67_{15}	75_{9}	72_{14}	67_{16}	280_{21}	193_{26}	231_{18}	224_{20}	246_{24}	202_{26}	66_{32}	347–356
	+ 5	77_{3}	78_{14}	82_{12}	93_{7}	82_{12}	78_{13}	332_{19}	238_{25}	270_{15}	270_{17}	291_{22}	246_{25}	79_{31}	339–356
	+ 0	90_{0}	91_{13}	95_{9}	94_{4}	97_{11}	94_{12}	405_{18}	269_{23}	329_{13}	316_{14}	351_{21}	278_{23}	91_{30}	325–364

Chicken/lean meat	+10	68_7	62_{17}	63_{17}	72_{10}	68_{15}	63_{17}	259_{21}	183_{26}	214_{18}	208_{19}	230_{24}	189_{26}	60_{31}	344–365
	+5	68_3	74_{15}	80_{14}	82_7	84_{14}	76_{14}	329_{20}	217_{24}	254_{15}	269_{17}	277_{22}	224_{24}	72_{30}	313–360
	+0	90_0	88_{14}	92_{10}	105_5	94_{12}	91_{13}	385_{18}	259_{23}	312_{13}	318_{14}	321_{20}	267_{23}	86_{30}	342–367
Soybean	+10	62_6	57_{14}	58_{13}	69_9	62_{13}	60_{14}	209_{23}	138_{25}	175_{20}	182_{18}	201_{16}	158_{20}	44_{27}	343–360
	+5	74_3	70_{13}	74_{10}	77_6	78_{12}	71_{12}	273_{21}	182_{24}	227_{17}	228_{14}	265_{15}	203_{17}	58_{27}	331–361
	+0	90_0	83_{12}	83_8	93_4	87_{10}	85_{11}	337_{19}	218_{22}	278_{14}	290_{11}	308_{13}	261_{16}	70_{26}	331–361
Legumes	+10	46_{26}	47_{26}	22_{53}	61_{18}	32_{44}	22_{54}	55_{64}	34_{65}	50_{61}	56_{59}	68_{58}	46_{62}	10_{67}	348–355
	+5	74_5	64_{20}	54_{33}	76_{10}	71_{18}	51_{35}	130_{58}	81_{62}	120_{52}	135_{48}	162_{44}	109_{53}	24_{66}	337–351
	+0	90_0	80_{19}	82_{13}	99_7	85_{16}	80_{17}	208_{53}	129_{59}	189_{43}	215_{37}	260_{31}	174_{45}	38_{64}	339–361
Groundnuts	+0	83_4	34_{42}	43_{36}	64_{24}	39_{39}	36_{40}	176_{38}	89_{45}	148_{36}	125_{41}	136_{41}	100_{43}	28_{47}	343–355
Double mixes	+10	70–82	74–81	60–96	81–86	61–78	59–94	54–100	55–100	56–100	58–100	59–100	57–100	54–100	
chemical score	+5	73–75	68–74	72–93	75–79	66–71	69–88	54–95	56–100	58–97	64–100	68–100	62–100	55–100	
range	+0	67–69	57–67	60–90	64–72	57–64	62–82	54–89	56–100	61–93	66–100	66–97	66–100	55–100	

Data sources: – Chatfield. C. Food Composition Tables for international use. FAO, 1953 (2nd edn.)
– Amino-acid Content of Foods. FAO. 1970
– Energy and Protein Requirements. FAO/WHO, 1973.

24

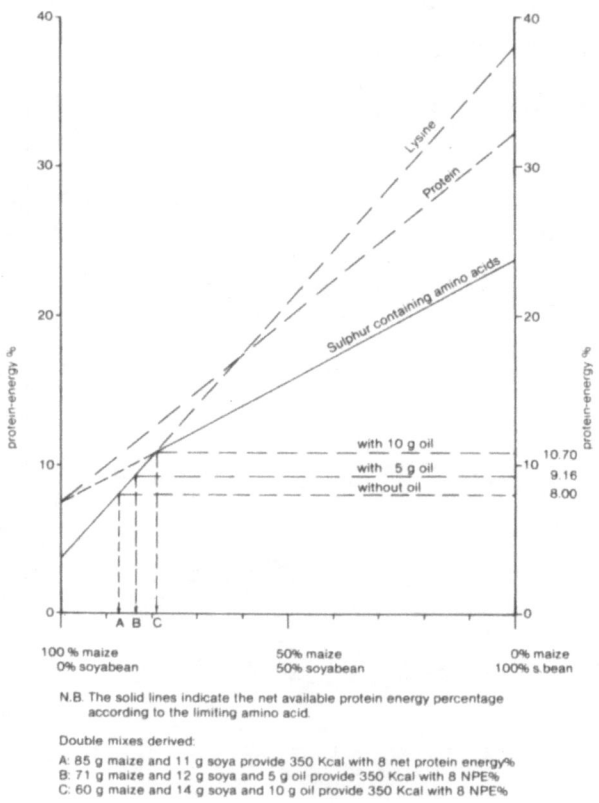

Figure 1. Double mixes of maize and soyabean. Protein-energy values of combinations of staple and supplement, mixed in varying proportions (as percentages of combined energy).

mentary food than irish potato and yam, while cassava flour needs most. Secondly, multiple mixes can easily and quickly be composed from the double mix proportions. Here the table of double mix proportions serves as an 'abacus' for the formulation of weaning mixes.

The principle is that when a portion (p) of a double mix is combined with the complement portion (1–p) of another mix, the combined multiple mix again provides 350 kcal and at least 8% net protein energy. The net protein level will not be less than 8.0%; it may be slightly over 8% if the two portions of double mixes had different limiting amino acids.

This principle can be used to vary the level of added oil, or to partially substitute ingredients by other ingredients. An example of varying the level of added oil is as follows: From Table 1 it can be read that the following double mixes are equivalent in energy value (350 kcal) and net protein energy percent (8.0%):

Table 2. Food composition references and basic data on the individual foods.

Food item	Food composition reference number (1)	Proximate composition per 100g edible portion (E.P.)				Source of energy factors applied	Available energy (kcal/100 g E.P.)	Lipid energy %	Protein energy %	Amino acid reference number (4)
		Water	Fat	Ash	Protein					
Oats (E.R. 50)*	18	10.0	7.5	1.7	13.0	(3)	387	16.2	11.6	11
Wheat flour (E.R. 72)	9	12.0	1.1	0.4	8.6	(2) = (3)	365	2.5	9.6	29
Rice (E.R. 67)	12	13.0	0.7	0.7	6.7	(3)	360	1.6	7.1	16
Millet meal (E.R. 90)	31	11.0	3.0	2.2	9.7	(2) = (3)	340	7.4	10.3	10
Sorghum meal (E.R. 90)	26	11.0	3.3	1.8	10.1	(2)	343	8.1	10.6	20
Maize (E.R. 100)	19	12.0	4.3	1.3	9.5	(3)	356	10.1	7.3	9
Irish potato	34	78.0	0.1	1.0	2.0	(3)	83	1.0	6.7	36
Sweet potato	36	70.0	0.4	1.0	1.3	(3)	117	2.9	3.1	37
Yam	41	72.4	0.2	0.9	2.4	(3)	106	1.6	6.3	42
Taro/Cocoyam	40	72.5	0.2	1.2	1.9	(3)	105	1.6	5.0	39
Banana	117	73.5	0.4	0.8	1.3	(2) = (3)	94	3.6	4.6	300
Plantain	118	68.2	0.5	0.9	1.2	(2) = (3)	113	3.7	3.6	300
Cassava flour	38	14.0	0.6	2.4	1.5	(3)	338	1.5	1.2	31
Egg	215	74.0	11.7	1.0	12.4	(2) = (3)	163	64.8	33.2	340
Dried skimmed milk	267	4.0	1.0	8.0	36.0	(2) = (3)	360	2.4	42.7	373
Dried whole milk	265	4.0	27.0	6.0	26.0	(2) = (3)	491	48.3	22.6	373
Fresh fish (average fat)	227	74.1	5.7	1.4	18.8	(2) = (3)	132	39.1	60.9	344
Chicken	204	65.6	12.6	1.6	20.2	(3)	200	56.9	43.1	323
Soybean	54	8.0	18.0	4.7	38.0	(3)	410	36.7	32.2	71
Legumes	63b	11.0	1.7	3.8	22.1	(2) = (3)	341	4.2	22.5	48
Groundnuts	52	5.2	43.3	2.5	25.6	(2) = (3)	547	66.3	16.3	57
Oil	277	0	100	0	0	(2) = (3)	884	100	0	–

Notes: (1) Source: Chatfield, C. Food Composition Tables for international use. FAO, Washington D.C., 1953 (2nd edn.); (2) Energy-yielding Components of Food and Computation of Calorie Values. FAO, Washington D.C., 1947; (3) Energy and Protein Requirements. FAO/WHO, 1973; (4) Source: Amino-Acid Content of Foods and biological data on proteins; * FAO, Rome, 1970 E.R. = Extraction rate of the cereal.

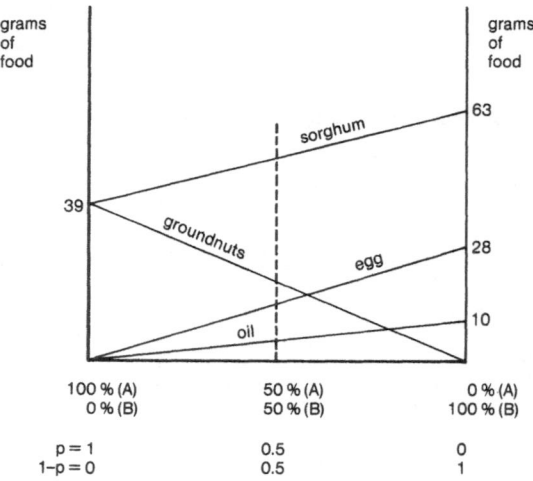

Figure 2. Proportions of foods obtained by combining two double mixes: (A) and (B).

63 g of sorghum and 28 g of egg and 10 g of oil
76 g of sorghum and 25 g of egg and 5 g of oil.

If one desires to know the double mix proportions with, say, 7 g of oil, it suffices to multiply the first double mix by a proportion of 0.4* and the second by a proportion of 1–0.4 = 0.6. The new mix contains 63 × 0.4 + 76 × (1–0.4) = 71 g of sorghum, 28 × 0.4 + 25 × (1–0.4) = 26 g of egg and 7 g of oil. An example of partial substitution of ingredients is as follows. Two double mixes from Table 1 are:

(A) 63 g of sorghum and 28 g of egg and 10 g of oil
(B) 39 g of sorghum and 39 g of groundnuts.

The range of combinations of sorghum, egg, groundnuts and oil is given by: {63 × p + 39 × (1–p)} g of sorghum and 28 × p) g of egg and {(1–p) × 39} g of ground-nuts and (10 × p) g of oil, where p varies between 0 and 1. This is visualized in Figure 2. The results for p = 0.5 for instance would be: 51 g of sorghum and 20 g of groundnuts and 14 g of egg and 5 g of oil. It will be appreciated that the latter figure concerns the added (visible) oil. There is another 10 g of invisible oil contained in the 20 g of groundnuts and 14 g of egg. Such a multiple mix can be combined at its turn with still another double mix from Table 1.

As a second major step, vegetables and/or fruits are added to the mix. These contribute little energy and generally take very well care of themselves as to their protein content. Such addition does not alter much the energy and net protein level of the resulting mix, so that complicated corrections are not necessary.

With each additional double mix, a degree of freedom is introduced in the

---

* In mathematical terms, 10 × p + 5 × (1–p) = 7 g of oil. This equation is solved by a value of p = 0.4.

multiple mix formula. The solution of the equations, or the multiple mix quantities selected, depends on a variety of possible criteria or constraints. These can have to do with factors as the resulting taste (e.g. not more than x g of groundnuts), availability of ingredients (e.g. either one or no egg), costs of the ingredients, level of added fat, level of total fat in the mix, bulk and consistency of the cooked mix, or any other aspect one might consider appropriate.

Several of these criteria require that some selected 'solutions' of multiple mixes be actually prepared and evaluated from various angles. Recipes could be developed that still maintain some degree(s) of freedom, by including an indication as to how far certain ingredient quantities can be varied if the user likes so.

References

1. Platt BS, Miller DS: The net dietary-protein value of mixtures of foods – its definition, determination and application. Proc Nutr Soc 18:vii–viii, 1959.
2. Miller DA, Payne PR: Problems in the prediction of protein values of diets. The influence of protein concentration. Brit J Nutr 15:11–19, 1961.
3. The health aspects of food and nutrition – a manual for developing countries in the Western Pacific Region of the WHO. (1969 1st edn) Manila (1972, 2nd edn) Taiwan.
4. Cameron M, Hofvander Y: Manual on feeding infants and young children. (1971, 1st edn; 1976, 2nd revised edn); Oxford University Press (1983, 3rd revised edn).
5. Platt BS: Tables of representative values of foods commonly used in tropical countries. London (1962).
6. Orr ML, Watt BK. Amino acid content of foods. USDA, Washington DC (1957).
7. FAO. Committee on Protein Requirements. Rome (1957).
8. Pellett PL, Mamarbachi D: Recommended proportions of foods in home-made feeding mixtures. Ecol Food Nutr 7:219–228, 1979.
9. Amino acid content of foods and biological data on proteins. FAO (1970).
10. Energy and protein requirements: Report of a joint FAO/WHO ad hoc expert committee. Geneva (1973).
11. Chatfield C: Food composition tables for international use. FAO (1953, 2nd edn).

The influence of mycotoxins on child health in the tropics

R.G. HENDRICKSE

Introduction

Mycotoxins are toxins produced by fungi, many of which are highly toxic to animals and man. Ergotism, caused by the alkaloids of Claviceps purpurea which contaminates grain, was known to the ancient Chinese, Greeks, Romans and Arabs and was an epidemic scourge in Europe from the middle ages to comparatively recent times. The origins of knowledge of this serious mycotoxicosis are losts in the mists of antiquity but mycotoxins and the diseases caused by them excited little interest in modern scientific literature until the discovery of aflatoxins in the early 1960s. Since then there has been an explosion of knowledge about many aspects of mycotoxins and the field is currently bewildering in its complexity [1]. The medical profession in general and clinicians ·in particular have, however, made little contribution to recent growth in knowledge about mycotoxins and, if the truth must be acknowledged, remain woefully ignorant about a subject that may have great implications for human health worldwide, but especially in the tropics where climatic, environmental and a variety of social factors produce conditions particularly favourable to the growth of many food moulds.

The primary objectives of this paper are to increase awareness of the prevalence and variety of mycotoxins in the human environment, draw attention to their potential danger to health and well-being and stimulate interest in systematic study of a subject which has been largely ignored by our profession. Recent experience of our group in Liverpool, working in collaboration with colleagues in Sudan and elsewhere in Africa, suggests that there is an urgent need for all who share a common purpose to promote good child health to direct their attention at mycotoxins which may constitute major hidden factors influencing the pattern of morbidity and mortality of children in the tropics.

Human exposure to mycotoxins

Almost all plant products can support fungal growth and subsequent mycotoxin formation. Human food may, therefore, be frequently directly contaminated by mycotoxins. Animals injecting mycotoxin contaminated feeds may pass on the toxins to humans via their milk and meat. Human exposure to mycotoxins may also occur by inhalation or skin contact in certain occupations. Breastfed babies may be exposed to mycotoxins in breast milk if their mothers eat mycotoxin contaminated food (see below).

Most of the available data on mycotoxins and mycotoxicosis have been obtained from veterinary medicine. There is now a long list of diseases in animals caused by specific mycotoxins and a number of other diseases strongly suspected to be caused by mycotoxins in which the specific mycotoxins responsible still await identification. Knowledge of human mycotoxicosis is growing but remains woefully incomplete. Extrapolation from veterinary work indicates that the potential for toxicity of mycotoxins in humans is great, but there are relatively few examples of human disease in which definite associations have been established with specific mycotoxins. This is perhaps not surprising, when cognisance is taken of the fact that risk of human exposure to mycotoxins has received much less attention from the medical profession than risk of animal exposure has from the veterinarians.

The mycotoxins for which there is evidence of human exposure and of well defined adverse effects, at least in animals, were listed by the WHO Task Group on Experimental Health Criteria for Mycotoxins as: aflatoxins; ochratoxins; and zearalenone. The trichothecenes were also included as they are produced by fungi which were associated with outbreaks of human alimentary toxic aleukia (ATA) some decades ago. Some more recently discovered mycotoxins which have been suggested to be related to disease in farm animals include: citreo-viridin; citrinin; cyclochlorotine; luteoskyrin; maltoryzine; patulin; P.R. toxin; rubratoxin; rugulosin; sterigmatocystine; and tremorgens [2].

Aflatoxins are the only mycotoxins which have been shown to be associated with well recognised effects on human health and our recent investigations suggest the possibility that their influence on child health may be more significant than previously suspected. We will return to aflatoxins after brief consideration of some of the other mycotoxins.

Ochratoxins

Ochratoxins are produced by several species of Aspergillus and Penicillium. The A. ochraceus group of fungi were found in all parts of the world in soil, insects, food such as rice, oats, wheat flour, chili and capsicum pepper, and in diseased plants and decaying vegetation. They were also frequently found in dried and salted fish products in the Orient. A large proportion of the A. ochraceus isolated from foods was toxigenic. Ochratoxins have been isolated from sorghum, hops, peanuts, pecan nuts, mouldy Japanese rice, black pepper, adzuki beans and ground pepper. (Data summarised by Harwig) [3].

Ochratoxins have proved nephrotoxic to all species of animals tested. A disease called mould nephrosis or mycotoxic nephropathy has long been recognised in Danish slaughter houses. The renal pathology includes tubular atrophy, interstitial fibrosis and hyalinised glomeruli. Ochratoxin residues can be detected in the kidneys, liver and adipose tissues of swine fed ochratoxin containing feed. Human exposure to ochratoxins may occur not only through consumption of mouldy plant material but also through eating animal products [3].

There is a form of human nephropathy that is endemic in parts of the Balkans and which has pathological features which are similar to ochratoxin nephropathy in pigs. The disease is chronic and is commonest in the age group 30–50 years affecting females more than males. In Bulgaria and Yugoslavia a high incidence of urinary tract tumours has been found to be closely correlated with the incidence and mortality of Balkan endemic nephropathy. Exposure to food borne ochratoxin A seems to be higher in areas with endemic nephropathy than in non-endemic areas. Notwithstanding these observations, the WHO Task Group on Environmental Health Criteria for Mycotoxins consider that 'there is, at present, no proof that ochratoxin A is causally involved in human diseases' [2].

There is currently virtually no information about the level of exposure of the child population in tropical countries to ochratoxins. There, however, is growing information about the prevalence of renal disease in childhood in the tropics and many of the diseases described behave atypically when compared with similar entities in non-tropical areas. In some instances specific endemic diseases have been identified as factors in atypical renal disease, e.g. quartan malarial nephrotic syndrome [4], but in many other instances the reasons for the peculiar clinical and/or pathological findings observed remain obscure. We need to consider the possibility that exposure to mycotoxins may influence the pattern and prevalence of renal disease in childhood in the tropics.

Zearalenone

Many species of Fusarium produce zearalenone which may be found as a natural contaminant of cereals, in particular, maize, in many parts of the world including Europe, Africa and North America. Zearalenone has been detected in cornmeal and cornflakes intended for human consumption. Very high levels of zearalenone have been detected in sour porridges and beers in Swaziland and Lesotho in Southern Africa. There are, however, no reports of adverse effects of these mycotoxins in man [2].

In animals, especially swine (probably the most sensitive of animals to activity of zearalenone), fed zearalenone under experimental conditions, a syndrome of oestrogenism develops within a week. The vulvas, mammae and nipples enlarge, and prolapse of the vagina may occur. The uteri are greatly enlarged and the ovaries atrophy. These changes revert to normal when zearalenone is removed from the diet [5]. Other effects in cattle that may be attributed to zearalenone or related mycotoxins include infertility and abortions. Congential skeletal defects have been reported in rats fed zearalenone.

Gynaecomostia is frequently observed in African men, the breasts enlarging to resemble those of females. Testicular atrophy in leprosy and cirrhosis of the liver are recognised associations in some cases but in many cases the cause of gynaeco-mastia remains obscure [6]. Ambiguous genitalia and problems of intersex appear to occur more frequently in parts of Africa than might be expected and it is interesting to speculate on the reasons for this. Hopefully, someone will be stimulated to examine possible relationships between zearalenone contents of diets and the problems of gynaecomastia and ambiguous genitalia in Africa.

Trichothecenes

These are a group of related chemical compounds produced by several species of Fusarium, Cephalosporium, Myrothecium, Trichoderma and Stachybotrys. Four trichothecenes have been detected as natural contaminants of some foods: T-2 toxin; Nivalenol; deoxynivaleno; and diacetoxyscirpenol [2].

Toxins of Fusarium cultures have been tested in many animals including mice, rats, guinea pigs, rabbits, dogs, cats and horses. Toxic effects characterised by necrotic mucosal lesions, extreme leukopaenia and haemorrhagic tendency have been observed in most animals. According to Joffe [7], the Fusarium species achieved notoriety during the closing stages of World War II as the cause of 'septic angina' or Alimentary Toxic Aleukia (ATA) in some districts of the U.S.S.R. ATA proved a very serious and in most cases lethal disease accom-panied by skin rash, necrotic angina, extreme leukopenia, multiple haemor-rhages, sepsis and exhaustion of the bone marrow. The cause of the outbreak was identified as consumption of mouldy grain which was overwintered in the field [2, 7].

No further outbreaks of this disease have been reported since the war. It is somewhat surprising that notwithstanding the relationships established between Fusarium Species and ATA in the U.S.S.R. the WHO experts are of the opinion 'There is no firm evidence connecting the recently identified trichothenes with alimentary toxic aleukia occurring in the past, or with other human disease' [2].

Aflatoxins

Aflatoxins (Figure 1) are produced by strains of Aspergillus flavus and Aspergillus parasiticus. These fungi occur worldwide but crops in tropical and subtropical areas are more liable to contamination since high temperatures and humidity provide optimal conditions for toxin formation. A. flavus grows best at 27° C in a relative humidity of 85% or more. There is abundant evidence that many foods which are commonly eaten in the tropics are contaminated by aflatoxins B_1, B_2, G_1 and G_2, e.g. ground nuts, maize, sorghum, millet, rice etc. [8].

In the early 1960s a mysterious disease killed over 100,000 turkeys in the U.K., it was designated Turkey 'X' Disease and became the subject of intense investigation. It soon became apparent that a cargo of groundnut meal imported from Brazil and incorporated in the turkey feed was responsible for the disease and further investigation identified aflatoxins as the toxic agents.

Subsequent investigations have shown that aflatoxins are extremely toxic to most animals and are among the most powerful carcinogenic agents known. Aflatoxins regularly produce hepatoma in many laboratory animals and can also cause other forms of malignancy.

The metabolic effects of aflatoxins observed in animals are protean and serious and include the following [2, 8]:
  inhibition of protein synthesis
  inhibition of enzyme synthesis
  inhibition of clotting factors synthesis
  depression of glucose metabolism (via 6-phosphate pathway)
  depression of fatty acid synthesis
  depression of phospholipid synthesis
  the feed-back control of cholesterol synthesis is lost
  immunosuppressive properties: reduced resistance to Pasteurella and Salmonella sp., viruses, coccidia and Candida albicans.

In all animals studied, the liver was the principal target organ for aflatoxin toxicity but different species vary considerably in their susceptibility to acute poisoning. The liver changes in aflatoxin poisoning include fatty infiltration, biliary proliferation, acute toxic necrosis and portal fibrosis [2, 8].

Direct evidence of aflatoxin toxicity in man is still rather meagre even though circumstancial evidence is strong and mounting. Malignant hepatoma is unusually common in many areas of the world where aflatoxins contaminate commonly eaten foods and these toxins are thought to be important in the pathogenesis of hepatoma. Aflatoxins have been incriminated in the etiology of cases of Reyes syndrome reported from New Zealand [9], Czechoslavakia [10], the U.S.A. [11] and Thailand [12, 13]. In the Czechoslovakia study aflatoxin B_1 was detected in the liver of all cases of Reyes syndrome but not in the livers of 25 other children who had died of other causes. Acute fatal hepatic necrosis and subacute

34

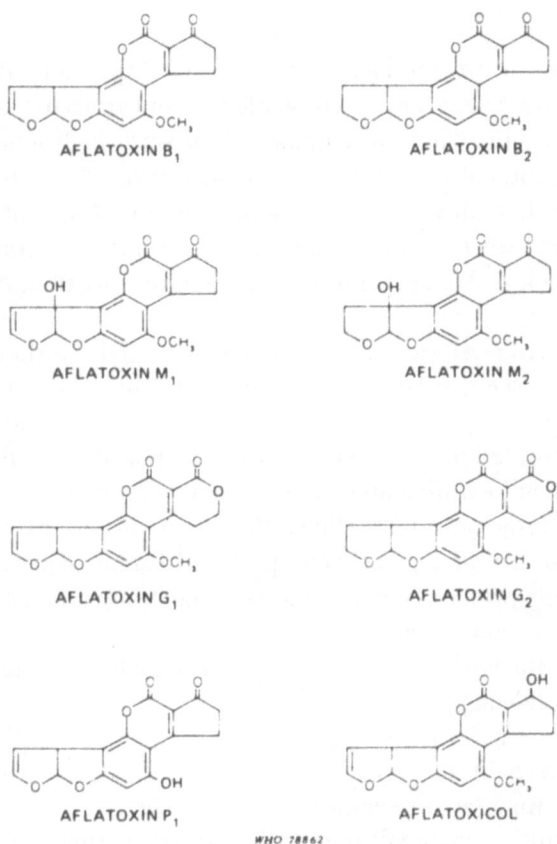

AFLATOXIN B₁   AFLATOXIN B₂

AFLATOXIN M₁   AFLATOXIN M₂

AFLATOXIN G₁   AFLATOXIN G₂

AFLATOXIN P₁   AFLATOXICOL

WHO 78862

Figure 1. The main classes of naturally occurring aflatoxins are B_1, B_2, G_1 and G_2, the B group being most toxic. Aflatoxins M_1 and M_2 are derived from B_1 and B_2 and excreted in breast milk. 17 aflatoxins have been identified.

progressive cirrhosis of the liver have been reported, mainly in children, in India [14, 15] and Africa [16] following consumption of grains heavily contaminated with aflatoxins.

It is apparent from animal experiments and from clinical observations in man that short exposure to large doses of aflatoxins produces acute toxicity which may be lethal while exposure to small doses of aflatoxins over a protracted period of time is carcinogenic. Virtually nothing is known about the effects of frequent exposure to moderate amounts of dietary aflatoxins which appears to be a common occurrence in many tropical countries.

Aflatoxins and kwashiorkor

The world distribution and seasonal fluctuations of aflatoxin contamination of food are similar to the geographical distribution and seasonal prevalence of kwashiorkor which tends to peak in the wet season in many areas. Kwashiorkor remains a disease of obscure etiology and pathogenesis inspite of intensive clinical, laboratory, and epidemiological research over many years [17, 18].

During the past three years we have been engaged in studies to determine the relationships between mycotoxins, in particular aflatoxins, in food and malnutrition in childhood with particular reference to the pathogenesis of kwashiorkor. Clinical and field studies in the Sudan have been augmented by study of autopsy liver specimens obtained in Nigeria, South Africa and Liberia from children who have died of kwashiorkor and other forms of PEM. The following is a summary of our experience to date. The methodologies employed were as previously described [19, 20] (Figures 2 and 3).

Food analysis

Aflatoxins have been detected frequently in a variety of commonly eaten foods

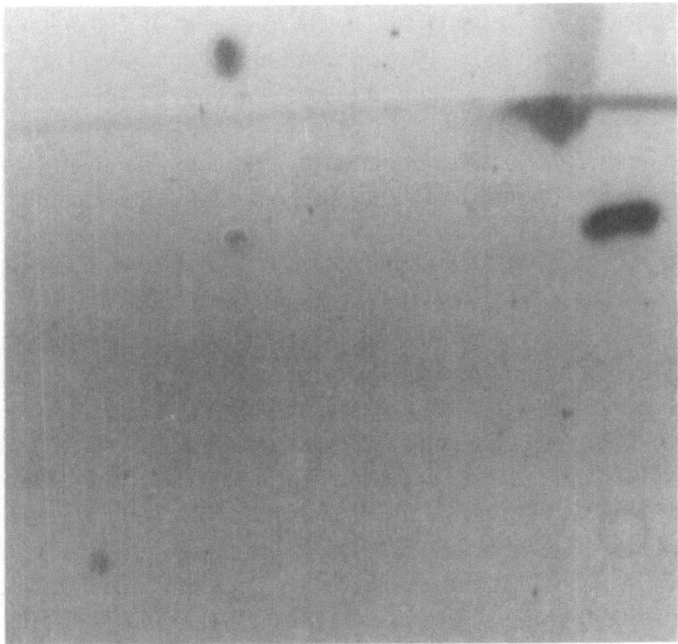

Figure 2. Identification of aflatoxins by two dimensional thin layer chromatography. (TLC) Photograph of a 10×10 cm TLC plate of serum extract containing aflatoxin B_1.

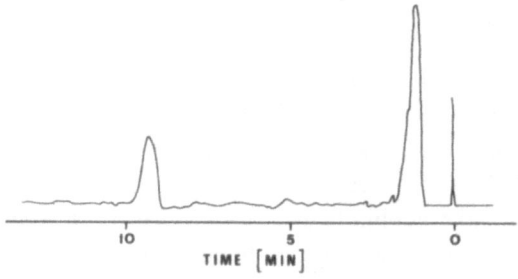

TIME [MIN]

Figure 3. Identification of aflatoxins by high performance liquid chromatography (H.P.L.C.) HPLC chromatogram of serum extract containing 240 pg aflatoxin B_1. Column: Spherisorb 5 μm ODS; mobile phase methanol-water (50:50); flow rate: 2 ml/min; fluorescence detector, excitation 365 nm, emission 418 nm.

obtained from local markets including the following: ground nuts (plain and limed), peanut butter, chickpeas, haricot beans, sorghum, dried ochra, wheat, millet, rice, lentils, dried tomatoes, dried meat, dried fish, and milk. Aflatoxins have also been detected in one or more food items from 80% of households tested and in 46% of composite meals 'food on the plate' ready for eating. The contamination rate in some commodities has been very high e.g. sorghum 51% samples positive, dried ochre 48% positive, foul musri (Egyptian Beans) 60% positive, dried meat 42% positive. The amount of aflatoxins detected in food samples has been very variable but levels in excess of 600 micrograms per kilogram have been recorded. Aflatoxins have also been found in milk and meals prepared for consumption by children in hospital.

Breast milk analysis. Variable amounts of aflatoxins M_1 and M_2 have been detected in just over one third of 99 samples of breast milk examined to date.

Serum and urine analysis. A total of 466 sera and 460 urines from children nutritionally graded according to the Wellcome classification [21] into controls, marasmus, marasmic kwashiorkor and kwashiorkor have been analysed for aflatoxins. The findings in this extended series are in broad agreement with our earlier reported findings on 252 Sudanese children [19]. Aflatoxins were detected more often and at higher concentrations in sera from children with kwashiorkor than in the other malnourished and control groups. Aflatoxicol a metabolite of aflatoxins B_1 and B_2 was detected in kwashiorkors (12%) and marasmic kwashiorkor (6%) but not in controls and only once in marasmus. Urinary aflatoxins were detected in 29% of all children in the study with similar excretion rates in the different nutritional groups. The pattern of excretion of individual aflatoxins, in particular M_2 and B_1 show some differences between controls and kwashiorkors. Aflatoxicol, was found in urines from children in all groups including controls who showed no aflatoxicol in serum.

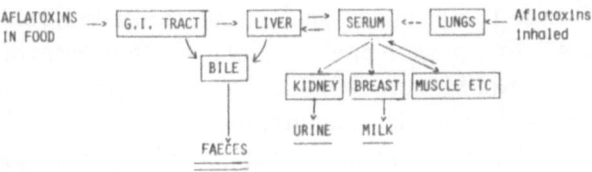

Figure 4. Schematic representation of aflatoxin absorption, metabolism and excretion. In normal health most aflatoxins injected appear to be rapidly excreted via the liver and biliary system.

Serial simultaneous estimations of aflatoxins in serum, urine and stool have been undertaken in 12 children. The results of this limited study provide clear evidence of rapid changes in aflatoxin metabolism which are reflected in qualitative and quantitative changes in aflatoxins in serum, urine and blood (Figure 4). Findings in three children are given in Table 1 and illustrate the lability of aflatoxin metabolism and underline the need for caution in interpreting findings based on examination of single samples for aflatoxins.

Autopsy liver studies

A total of 19 autopsy liver specimens from children dying from kwashiorkor, marasmic kwashiorkor or marasmus have been analysed for their aflatoxin content. The specimens were forwarded to us by colleagues in three widely separated geographical locations viz: Durban, South Africa; Lagos & Ibadan in

Table 1. Serial aflatoxin estimations in sera, urines and faeces (pg/ml).

Patient		Hours			
		0	6	12	24
No. 620	Serum	$M_1$3182, $B_1$4440,	$M_1$3373, $M_2$11,	$M_1$2068,	$M_1$1152,
Female		$B_2$501	$B_1$725	$M_2$11	$M_2$11
Marasmic/		Aflatoxicol 220		$B_1$150	$B_2$41
Kwash.	Urine	Aflatoxicol, 2627	$B_1$1538	$M_1$7609	–
	Faeces	–	–	No stool	No stool
No. 617	Serum	$M_1$85, $B_1$450, $B_2$3,	–	–	–
Female		$G_1$2721, $G_2$2			
Marasmic/	Urine	–	$M_1$185, $B_1$385,	$B_2$90	$B_2$90
Kwash.			Afl. 385		
	Faeces	–	$B_2$149	–	–
No. 624	Serum	–	–	–	–
Male	Urine	–	$M_2$31	$B_1$377	–
Marasmus	Faeces	$G_1$4372	–	$G_1$9028	$G_1$243

Nigeria and Liberia. The results of analysis summarised in Table 2 show that Aflatoxin B_1 or Aflatoxicol were present in all livers from cases of kwashiorkor, Aflatoxicol or Aflatoxin M_1 were found in five of six cases of marasmic kwashiorkor and no aflatoxins were detected in three cases of marasmus.

Our findings provide firm evidence that children in the Sudan are exposed to aflatoxins in their diet and these toxins can be detected in the serum and urine of a high proportion of the population of young children. Our serial studies indicated that single sample analysis is likely to underestimate the true exposure rate to aflatoxins. The more frequent detection and higher mean concentrations of aflatoxins in the sera of children with kwashiorkor than in normal controls might reflect greater exposure to aflatoxins in the kwashiorkor group, or they may be the result of impaired ability to transport and excrete these substances consequent on the metabolic derangements associated with kwashiorkor. The detection of aflatoxicol, and metabolite of aflatoxins B_1 and B_2 in children with kwashiorkor and marasmic kwashiorkor but not in controls or marasmic children indicates some fundamental difference in the metabolism of aflatoxins in the different categories of children.

The livers examined were from three widely separated geographical locations where the children have different ethnic, social and cultural backgrounds. The detection of aflatoxins in the livers of fatal cases of kwashiorkor and marasmic kwashiorkor in all three locations extend and confirm results of clinical and epidemiological investigations in a fourth location, the Sudan, which establish associations between aflatoxins and kwashiorkor though the nature of this association remains obscure.

The hypothesis that aflatoxins (and possibly other mycotoxins) have a causal role in the pathogenesis of kwashiorkor is attractive as it provides a rational basis for many of the epidemiological, clinical and biochemical observations on kwashiorkor which have defied explanation to date. To take but two examples: Reports of kwashiorkor in entirely breastfed infants appeared many years ago [22] but were disregarded as they could not be reconciled with the nutritional theories for the etiology and pathogenesis of kwashiorkor. Aflatoxins are ex-

Table 2. Aflatoxins in autopsy liver samples (pg/g).

Diagnosis	Country of origin			Total cases	No. positive	B_1	Aflatoxicol	M_1
	Nig.	S. Af.	Lib.					
Kwashiorkor	2	6	2	10	10	9 (391–8350)	1 (188)	–
Marasmic/ kwashiorkor	3	3	–	6	5	–	4 (108–8500)	1 (15)
Marasmus	2	1	–	3	0	–	–	–

Nig. = Nigeria; S. Af. = South Africa; Lib. = Liberia.

creted in animal and human milk if mothers are exposed to these toxins in their diet. If aflatoxins are causally related to kwashiorkor then the occurrence of the disease in breastfed babies would have a rational explanation. There is clinical and pathological evidence which indicates that children with kwashiorkor seem to be less susceptible to falciparum malaria than normal children [23]. This observation has prompted us to investigate the influence of aflatoxins on malaria in experimental animals. Our first series of experiments supervised by Professor B.G. Maegraith produced results which indicate that aflatoxins suppress P. berghei infection in mice. These findings have opened up an exciting new field for further study.

The toxicity of aflatoxins is modified by many factors, some of which also have a direct bearing on kwashiorkor. The very young are at greater risk from aflatoxins than older age groups. One factor which contributes to this is the larger food consumption per kg bodyweight of infants so that any level of aflatoxin contamination of food will be more significant for the child than the adult. It has also been established that a high protein intake protects while a deficient protein intake increases susceptibility to aflatoxins. In experimental animals Vitamine A deficiency is associated with a high mortality from aflatoxins. Aflatoxins are less toxic to animals fed selenium. Toxicity is also modified by the methionine, choline and fat contents of diets [2, 8].

Whatever the final explanation of the nature of the association between aflatoxins and kwashiorkor may prove to be, children with kwashiorkor are clearly at greater risk from aflatoxins than normal children. A situation can be envisaged in which following some initial insult to the liver, impaired ability to handle and excrete aflatoxins creates a vicious cycle in which aflatoxins accumulate as the ability to metabolise and eliminate these substances declines.

Conclusion

Mycotoxins are widespread throughout the world and human exposure to mycotoxins is greatest where climatic conditions favour fungal growth and social and economic conditions determine that populations must eat whatever foods are available in order to survive irrespective of the quality of the foods. This state of affairs exists in all the tropical developing countries and the children in these countries represent those at greatest risk from mycotoxicosis. The current paucity of scientifically acceptable evidence of diseases in man attributable to specific mycotoxins is no cause for complacency in our attitude to environmental hazards most of which have proved to be lethally toxic when tested on animals. Animals in the developed countries of the world are currently better protected from mycotoxin contaminated food than people in the tropical developing world. On scientific, economic and moral grounds, the influence of mycotoxins on human health is deserving of much greater attention than has been directed at it by the medical profession to date.

40

Acknowledgment

The principle collaborators in the studies on aflatoxins referred to were: J.B.S. Coulter, S.M. Lamplugh, S.B.J. Macfarlane and T.E. Williams, School of Tropical Medicine, Liverpool and M.I.A. Omer, G.I. Suliman and G.A. El-Zorgani, Khartoum, Sudan. The research was supported by Oxfam, I.D.R.C., Canada and the O.D.A. of H.M. Government.

References

1. Purchase IFH (ed): Mycotoxins. Elsevier, Amsterdam-Oxford-New York, 1974.
2. WHO: Environmental health criteria. II – Mycotoxins. Geneva, World Health Organisation, 1979.
3. Harwig J: Ochratoxin A and related metabolites. In Purchase IFH (ed) Mycotoxins. Elsevier, Amsterdam-Oxford-New York, 1974, pp 345–364.
4. Hendrickse RG, Adeniyi A: Quartan malarial nephrotic syndrome in children. Kid Int 16:64–74, 1979.
5. Mirocha CJ, Clyde M Christensen: Oestrogenic mycotoxins synthesized by fusarium. In: Purchase IFH (ed) Mycotoxins. Elsevier, Amsterdam-Oxford-New York, 1974, pp. 129–147.
6. Gelfand M: The sick Africa. JUTA, Cape Town, 1957.
7. Joffe AZ: Toxicity of fusarium poae and F. sporotrichioides and its relations to alimentary toxic aleukia. In: Purchase IFH (ed) Mycotoxins. Elsevier, Amsterdam-Oxford-New York, 1974, pp. 229–260.
8. Goldblatt LA: Aflatoxin. Academic Press, New York, 1969.
9. Becroft DMO, Webster DR: Aflatoxins and Reye's disease. Br Med J 117, 1972.
10. Dvorackova I, Brodsky F, German J: Aflatoxin and encephalitic syndrome with fatty degeneration of viscera. Nutr Rep Int 10:89–102, 1974.
11. Chaves-Carballo E, Ellefson RD, Gomez MR: An aflatoxin in the liver of a patient with Reye-Johnson syndrome. Mayo Clin Proc 51:48–50, 1976.
12. Olson LC, Bourgeois CH, Cotton RB, Harikul S, Grossman RA, Smith: Encephalopathy and fatty degeneration on the viscera in north eastern Thailand. Clinical syndrome and epidemiology. Pediatrics 47:707–716, 1971.
13. Shank RC, Bourgeois CH, Keschamras N, Chandavimol P: Aflatoxins in autopsy specimens from Thai children with an acute disease of unknown aetiology. Food Cosmet Toxicol 9:501–507, 1971.
14. Amla I, Kamala CS, Gopalakrishna GS, Jayaraj AP, Sreenivasamurthy V, Parpia HAB: Cirrhosis in children from peanut meal contaminated by aflatoxin. Am J Clin Nutr 24:609–614, 1971.
15. Krishnamachari KAVR, Ramesh V, Bhat VN, Tilak TBG: Investigations into an outbreak of hepatitis in parts of Western India. Ind J Med Res 63:1036–1049, 1975.
16. Serck-Hanssen A: Aflatoxin-induced fatal hepatitis? A case report from Uganda. Arch Environ Health 20:729–731, 1970.
17. Alleyne GAO, Hay RW, Picou DI, Stanfield JP, Whitehead RG: Protein energy malnutrition. Edward Arnold, London, 1976.
18. Coward WA, Lunn PG: The biochemistry and physiology of kwashiorkor and marasmus. Br Med Bull 37(1):19–24, 1971.
19. Hendrickse RG, Coulter JBS, Lamplugh SM, Macfarlane SBJ, Williams TE, Omer MIA, Suliman GI: Aflatoxins and kwashiorkor: a study in Sudanese children. Br Med J 285:843–846, 1982.
20. Lamplugh SM, Hendrickse RG: Aflatoxins in the livers of children with kwashiorkor. Ann Trop

Paediat 2:101–104, 1982.
21. Wellcome Trust Working Party: Lancet ii:302, 1970.
22. Trowell HC, Davies JN, Dean RFA: Kwashiorkor. Edward Arnold, London, 1954.
23. Hendrickse RG: Nutrition and infection in Nigeria. Ciba Foundation Study Group, No. 31., pp 98–111, 1967.

Bodily growth in thalassemia

V.S. TANPHAICHITR, C. TUCHINDA, V. SUVATTE and S. TUCHINDA

1. Introduction

Thalassemia is a genetically determined anemia prevalent in Mediteranean countries, the Middle East and South East Asia. It is an inherited disorder of the synthetic rate of globin chains resulting in unbalanced production of α- or β-chains [1]. In Thailand both α- and β-thalassemia are wide spread, and there is more than one subtype in each variety [2]. Besides, hemoglobin variants, i.e. HbE which is a β-chain variant with lysine replacing glutamic acid at position 26 and Hb Constant Spring which is an α-chain mutant with 31 amino acid residues elongating from the C-terminal of the normal α-chain are also common [3, 4]. These abnormal genes in different combinations result in a spectrum of syndromes ranging from asymptomatic heterozygotes to lethal Hb Bart's hydrop fetalis.

In Thailand the incidence of thalassemia and hemoglobinopathies are as follows: α-thalassemia, 20–30%; β-thalassemia, 5%; HbE, 13%; Hb Constant Spring, 4% [2, 3, 4]. Thus approximately 1% of the Thai population are estimated to suffer from thalassemia syndrome. As already mentioned Hb Bart's hydrop fetalis, homozygosity of α-thalassemia-1, is totally lethal either in utero or shortly after birth. The other common forms of thalassemia syndrome in Thailand are β-thalassemia major, β-thalassemia/HbE disease and HbH disease. Among these, β-thalassemia major which is homozygosity of β-thalassemia is the most servere form. The patients are expected to die in childhood unless they are kept alive by constant transfusion. β-thalassemia/HbE disease is moderately severe whereas HbH disease is the mildest form. The latter consist of the classical HbH and HbH + Constant Spring diseases. Classical HbH occurs from double heterozygosity between α-thalassemia-1 and α-thalassemia-2 while the HbH + Constant Spring disease occurs from α-thalassemia-1 and Hb Constant Spring [3].

2. Health consequence of thalassemia

The general health in thalassemia is poor due to anemia from chronic hemolysis and ineffective erythropoiesis, leading to tissue hypoxia. In response, there is gross bone marrow hyperplasia. If it is severe enough, bone changes will occur which include characteristic thalassemic facies and generalized skeletal osteoporosis with thinning of the cortex. Pathological fracture of the long bones and vertebral collapse may occur. Extramedullary erythropoiesis produces the enlargement of spleen and liver. Massive splenomegaly with secondary hypersplenism results in thrombocytopenia, leukopenia and accelerated red cell destruction [1]. Repeated blood transfusion and increased intestinal iron absorption lead to hemosiderosis. Iron overload occurs even in the cases that receive no or minimal blood transfusion. Besides, after splenectomy, iron loading is even augmented [5]. These lead to malfunction of affected organs, including liver and endocrine glands. Thus thalassemic patients suffer from anemia, consequences of splenomegaly, growth failure, iron overload, and intercurrent infection [1, 6]. However, in mild thalassemic cases, especially HbH disease, may clinically appear normal.

3. Bodily growth in thalassemia

Johnston and Krogman [7] have shown that growth patterns in children with β-thalassemia major alter in two ways: a retardation in their normal growth expectation and a retardation in their rate of growth. Similar findings are also observed by Constantoulakis et al. [8] therefore we are interested to assess growth in Thai children with different forms of thalassemia.

Two hundred and forty-eight thalassemic children aged ranging from 9 months to 15 years were included in our study. They consisted of 53 cases of HbH disease, 112 cases of β-thalassemia/HbE disease prior to splenectomy, 60 cases of β-thalassemia/HbE disease post splenectomy and 23 cases of β-thalassemia major. Height, body weight and upper arm circumference (UAC) were measured by standard technique [9]. Standards of height for age and weight for age were taken from Khanjanasthiti [10] and Chavalittamrong [11] whereas standard of UAC for age was taken from Jelliffe [9]. Percent standards of these parameters in each patient were calculated by comparing with the corresponding standard values. Table 1 shows the means ± SEM of weight, height and UAC for age in five groups of thalassemic children. The anthropometric parameters of children with HbH disease were less affected than the other groups. In children with β-thalassemia/HbE disease, prior to splenectomy their anthropometric parameters were less affected than those after splenectomy. This was probably due to the clinical severity of the latter group. The less affected anthropometic measures in the group of β-thalassemia major is related to the fact that their ages were younger than the other groups. This is consistent with the reports of Johnston et al. [12] and Constantoulakis et al. [8] that the growth velocity in β-thalassemia major decreased at about age six years for males and eight years for females.

It is well established that protein-energy status can be assessed by anthropometric measurement [9]. UAC is the composite measures of triceps skinfold thickness and upper arm muscle circumference which represent fat store and muscle mass, respectively. Though body weight is a gross quantitative measurement of body composition, it provides clinically significant information on protein-energy status. Degree of protein-energy malnutrition (PEM) in each patient based on weight for age and UAC for age was graded according to the following criteria: 90–100% of standard values are normal and 75–89%, 60–74%, and less than 60% of the standard values are considered to be mild (first degree), moderate (second degree), and severe (third degree) PEM [10]. Degree of PEM based on height for age was catagorized as follows: 95–100% of standard is normal and 90–94%, 85–89%, and less than 85% are considered to be mild, moderate and severe PEM, respectively [10].

Based on weight for age, height for age and UAC for age, the prevalence of PEM in 248 thalassemic children were 54.1%, 68.2% and 72.6%, respectively (Table 2). However, most of them were confined to mild and moderate PEM.

PEM can be either primary or secondary in origin. The primary PEM is caused by inadequate supply of food quantitatively and/or qualitalively. In secondary PEM, other illness or treatment affects protein-energy status of subjects by several mechanisms which include inadequate intake, impaired ingestion, defective absorption, faulty transport, impaired utilization, increased requirement and increased excretion of the nutrients [13].

Moderate to severe anemia were detected in all of the thalassemic patients except HbH disease (Table 3). Kattamis et al. [14] have shown that the growth of thalassemic children during the first decade largely depends upon the maintenance of fairly high hemoglobin levels. This implies that hypoxia is the main

Table 1. Weight for age, height for age and UAC for age in thalassemic children.

Subject			Mean ± SEM, % standard		
Group	Sex	No	Weight	Height	UAC
HbH disease	F	27	93.7 ± 1.9	94.2 ± 0.9	89.3 ± 1.3
	M	26	92.1 ± 2.0	93.9 ± 0.8	86.5 ± 1.5
β-thalassemia/HbE	F	56	85.8 ± 2.0	91.1 ± 1.0	83.3 ± 1.2
	M	56	89.3 ± 1.9	93.7 ± 0.7	84.6 ± 1.1
β-thalassemia/HbE	F	36	82.8 ± 2.1	90.1 ± 0.9	84.5 ± 0.9
post splenectomy	M	24	82.9 ± 2.9	89.8 ± 1.2	81.1 ± 1.7
β-thalassemia	F	5	92.3 ± 6.2	92.2 ± 2.5	84.9 ± 5.8
major	M	18	87.3 ± 3.3	91.3 ± 1.0	80.3 ± 2.0

factor retarding growth. In older children iron overload may be responsible for the delayed growth spurt at puberty. The impaired growth related to anemia is also evidenced in our study. Children with HbH disease had only mild anemia (Table 3). Their anthropometric measures were also better than the remaining groups (Table 1). It should be noted that children with HbH disease seldom recieve blood transfusion. Thus their risk to develop iron overload is less than other forms of thalassemia.

4. Growth hormone in thalassemia

Though the etiology of growth retardation in thalassemia has been ascribed to chronic hypoxia associated with anemia as already discussed hormonal insufficiency may be another contributing cause. This is suggested by the findings of hemosiderosis of endocrine glands at necropsy [15]. McIntosh [16] had shown the wide spread impairment of endocrine functions in β-thalassemia major. Thus we were interested to assess the endocrine functions in 4 children with β-thalassemia major and 14 children with β-thalassemia HbE disease. Their age ranged from 5 to 15 years. In this study linear growth was expressed as height age at which the

Table 2. Prevalence of PEM in 248 thalassemic children.

Parameter	PEM, % of total subjects*			
	mild	moderate	severe	total
Weight for age	38.3	13.0	2.8	54.1
Height for age	38.3	22.6	7.3	68.2
UAC for age	60.1	12.1	0.4	72.6

* Aged ranging from 9 months to 15 years.

Table 3. Hematocrit levels in thalassemic children.

Subject			Hematocrit %, Mean ± SEM
Group	Sex	No	
HbH disease	F	27	31.5 ± 0.6
	M	26	30.3 ± 1.2
β-thalassemia/HbE	F	56	21.8 ± 0.7
	M	56	23.3 ± 0.6
β-thalassemia/HbE	F	36	23.8 ± 0.1
post splenectomy	M	24	24.3 ± 0.7
β-thalassemia major	F	5	16.2 ± 2.4
	M	18	17.4 ± 1.6

patient's age would be at the 50th percentile for normal Thai children. Weight age was determined accordingly [10, 11]. Bone age was determined from roentgenograms of the wrist and hand using the standard of Greulich and Pyle [17]. Serum thyroxine level was determined by radioimmunoassay. Growth hormone release was induced by intramuscular injection of 1 mg glucagon. Blood samples were drawn before and at 30, 45, 60, 90, 120, 180 and 210 minutes after glucagon administration. Growth hormone was measured by a double antibody technique [18]. All tests were carried out before blood transfusion to eliminate the possibility of transfused hormones.

Table 4 shows that weight age, height age and bone age in children with β-thalassemia/HbE disease and β-thalassemia major were lag behind their chronological age. These indicate the impairment of their growth.

Two most important hormones needed for normal growth are thyproid and growth hormone. Our study shows that there is no impairment of thyroid function based on serum thyroxine levels (Table 4). This is also supported by clinical euthyroid. Besides, their bone age is almost corresponding to height age and weight age. In classical hypothyroidism profound retarded bone age as compared to height age is observed whereas weight age is higher than height age and bone age.

Impaired growth hormone release in both groups of thalassemic patients was evidenced by the low serum growth hormone levels at 120 minutes after glucagon administration (Table 4). Thus the growth retardation in thalassemic cases should, at least in part, due to impairment of pituitary function. Iron overloading of pituitary is generally believed to be responsible for this defect. Sonakul et al. [19] reported the pathological findings in 24 β-thalassemia/HbE disease. Hemosiderosis of parenchymal and reticuloendothelial tissues was detected. The organs involved include the spleen, liver, pancreas, lymph node, adrenal, kidney, alimentary tract and heart. However, hemosiderosis in pituitary was not as severe as other organs (Pacharee P, personnel communication). Thus anemia might be

Table 4. Mean ± SEM of growth parameters, serum thyroxine and growth hormone levels in thalassemic children.

Parameter	β-thal/HbE n = 14	β-thal major n = 4
Chronological age, yr	8.7 ± 2.8	12.8 ± 2.1
Weight age, yr	5.7 ± 2.9	7.8 ± 1.3
Height age, yr	5.2 ± 2.8	8.2 ± 1.3
Bone age, yr	6.3 ± 4.3	9.5 ± 0.7
Thyroxine[a], μg/dl	7.8 ± 1.3	7.2 ± 1.7
Growth hormone[b], ng/ml	5.8 ± 4.7	4.2 ± 2.5

[a] Normal level is 4–9 μg/dl.
[b] Determined at 120 minutes after glucagon stimulation test; normal level is above 20 ng/ml.

responsible for the defective growth hormone release in addition to hemo-siderosis and the gland is impaired functionally more than that seen anatomically.

5. Conclusion

Impaired growth is observed in thalassemic patients. The severity is more pro-nounced in β-thalassemia major and β-thalassemia/HbE disease. Their growth failure is due to chronic hypoxia caused by anemia and impaired growth hormone release. However, inadequate dietary intake and intercurrent infection may also be the contributing factors affecting their nutritional status and growth.

Acknowledgement

This work was supported in part by a grant from the Thai National Research Council.

References

1. Weatherall DJ, Clegg JB: The thalassemia symdrome. Oxford, Blackwell, 1972 (2nd edn).
2. Wasi P, Na-Nakorn S, Pootrakul S, Sookanek M, Disthasongchan P, Pornpatkul M, Panich V: Alpha- and Beta-thalassemia in Thailand. Ann NY Acad Sci 165:60–82, 1969.
3. Wasi P: Haemoglobinopathies including thalassemia. Part 1: tropical Asia. Clin Haematol 10:707–729, 1981.
4. Wasi P, Na-Nakorn S, Suingdumrong A: Studies of the distribution of haemoglobin E, thalas-semias and glucose-6-phosphate dehydrogenase deficiency in north-eastern Thailand. Nature 214:501–502, 1967.
5. Pootrakul P, Rugkiatsakul R, Wasi P: Increased transferrin iron saturation in splenectomized thalassemic patients. Brit J Haematol 46:143–145, 1980.
6. Tanphaichitr VS, Suvatte V, Mahasanda C, Tuchinda S: Host defense in thalassemias and the effects of splenectomy I. Incidence of mild and severe infections. J Med Assoc Thailand 61:66, 1978.
7. Johnston FE, Krogman WM: Patterns of growth in children with thalassemia major. Ann NY Acad Sci 119:667–679, 1964.
8. Constantoulakis M. Panagopoulos G, Augoustaki O: Stature and longitudinal growth in thalas-semia major. A study of 229 Greek patients. Clin Pediatr 14:355–368, 1975.
9. Jelliffe DB: The assessment of nutritional status of the community. World Health Organization, Geneva, 1966.
10. Khanjansathiti P: The anthropometric nutritional classification in Thai infants and preschool children. J Med Assoc Thailand 60:1–20 (suppl 1), 1977.
11. Chavalittamrong B, Vachakonon R: Height and weight of Bangkok children. J Med Assoc Thailand 61:1–28 (suppl 2), 1978.
12. Johnston FE, Kieth P, Hertzog BA, Malina RM: Longitudinal growth in thalassemia major, Am J Dis Child 112:396–401, 1966.

13. Tanphaichitr V, Kulapongse S: Diagnosis and management of adult protein-calorie malnutrition. In: Eng AS, Garcia-Webb P (eds) Clinical biochemistry, principles and practice. Singapore, Second Asian Pacific Congress of Clinical Biochemistry, 1983, pp 101–110.

14. Kattamis C, Touliatos N, Haidas S, Matsaniotis N: Growth of children with thalassemia: effect of different transfusion regimens. Arch Dis Child 45:502–505, 1970.

15. Bhamarapravati N, Na-Nakorn S, Wasi P, Tuchinda S: Pathology of abnormal hemoglobin diseases seen in Thailand I. Pathology of β-thalassemia hemoglobin E disease. Am J Clin Pathol 47:745–757, 1967.

16. McIntosh N: Endocrinopathy in thalassemia major. Arch Dis Child 51:195–201, 1976.

17. Greulich WW, Pyle JS: Radiographic atlas of skeletal development of hand and wrist. Standford, Calif., Standford University Press, 1959.

18. Lodeweychx MV: The glucagon stimulation test: effect on plasma growth hormone, J Pediatr 85:187–191, 1974.

19. Sonakul D, Sookanek M, Pacharee P: Pathology of thalassemia disease in Thailand. J Med Assoc Thailand 61:72, 1978.

Ecological evaluation of human development: The case of the child in the tropics

L. SINISTERRA

Definition and rationale

We understand as ecological the type of approach to the study of biological events which gives special importance to the dynamics of the relationships between the living organism and its surrounding environment as primary cause for adaptations and changes of one to the other. The successful adaptation of the two members of the equation will be key in survival and progress of the living organism.

In the case of human beings, it is justifiable to take an ecological attitude to study the process of growth and development of children, for in this case the two members of the equation and their mutual interaction are very dynamic in nature. The favorable environment will concur in a positive manner to the stimulus for the child to grow.

Ecological relations of the living organisms

It is appropriate te remember that Ecology is a young science which attempts to classify the relationships of living organisms and their environment. The first chapter of this science studies plants and their relationships with the physical environment which constitutes the subject matter of Plant Ecology. In this we see how plants have a total dependence on the conditions and characteristics of the inmediate physical environment. A large amount of sun light will promote an intense photosynthesis. If water and abundant nutrients exist in the top soil next to the roots of our plant, the complete process of growth and maturation will successfully occur, and stem, branches, leaves, fruits and flowers will grow vigorous and robust. If one or more of these factors is limited, the plant will show it in the quality of its frail structures.

In the next we find studies of the relationships existing between animals and their environment which constitute the subject matter of Animal Ecology. Looking at this process in more detail we observe that animals have a little more autonomy in relation to their environment. Although animals have an imperative need for water, for example, in most cases they can move around and reach the water they need. They also have an essential need for foods, and in most cases they can obtain them through the use of their own resources.

At this point, it is of interest to note that all of the resources, which are indispensable for growth and survival of plants and animals, are completely within reach of all of the members of the different species of the vegetable and animal kingdoms and that the only restriction for their access to them is the limitation derived from the physical capacity or the biological fitness. This is why for plants and animals survival is a privilege of the better fit members of the respective community which will be the ones responsible for the perpetuation of the species.

The ecological relations of the human beings

Relations of human beings with their environment (physical, social) are always characterized by the different tints of social interactions derived from the stratum in which the human being was born. Children who belong to the upper socio-economic groups have access to all kinds of resources and facilities. The pregnant woman in these groups can afford to reduce her physical activity and to increase her diet, both under the scientific direction of her obstetrician. Her delivery will be taken care of under the best conditions of technical care and hygiene. The child's intellectual and nutritional diet will be immediately instituted under adequate supervision and will be designed to supply all of the emotional and biological needs of the newborn. Custody, care and stimulation of the child will occur under the most advanced methods of child-rearing practices. In case the mother's attention is distracted by activities other than full-time supervision of the child, she can afford payment of a qualified person (maid, wet-nurse, nurse) to take full or partial responsibility for the care of the child. Later on, the child will receive medical attention, vaccines, education and adequate food which will allow him or her to grow optimally in both a physical and psychological context.

In contradistinction to the previous development of events, the child born in a family of the lower socio-economic groups is subjected from conception to limitations derived from the social conditions in which the family lives. The mother will continue working until very close to delivery, because she must contribute to the family income. Frequently, she will not be able to increase her diet and, as a consequence, the child may be born with low birth weight or small for gestational age with all of the consequences implied for growth and maturation of his tissues and organs including his brain.

As part of the picture of poverty, the child is not likely to have access to adequate medical care as required by his health necessities. The food received by

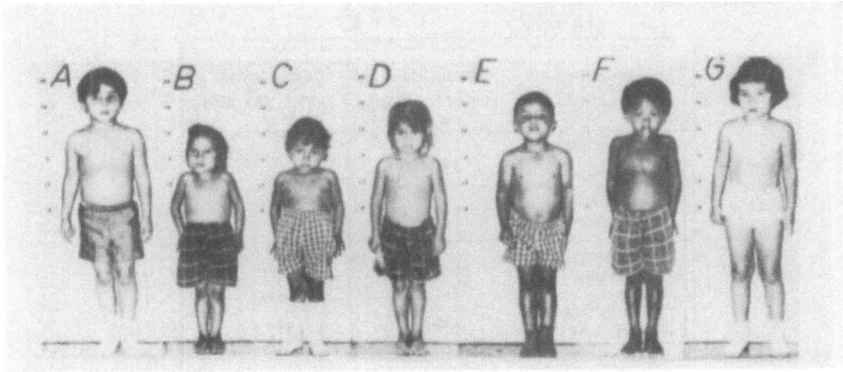

Figure 1. Children of the research project; all the children are 4 years old.

the child will probably not be adequate in quality and quantity. The living quarters of the family will be poor, and water and housing conditions will be of the kind which induces repeated infections and makes an inappropriate ecological niche for proper nurturing of the child. Consequences of these conditions in terms of physical growth can easily be seen in Figure 1 of several 4-year-old children of our program [1]. The boy and the girl at the extremes of the picture belong to the upper socio-economic group while the other five children come from the economically depressed family contexts, the girl in the middle has the stature corresponding to the average of the poor children. The boy and the girl at her right and left are one standard deviation away from the average and the two other children farther away are at two standard deviations from the average. This is then a distribution curve of children's statures which is very representative of the actual situation of the social groups in Colombia. We can then establish the relationship between physical (height and weight) parameters of the growth of children and data on the socio-economic conditions of the families to which they belong. We see Table 1 how educational levels of the parents are remarkably different: fathers of the upper group have an average of 14.5 years of formal education against 3.3 years for the lower class father; for mothers it is 10.4 years against 3.0 for the poor mothers. As is to be expected, income of the two groups is 12 times higher for the more educated group.

It is then clearly seen how the ecological niche surrounding the growing preschool child conditions his/her physical growth in a close cause-effect kind of relationship. For all of us in the medical profession this initial evidence must help us to recognize the need to expand our clinical knowledge to include considerations for the characteristics of the surrounding family environment (Ecology), if we want to participate in the orientation of official policies for the solution of the impact of poverty on the human being.

Table 1. Characteristics of the families.

SOCIOECONOMICS CHARACTERISTICS	REFERENCE GROUP (No.=60) a	EXPERIMENT GROUP (No.=300) b
NUMBER OF PERSONS IN HOUSE	4.9	7.5
YEARS EDUCATION OF FATHER	14.5	3.3
YEARS EDUCATION OF MOTHER	10.4	3.0
TOTAL MONTHLY INCOME(IN U.S.$)	560	44
FOOD EXPENDITURE % OF INCOME	22 %	74 %
PERSONS PER SLEEP ROOM	1.2	4.7
ELECTRICITY OR GAS FOR COOKING	100 %	6 %
POTABLE WATER AT HOME	100 %	4 %

a. UPPER CLASS CHILDREN.

b. LOWER CLASS CHILDREN.

Human ecological relations in tropical America

In tropical America in addition to the implications of poverty on growth and development of children, we must include some consideration for the historical series of events which caused all of the population changes and forced displacement as a consequence of the arrival of Europeans.

Before the arrival of the Spaniards at the end of the XVth century, America was a peaceful continent with a small number of Indians scattered over its immense extension. Some of them were more culturally advanced as in the case of the Aztecs in Mexico, the Mayas in Central America and Incas in Peru. For the rest, most of the populations were scattered small groups living in peaceful agricultural and artisanal societies.

The arrival of the buccaneer conqueror had a tremendous impact on the native society of the local Indians. The social habits of the newcomers were soon copied, for their adoption had the connotation of power and success. Often times the adoption of these new habits was the result of the imposition of laws decreed by the distant King under suggestions of the newly created 'aristocracy' who, in final analysis, were not much more than bandits and criminals who had become heroes as a result of their temerity in facing the risks of navigating to a very distant America. By an ordinance of 1530, for example, it was forbidden for Indians to ride on horses and mules for they were considered to be inferior to those animals which should only be used by the whites. A law signed by His Majesty in 1571 made it a crime for blacks to wear anything made of gold or silk.

Furthermore, the import of African slaves was a most unfortunate blow to the traditionally simple Indian society as well as to the blacks themselves. Their incorporation into everyday life, together with the authoritarian presence of the white group, disrupted traditions and beliefs of the local group and 'dialogue' among the different ethnic groups was only limited to the whip wielded by the ascendent whites for a very long time. In the last 150 years that our countries have been independent, progress in the direction of social harmony has moved very slowly and at this moment is far from ideal.

Ethnic adaptation to the tropical climates: Racial gradients

As is well known, in the tropical regions of the world in terms of ambient temperature, there are no seasons, and the local climatic conditions are mostly determined by the altitude above sea level. Sea level lands in the tropics are hot and have a very humid climate, and temperatures range between 30 and 35° C all year round. Colombian blacks live mostly in these kind of lands: around 80% of the 5 million Colombian blacks live in lands at or below 1,000 meters.

These low lands of Colombia are mostly covered by dense tropical jungle and are located in the Amazonian region and close to the coasts of the Pacific and Atlantic (Caribbean) oceans. Our black population lives in these regions mostly for social and survival reasons: these lands were the best haven when the majority of them escaped from the oppressive whites around the middle of the XIXth century. The settling of blacks around and close to the Colombian coasts has been the reason for the assertion that Colombia is surrounded by a 'black belt', as can be seen in Figure 2.

On the other hand, Indians had traditionally settled in the high lands away from the jungle and its innumerable dangerous beasts and snakes. Most of their lands are located above 2,000 meters, and temperatures oscilate around 10° C throughout the year.

With this distribution of the population, it is not difficult to establish something we could call a 'racial gradient' where Indians reside predominantly in the high lands at the cold end of the gradient and blacks live mostly in the low lands or hot end of the gradient. As shown in Figure 3, the Colombian racial groups of whites, mestizos and mulattos are ubiquitously located throughout the country.

It is also of some interest to note that altitude above sea level determines the different types of agricultural production in the tropics. For example, wheat, potatoes and barley grow only on lands above 2,000 meters where the low temperatures regulate their production. Low lands with high temperatures and humidity are favorable for the production of cassava, beans, rice and plantains. In Figure 4, we can observe a schematic diagram of the distribution of the agricultural production of the tropics as a function of the altitude.

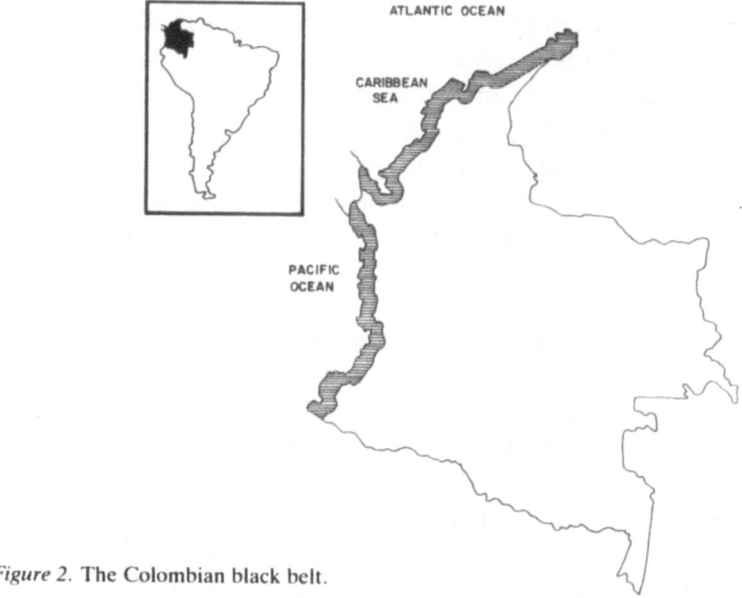

Figure 2. The Colombian black belt.

The human eco-system in tropical America

What we have described up to this point is valid for Colombia and also for most of the Latin American countries close to the tropics.

The cultural patterns and characteristics of the different human ecosystems are quite different from each other, and the ways children are educated, stimulated and ultimately raised differ significantly. This is what characterizes the family

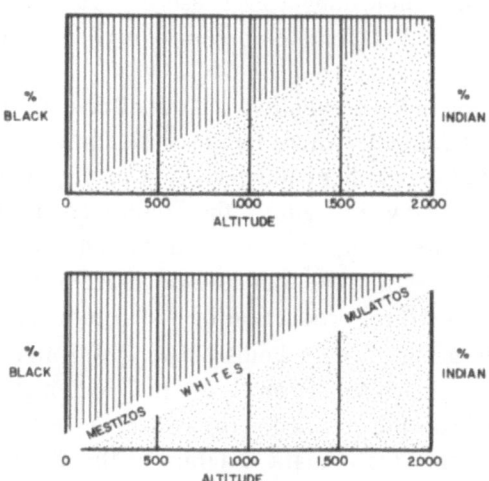

Figure 3. Racial gradient human thermic floors.

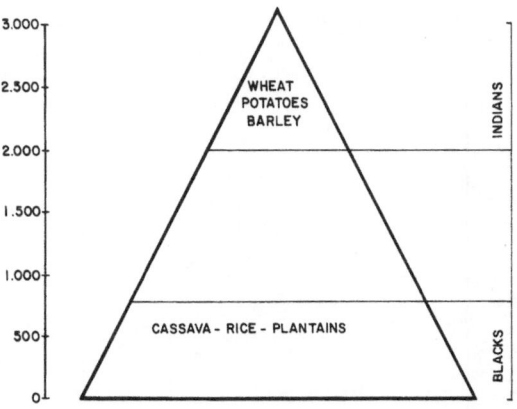

Figure 4. Agricultural production of the tropics.

ecological niche which induces marked differences, physical as well as behavioral, in the children of these groups.

Indians have close families with primary authority invested in the father. Deep
respect for traditions and a very conservative attitude are typical of the Indian
culture. Children from a very early age are supposed to help in the family work,
and education is of secondary importance. Malnutrition is very frequent and
upper respiratory infections complicate their lives and result in a high mortality.

Black families on the other hand have a very open social life. High temperatures favor outdoor life, and children move around nude and barefooted. Malnutrition is less frequent but gastro-intestinal infections with diarrhea and dehydration are frequently seen and contribute to the high death rate observed.
Interest in educating their children is reduced in black families to the acquisition
of elemental abilities in writing and arithmetic.

Rural-urban migration in Latin America

The final major factor affecting child health in tropical America is undoubtedly
migration from the rural to the rapidly growing urban towns. In Figure 5 it can be
seen that Latin America's urban population will grow 235% in the last 25 years of
the present century, while the rural population will grow a bare 20% during the
same period.

In Colombia, with about 26 million people, almost 70% of the population (18
million) live in the urban sector. Towns in Colombia have grown from 4 to 18
million people in the last 30 years, but the increment in public services, water
supply, sewage, electricity, schools, medical services, etc., has not kept up and a
deterioration of the 'quality of life' has ensued. Migrants from all over the country
arrive in towns bringing with them some of their farm implements and domestic

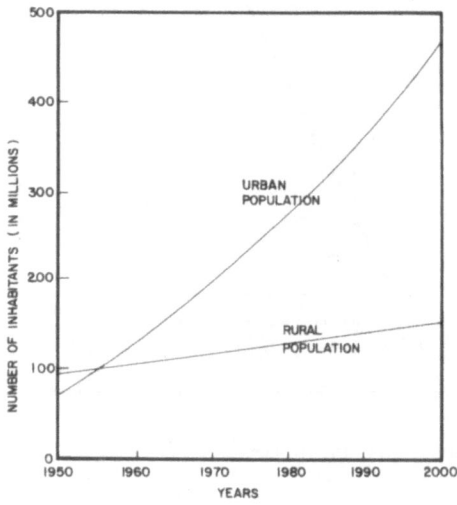

Figure 5. Latin American population growth; urban and rural increment 1950–2000.

animals, horses, dogs, chickens, pigs, etc., contributing to the so called process of 'ruralization of towns' [2].

In summary, then, the health of children in tropical America has to be carefully scrutinized because family conditions vary drastically among the various groups. Indians, blacks and migrants inhabit social and ecological niches which produce children in completely different psychological and physical conditions.

Human development studies in Colombia

From its inception in 1950, the Medical School of the University of the Valley, Cali, Colombia, decided to characterize and define the profiles of the local human health conditions. One of the initial findings was the high prevalence of infantile malnutrition with all its complications and high infant mortality rate. An early product of the identification of the problem of child health and poor nutrition in this part of the tropical world, was the development of a nutritional supplement based on a vegetable mixture, Colombiharina, the result of mixing soybean and rice, with vitamins and minerals added [3]. It was early seen that in this infantile population receiving a deficient diet and poor education, mental development was retarded almost as much as physical development [4].

Early in 1970 we started a comprehensive program of educational, medical and nutritional intervention in poorly nourished children. The experimental design can be seen in Figure 6. Three hundred 3-year-old children of lower socio-economic families and 60 children of the same ages but belonging to the upper social groups were included in the program, which lasted four years with direct

experimental design						
NUTRITION, HEALTH AND EDUCATION PRESCHOOL PROJECT CALI COLOMBIA						

GROUPS	N. 1.971	treatment years				N. 1974
		1.971	1.972	1.973	1.974	
T4	60	enh	enh	enh	enh	53
T3	60		enh	enh	enh	50
T2	60			enh	enh	51
TI	60				enh	50
HS	60	UPPER	CLASS	COMPARISON	GROUP	52
TI (a)	20	nh	nh	nh	enh	16
TI (b)	20		nh	nh	enh	17
TI (c)	20			nh	enh	16
	360					315

e = EDUCATION
n = NUTRITIONAL SUPPLEMENTATION
h = HEALTH CARE

Figure 6. Schematic of Cali project design.

stimulation of the children and another two years of indirect observation.

Results of the initial portion of the program were published in 1978 [5], and the most informative graph of this publication can be seen in Figure 7. It is easy to appreciate that children who started to participate at age three showed the most spectacular results of psychological gains. It is also clear that there is a significant difference in psychological development between the upper and lower class children as a whole.

The continued observation of these children for another two years [6] after termination of the pre-school intervention showed a clear reduction of the effects initially obtained, both psychological and physical, with a lessening of treatment effects and a progressively widening gap between these children and those from the higher socio-economic group (Figure 8). These results demonstrate the difficulty of sustaining cognitive gains in the poverty setting in which these children live. The home, the community in general and, unfortunately, also the public schools have become increasingly less adequate as providers of the stimuli necessary for what could be considered normal intellectual growth. This is then the result of a competition between the official educational system, very inadequate and inefficient, and the home and community environments (ecological niche) which appear as the strongest factors shaping the characteristics of the tropical American child of the lower classes.

A sub-sample of these same children were also evaluated for physical working capacity, with the utilization of the treadmill [7, 8]. Measurements taken provided information about the energy liberating processes in the skeletal muscles involved in the work as well as the functional capacity of the circulation. Results obtained can be seen in Table 9, which shows how children of the upper classes

60

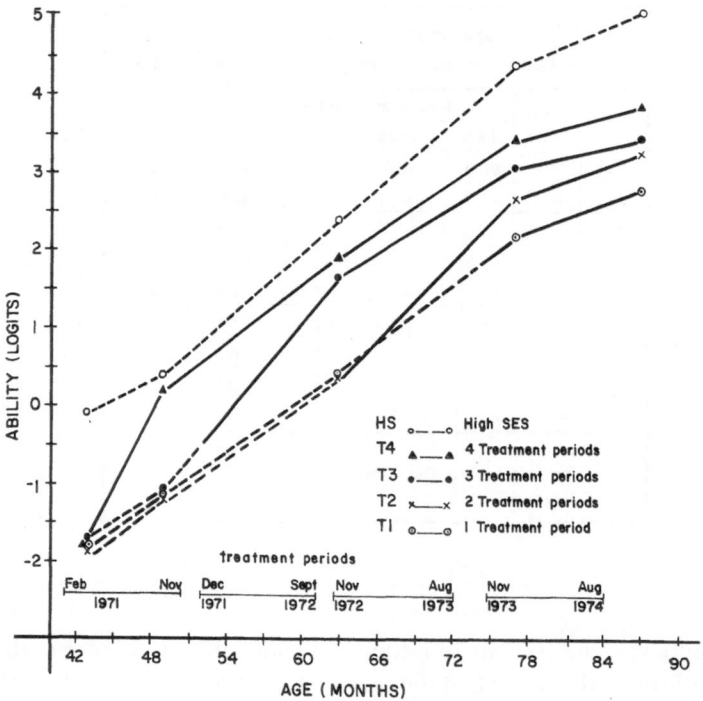

Figure 7. Growth of general cognitive ability of study children from 43 months of age to 87 months, the beginning of primary school.

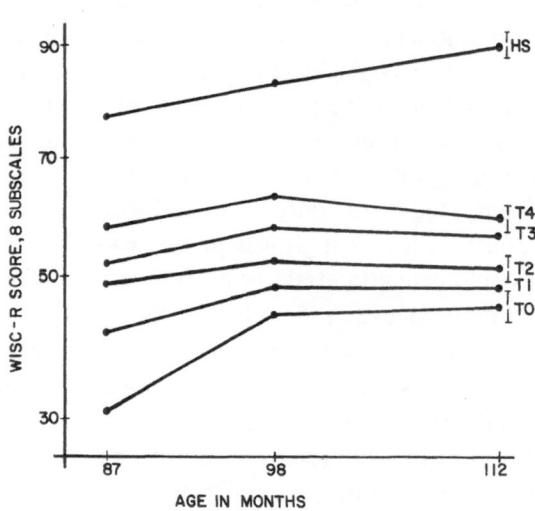

Figure 8. Progress of cognitive development of experimental and comparison groups in the period following preschool intervention.

GROUP NUMBER[e]	DISADVANTAGED[a]			PROBABILITY[b] (1-3)	ADVANTAGED[cd]		PROBABILITY[b] (1-5)
	1	2	3		4	5	
BODY WEIGHT, KG.	17.5 ± 1.5	16.9 ± 1.2	15.0 ± 1.3	<0.002	23.8 ± 4.2	21.6 ± 3.1	<0.0001
HEIGHT, CM	105.6 ± 3.0	105.7 ± 3.2	101.8 ± 4.3	<0.05	120.5 ± 5.3	120.0 ± 6.2	<0.0001
WEIGHT/HEIGHT, KG·M⁻¹	16.5 ± 1.2	16.0 ± 0.9	14.7 ± 0.8	<0.002	19.7 ± 2.9	18.0 ± 1.7	<0.0001
MAX HEART RATE, BEATS·MIN⁻¹	197 ± 11	195 ± 9	196 ± 10	NS	197 ± 5	192 ± 6	NS
$\dot{V}_{O_2}$ MAX (STPD), ML·MIN⁻¹	603 ± 71	584 ± 108	500 ± 97	<0.05	901 ± 112	912 ± 207	<0.0001
$\dot{V}_{O_2}$ MAX (STPD), ML·KG⁻¹·MIN⁻¹	34.6 ± 3.7	34.5 ± 5.6	33.2 ± 5.0	NS	38.1 ± 2.4	41.7 ± 4.3	<0.01
O$_2$ PULSE, ML/BEAT	3.1 ± 0.4	3.0 ± 0.6	2.6 ± 0.5	NS	4.6 ± 0.7	4.8 ± 1.1	<0.0001
$\dot{V}_E$ MAX (BTPS), LITER·MIN⁻¹	29.7 ± 4.9	27.5 ± 4.7	27.1 ± 6.6	NS	44.1 ± 6.0	39.7 ± 7.1	<0.0001

[a] UNDERNOURISHED AT AGE 3. [b] ONE WAY ANALYSIS OF VARIANCE. [c] NEVER EXPOSED TO UNDERNUTRITION. [d] NO STATISTICALLY SIGNIFICANT DIFFERENCE BETWEEN GROUPS 4 AND 5. [e] GROUP 1 - DIETARY REPLETION AT SCHOOL (n=10); GROUP 2 - DIETARY REPLETION AT HOME (n=10); GROUP 3 - NO DIETARY REPLETION (n=10); GROUP 4 - COLOMBIANS (n=6); GROUP 5 - AMERICANS (n=6). NS = NOT STATISTICALLY SIGNIFICANT.

Figure 9. Means and standard deviations of anthropometry and maximum physiologic responses of disadvantaged Colombian and advantaged Colombian and American six-year-old children.

have a much higher capacity to utilize oxygen, undoubtedly as a result of the larger quantity of muscle available for maximal work. This reduction on the physical potentiality of the lower-class child of tropical America may interfere with his curiosity and exploratory capacity, limiting his opportunities for learning and contributing in this way to his slower mental progress.

Present research programs in Cali

As a continuation of the research programs developed in the previous decade, we are now taking two lines of action which we hypothesize can contribute information about our main scientific purpose of defining strategies for fighting human underdevelopment of the tropical American child. These two lines are: (1) to develop a sound experimental integral care program for control of pregnancy, delivery and early stimulation of the child with very active participation of the family group and (2) to promote Primary Health Care Programs at the official level with very special participation of the Nurse and of the auxilliaries and community promotors as the field action group. Their main purpose will be the health of mother and child.

References

1. Sinisterra L: La Ecología del desarrollo humano: Ampliación del impacto de la educación médica. Bol Of Sanit Panam 85(4): 1978.
2. Sinisterra L: La atención y el manejo del niño. Evolución hacia el cuidado integral del niño y su familia. Courrier 31:593, 1981.
3. Sinisterra L: A vegetable protein mixture for the prevention and treatment of preschool malnutrition: Colombiharina, VIIIth Intl Nutr Congr, Prague, 1969, p 100.
4. Sinisterra L: Nutrition and early mental development. J Educ Res Editorial, Sept., 1970.
5. McKay H et al.: Improving cognitive ability in chronically deprived children. Science 200:270, 1978.
6. Sinisterra L et al.: Response of malnourished preschool children to multidisciplinary intervention. Proceedings of the International Nutrition Conference: Behavioral effects of energy and protein deficits. NIH Publication 79–1906, August, 1979, p 229.
7. Spurr GB: Nutritional status and physical work capacity. Yearbook of phys anthropol 25:1–34, 1983.
8. Spurr GB et al.: Childhood undernutrition: implications for adult work capacity and productivity. In: LJ Folisbee, JA Wagner, JF Borgia, BL Drinkwater, JA Gliner, JF Bedi (eds) Environmental Stress, Individual Human Adaptations. New York, Academic Press, 1978, pp 165–181.

Session II

Diarrhoeal diseases

Chairman: O. RANSOME-KUTI

Rice based oral rehydration therapy in acute diarrhoea: a superior therapy and a medium for calorie supplementation

A.M. MOLLA, S.A. SARKER, A. MOLLA, M. KHATOON
and W.B. GREENOUGH III

Summary

A randomised control study was carried out in 27 children between the ages 2 and 5 years with acute watery diarrhoea by using 80 g rice powder per litre of ORS with electrolyte concentrations as recommended by WHO, and 25 matched patients, who were treated by WHO standard ORS, acted as controls. During the first 24 hours of treatment, the patients of both groups received only ORS and no food. During a subsequent 48-hour period, patients received ORS according to random allocation and were offered measured amounts of food ad libitum. The efficacy of ORS was assessed by calculating the amount of ORS consumed, reduction in stool output and vomiting, biochemical changes and gain in body weight, and the calorie balance from only ORS during the first 24 hours and from ORS plus food during the subsequent 48 hours was calculated. Patients treated by rice ORS consumed 50% less ORS, their stool output and vomiting were reduced by 50% and 75% respectively. The gain in body weight was similar in both groups, and the calorie balance from only ORS was significantly higher in the rice ORS group.

Introduction

The immediate effect of diarrhoea is fluid and electrolyte malnutrition (FEM), but the delayed and disastrous effect is protein energy malnutrion (PEM). PEM diarrhoea involves factors such as (a) decreased intake of food due to anorexia or withholding food, (b) loss or malabsorption of nutrients through faeces and (c) increased catabolism. Fluid electrolyte loss is adequately and correctly treated by oral rehydration therapy, but the PEM following diarrhoea is not taken care of by the ORS available at present. Hence research on ORS continues in order to simplify and improve ORS so that simultaneous rehydration and calorie supplementation can be achieved.

For this reason, glucose alternatives have been tried. One successful alternative was 40 g of sucrose instead of 20 g glucose in one litre of ORS [1, 2]. Other alternatives of glucose have also been tried [3]. Any attempt for calorie supplementation has always been penalised by invariable osmotic problems. Recently, however, a suitable and successful substitute was found: 30 g rice has been used instead of 20 g glucose in one litre of ORS with equal success as glucose or sucrose ORS [4]. Rise, however, has several advantages:

(a) it is cheap and available.

(b) being a staple, it is readily acceptable.

(c) it is digested by intraluminal enzymes and liberates glucose molecules slowly and thus eliminates osmotic problems such as diarrhoea and vomiting.

(d) it contains higher amounts of cereal, and more calories can be packed through ORS.

In a subsequent study, a higher (50 g) amount of rice was used in ORS and was proved to be not only successful but superior to glucose-based ORS [5]. This was further confirmed in a larger number of patients with acute diarrhoea using 80 g of rice powder per litre of ORS [6]. The present study was designed to test the efficacy of using the highest amount of rice powder (80 g) as a rehydration therapy and digestibility without making it too thick to drink.

Patients and methods

The balance study was carried out in the Metabolic Study Unit of the International Centre for Diarrhoeal Disease Research, Bangladesh (ICDDR,B). A total of 52 children aged between 2 and 5 years with less than a 24-hour history of diarrhoea, no signs of systemic illness and having moderate to severe degree of dehydration were included in this study. Prior consents were obtained from the parents or guardians of the patients. Patients were allocated to the WHO ORS or rice ORS therapy according to random number. Those with severe dehydration received initial rehydration through intravenous solution, and patients with moderate dehydration were treated directly with oral rehydration solution.

Before starting oral rehydration therapy, each patient was fed an unabsorbable charcoal marker. The appearance of the marker was taken as the zero hour, and the study was conducted for 72 hours. Patients were randomized, but the ORS could not be hidden because of its distinctive colour. During the first 24 hours nothing but ORS was allowed; during the second 48 hours measured amounts of familiar Bangladeshi food was offered ad libitum. Accurate record was maintained of the stool, urine or vomitus and of ORS or any other fluid or food consumed during the whole study period. The glucose content from the aliquote of 24-hour stool was determined before and after hydrolysis. Calorie intake was measured and calculated from homogenized samples of stool, vomitus and food.

No antibiotic was given until the study was over. The efficacy of both solutions was calculated by measuring the amount of ORS consumed, reduction in purging rate and vomiting during each 24-hour period. Calorie intake, absorption and balance were calculated during the first 24 hours and the subsequent 48 hours separately. Since purging in many patients became very low, data of only the first 24 hours and the second 24 hours were considered in most cases.

Results

25 patients were treated by WHO ORS and 27 patients by rice ORS. Most patients were positive for vibrio cholerae and were suffering severe dehydration on admission. The clinical characteristics of the study patients are presented in Table 1. Patients were very closely matched as judged by age, body weight, adm serum sp gr., duration of diarrhoea and degree of dehydration. Table 2 compares the efficacy of both solutions. It is clear that patients treated by rice ORS consumed lower amounts of ORS during the 48 hours of therapy, passed lower amounts of stool and gained similar body weight. Vomiting in the rice ORS group was reduced by 75%, and the reduction of serum specific gravity was more pronouned in the rice ORS group. The differences between the two groups were significant as is illustrated in Table 2; the biochemical changes brought about by the two types of ORS are shown in Table 3. Biochemical parameters were corrected and maintained by both ORS. The stool sugar content in the rice ORS group after hydrolysis was not significant. The calorie intake, absorption and balance are presented in Table 4. The calorie balance during the first 24 hours was significantly higher in the rice ORS group, but during the second 48 hours it was not significantly different in either group. The absorption of calories from both solutions was not significantly different in either group, but the rice ORS patients

Table 1. Clinical characteristics of children with diarrhoea (mean ± SD).

Criteria	WHO ORS Gr (25)	Rice ORS Gr (27)
Age (months)	43.8 ± 14.9	40 ± 17.7
Adm. Wt. (kg)	10.8 ± 2.5	11.1 ± 2.3
Adm. Hct	44.2 ± 4.36	40.81 ± 5.14
Adm. Sp. gr.	1.0314 ± 0.0031	1.0300 ± 0.0037
Dur Diarrh (h)	11.0 ± 6.9	11.4 ± 6.8
Dehydration		
Mild	0	0
Moderate	29.6	29.6
Severe	66.6	70.4
Total patients/cholera	25/21	27/71

Table 2. Comparison of efficacy of the glucose and rice ORS in children with acute diarrhoa (mean ± SD).

Particulars	Glucose ORS	Rice ORS	P
Amount of ORS (ml/kg/day)			
1st 24 h	302 ± 145	171.8 ± 118.7	<0.001
2nd 24 h	126.7 ± 70.2	76 ± 63.5	<0.001
Purging rate (ml/kg/day)			
1st 24 kg	210 ± 157.7	105 ± 75.5	<0.005
2nd 24 h	89.8 ± 57	68 ± 73	<0.02
Amount of Vomitus (ml/kg/day)			
1st 24 h	22 ± 26.3	4.7 ± 9.2	<0.005
2nd 24 h	5.7 ± 7	3.8 ± 4.7	
% gain in body wt.			
1st 24 h	4.9 ± 5.8	5.4 ± 3.9	NS
2nd 24 h	6.4 ± 4.2	5.0 ± 3.9	NS
Change in sp. gr.			
Adm	1.0314 ± 0.0031	1.0300 ± 0.0037	
1st 24 h	1.0289 ± 0.0071	1.0254 ± 0.0023	<0.02
Change in Hct %			
Adm	44.2 ± 4.36	40.81 ± 5.14	
1st 24 h	35.76 ± 4.74	34.21 ± 4.99	

had a significantly higher calorie balance during the first 24 hours when both groups were on ORS only.

Discussion

Previous studies have shown that both 30 g or 50 g rice powder used along with WHO recommended salts were as effective as or superior to WHO ORS [4, 5]. Further information was necessary in order to establish the superiority of rice based ORS with respect to reduction in stool output, vomiting, capability of correcting biochemical abnormality and, most importantly, digestibility as judged by stool glucose content before and after *in vitro* hydrolysis. This metabolic balance study has very clearly demonstrated that even when 50% less ORS is consumed, rice based ORS is capable of reducing stool output by 50%, vomiting by 75% while the gain in body weight is similar. Biochemical changes, like the correction of acidosis and electrolyte balance, are equally efficient and the glucose content after hydrolysis; though higher in rice ORS group, it is not significant and did not affect the efficacy or calorie balance significantly. This is an additional and most important advantage especially when none of the antisecre-

Table 3. Biochemical changes during 1st 24-h therapy in children (mean ± SD).

Particulars	Glucose ORS		Rice ORS	
	Adm	24 h	Adm	24 h
Electrolytes				
Na⁺	134.3 ± 5.1	135 ± 7.3	136.5 ± 4.9	138.4 ± 4.3
K⁺	4.3 ± 0.7	4.6 ± 1.4	4.5 ± 0.8	4.0 ± 0.7
Cl⁻	103 ± 6.0	104 ± 5.1	105 ± 5.1	106 ± 6.0
TCO_2	12.1 ± 3.2	17.8 ± 2.4	13.9 ± 3.1	18.0 ± 3.9
Stool sugar (mMol/l)				
Before hydrolysis	4.4 ± 1.5	3.0 ± 8.3	4.0 ± 8.6	$6\,2 \pm 8.4$
After hydrolysis	11.6 ± 22.1	5.3 ± 17.0	14.8 ± 38.0	29.2 ± 54.0

Table 4. Calorie balance in children during 1st 24 h of therapy (mean ± SD).

Particulars	Glucose ORS		Rice ORS		P
	0–24 hr[a]	25–72[b]	0–24 hr[a]	25–72[b]	
Intake (kcal/kg/day)	22.3 ± 14.6	85.2 ± 24.6	45.6 ± 27.8	86.5 ± 36.6	<0.001
Output (kcal/kg/day)	9.0 ± 7.2	10.1 ± 9.2	14.3 ± 15.6	14.2 ± 13.8	NS
Calorie Intake only from ORS (kcal/kg/day)	8.6 ± 8.0	–	18.5 ± 13.2	–	<0.002
Co-efficient of absorption of calories (%)	55.6 ± 35.6	–	64 ± 40.8	–	NS
Calorie balance only from ORS (kcal/kg/day)	13.4 ± 12.4	–	32.2 ± 24.6	–	<0.001

[a] ORS only.
[b] ORS + Food.

tory drugs so far tested has proved to be satisfactory. Diarrhoea causes anorexia but the reduced calorie intake is also partly due to withholding food by the relatives as a measure to control diarrhoea. While the preaching of simultaneous feeding during diarrhoea therapy will take time to be effective, evolution of a calorie dense ORS to provide extra calories during therapy for diarrhoea will provide an excellent opportunity and tool for effective interruption of the diarrhoea malnutrition cycle.

References

1. Hirschhorn N, Kinzie JL, Sachar DB et al.: Decrease in net stool output in cholera during intestinal perfusion with glucose containing solution. N Engl J Med 275:176–181, 1968.

2. Sack RB, Casella J, Mitra R et al.: The use of oral replacement solutions in the treatment of cholera and other severe diarrhoeal disorders. Bull WHO 43:351–360, 1970.

3. Sack DA, Islam S, Brown KH et al.: Oral therapy in children with cholera a comparison of sucrose and glucose electrolyte solution. J Pediatr 96:20–24, 1980.

4. Molla AM, Sarker SA, Hossain M, Molla Ayesha, Greenough WB III: Lancet i:1317–1319, 1982.

5. Patra FC, Mahalanabis D, Jalan KN, Sen A, Banerjee P: Is oral rice electrolyte solution superior to glucose electrolyte solution in infantile diarrhoea? Arch Dis Child 57:910–912, 1982.

6. Molla AM, Masud A, Makhduma K, Greenough WB III: Trial of a calorie dense rice ORS in acute diarrhoea (unpublished).

Acute infantile gastroenteritis in Hong Kong

CHAP-YUNG YEUNG

Introduction

Acute infantile gastroenteritis was declared by the WHO in 1980 as one of the four global diseases [1]. The condition has resulted in high mortality and severe morbidity in developing countries [2]. Although it has not produced equally severe sequelae in the developed world, it still remains one of the most distressing health problems in infant health care programmes [3]. Hong Kong is situated between the developing and the developed world and is in a unique position to witness a continued change of the clinical pattern of gastroenteritis occurring in our community. Statistics from our department reveal that infantile diarrhoea is among the leading causes of peadiatric admissions and has been increasing in incidence over the past 12 years (Table 1).

Materials of this study

Children with diarrhoea admitted to our service at Queen Mary Hospital in 1981 and 1982 form the basis of this report. The records of the children admitted in 1971 and 1972 were analysed to demonstrate the difference in clinical pattern of the condition 10 years earlier.

During the past few years, there has been a significant improvement in laboratory techniques including identification for campylobacter, demonstration of enterotoxins in E. coli, and electron microscopic and ELISA techniques for identification of rotavirus infection. The scarcity of campylobacter and absence of rotavirus infections in the past, therefore, may not be representative of the real picture of that time. However a number of issues of interest will be discussed in the present paper.

Results and comments

A total of 822 patients were admitted in 1981/82 because of acute diarrhoeal illness. Of these, 58% (477/822) were males and 16.8% were infants under 1 month, half (51.9%) of them were less than 6 months old (Table 1). It can be noted that there has been a significant increase of admission of children with gastroenteritis in 1981/82 over that of 71/72 (Table 1).

It is distressing to note that a high proportion of our children with diarrhoea (1981/82) had a rather prolonged illness: 36% of the young infants had their diarrhoeal course lasting more than 7 days, and 14.2% had a protracted course beyond 2 weeks. Nearly half (45%) of the cases occurred in the winter months of November, December and January. Rotavirus infection was the single most prevalent infective agent associated with the diarrhoeal disease during the winter months, with the peak incidence of nearly 60%. Salmonella infection topped the list of bacterial gastroenteritis, followed closely by campylobacter, with Shigella ranking third in frequency (Table 2).

It is interesting to note that there were a number of significant changes in the clinical pattern of diarrhoeal illnesses in 1981/82 compared to that of 1971/72. Firstly the disease has become much more prevalent in number in 1981/82 but the proportion of infants under 3 months has reduced to less than half compared to 1971/72. Cases clustered around summer and early autumn 12 years ago but have become more prevalent in winter months recently. A third of the patients ran a very prolonged course or illness over 2 weeks in 1971/72 while the incidence has reduced to only 12% in recent years. Like other developing countries, gastroenteritis resulted in high mortality in 1971/72 (35/445) with the corrected mortality at about 5% (22/445). By 1981/82, despite of a significant increase in the incidence of diarrhoeal illnesses, there was only one death due to the condition.

Table 1. Incidence of gastroenteritis admitted to the paediatric service of Queen Mary Hospital.

Infant		1971/72	1981/82
Sex:	Male	93 155	220 257
	Female	75 122	129 216
Age:	< 1/12	186 (38.1)	138 (16.8)
	< 3/12	142 (67.2)	141 (33.9)
	< 6/12	81 (83.8)	140 (51.9)
	<12/12	36 (91.2)	188 (73.8)
	<24/12	21 (95.5)	127 (89.3
	<5 yr	10 (97.5)	49 (95.2)
	<5 yr	12 (100)	39 (100)
Mortality		35/445	5/822
Corrected mortality		22/445	1/822

( ) = cumulative percentage

There had been a number of claims from indirect survey to indicate the association between decreasing incidence of breast feeding with increasing frequency of gastro-enteritis in young infants [4, 5]. A similar trend was also observed in Hong Kong. However, there was also a marked decrease in the mortality. This does not appear to be a direct benefit of reduced breast feeding practices, but is probably related to the continued improvement in health care deliverance and social conditions as Hong Kong has continued to develop and progress to a 'near-developed' state over these years.

Specific conditions causing gastroenteritis

The following sections briefly discuss some of the features of specific aetiologic conditions causing gastroenteritis in our children.

Salmonella gastroenteritis

Excluding typhoid and paratyphoid, salmonella species still remain the commonest bacteria causing diarrhoea in children. The age and seasonal distribution of this condition is similar to those reported elsewhere [6]. However, there are two unusual features which are seldom encountered in other series. First of all, there was a fairly high incidence of Salmonella septicaemia (Table 3). Contrary to usual belief, three of the six infants with septicaemia were over 6 months, and half of these septicaemic infants were inflicted by the highly disabling condition of meningitis also.

Although the one who died of meningitis did not develop symptoms of diarrhoea, rather, he had constipation, he also had positive stool culture for the same

Table 2. Gastroenteritis: Micro-organism

	1971/72	1981/82
Salmonella	39	54
Campylobacter	?	45
Shigella	24	42
Staph. aureus	34	3
Yersinia		2
EPEC	99	–
Rota-virus	?	68 (132)
Adenovirus	?	11 (21)
27 n.m. virus	?	6 (11)
N.O.S.	249	591
Total	445	822

salmonella species suggesting that the portal of entry was most likely from the gastrointestinal tract. The incidence of septicaemia in our series is certainly much higher than those reported by others. This indicates the need for vigilant observation and search for septicaemic state in cases of Salmonella gastroenteritis in children. A review of the experience in 1971/72 also shows that Salmonella gastroenteritis in those days carried a very high mortality (7 out of 39). And again the severe outcome of the disease associated with septicaemia and death were not confined to infants of less than 3 months; four of the 7 deaths were older than 4 months of age (Table 4).

Campylobacter gastroenteritis

Improved technique of identification for campylobacter species was only introduced to our microbiology laboratory by late 1980. Since then campylobacter fetus ssp. jejuni has been identified to be the second commonest bacteria associ-

Table 3. Salmonella septicaemia.

Infant		Clinical feature		Salmonella species	Outcome
Sex	Age	Diarrhoea	Other features		
M	4 wk	+ +	Lethargic, jaundiced	S. Typhimurium	Well
F	6½ mo.	+ +	Fever, vomit, toxic	S. Johannesburg	Well
M	18 d.	+ +	Jaundice, lethargic	S. Gr. E.	Well
F	3 m.	+	Meningitis with cerebral infarcts	S. San Diego	Cerebral palsy
M	6 m.	−	Meningitis	S. Derby	Well
M	8 m.	−	Meningitis + infected subdural effusion	S. Newport	died

Table 4. Salmonella G-E deaths 71/72.

Salmonella	Sex	Age	Primary cause	Secondary	Feeding
Derby	F	5½ m	GE	−	A+B
B	F	2½ m	GE	Septicaemia	A
B	F	6 m	GE	−	B
Typhimurium	M	4 m	GE	Septicaemia	A+B
Typhimurium	F	3½ m	GE	−	A
Typhimurium	F	3 m	GE	Septicaemia	A
Typhimurium	M	4 m	GE	−	A

Incidence: 7/39.
A = Artificial; B = Breast

ated with diarrhoeal illness in infants of Hong Kong. A detailed account of its clinical feature is reported elsewhere [7]. Suffice it is to mention here that blood and mucus in the stool is a very frequent feature suggesting a degree of invasiveness of the organism, yet the disease seems to be fairly self-limiting. Of the two infants who developed septicaemia, one was treated with antibiotics but both had favourable outcome with complete recovery.

Shigella gastroenteritis

Shigella ranked third in frequency among bacterial related diarrhoea in this series. The commonest subspecies was S. Flexneri (24/42) followed by S. Sonnei (14/42) and Boydii (4/42). This disease differs significantly from Salmonella and Campylobacter infections in that the majority of children affected were older ones rather than infants less than 2 years (Table 5).

Rotavirus gastroenteritis

Rotavirus gastroenteritis has gained a significant prominence among diarrhoeal children in Hong Kong due mainly to recently established technique of identification as well as an increasing incidence of viral infections among children in general, compared to 12 years ago. There has also been a tendency of increasing incidence of rotavirus infections among our children over the past 3 years. At one time during last winter, the incidence of positive rotavirus identification approached 60% of all patients with diarrhoeal illness in our unit [8]. Among these there were a high number of nose-comial infections as well. A representative sample of 30 infants taken from the present series showed that the clinical features were very similar to those reported in the literature [9]. Although severe dehydration had not been a prominent feature among our children, there is a

Table 5. Shigella gastroenteritis (81/82).

Sex (male:female) = 28:14	
Age: <1/12	2
<6/12	6
<12/12	4
<24/12	4
2–5 yr	13
5 years	13
Organisms S. flexneri	32
S. sonnei	9
S. boydii	1

tendency for these infants to require relatively long period of intravenous fluid/ electrolyte therapy because of protracted vomiting and loss of appetite [8].

Entero-pathogenic E. coli (EPEC) gastroenteritis

During this study period, an outbreak of EPEC gastroenteritis was encountered in a maternity hospital. This is a hospital in which minor and major outbreaks of EPEC gastroenteritis have been recurring every 3 to 4 years ever since the department was first involved in the care of the sick newborn 20 years ago. Policies and management plan for each outbreak differed according to the different paediatricians in charge of that time. There was varying mortality associated with different outbreaks. The strategy of management for the 1982 outbreak was based on experience drawn between 1968 to 71 when similar epidemics occurred among two different hospitals treated with two different regimes with very different outcomes [10]. Encouraged by this past experience, a neomycin prophylaxis regime was introduced with an attempt to control the spread of the epidemic.

Upon identification of 10 out of the initial 12 infants who developed diarrhoea within 48 hours from ward A who were carrying EPEC 0126, all infants in that ward were treated with neomycin 15 mgm q 8 h for 5 days prophylactically, beginning the 3rd day following the initial outbreak of the diarrhoeal illness. The ward was closed from 3rd day onwards while other postnatal wards were closely monitored for the spread of the disease. It can be noted from the Table 6 that there were further 5 children who developed symptoms of diarrhoea in this ward in the ensuring 2 days, of whom 1 was stool positive for the same EPEC.

The disease kept on spreading to other wards (C, P, N) on day 3, and by the fourth day, ward B was also affected. Once a case of diarrhoea occurred in any of these wards, all infants in the same ward were covered with a similar regime of neomycin prophylaxis. This practice was continued for a full 14 days for all subsequent neonatal admissions.

It is of interest to note there were a total of 12 positive cultures among 24 infants who developed the diarrhoeal illness (Table 7). As the hospital laboratory could not cope with identification of stool samples from all infants and mothers, it was not known as to the extent of the spread of the EPEC carrier states in these patients. However, it was extremely gratifying to see that the disease was controlled fairly promptly from spreading and there was not a single death. In contrast, the outbreak in 1979 lingered on for months and carried a high mortality although it was infected by a different strain of EPEC at that time.

Discussion

This study has demonstrated the marked change in the clinical pattern of gastroenteritis in children of our community which has also witnessed a dramatic progress in various economic and social programmes, evolving from an underdeveloped to a 'near-developed' society. Formerly, the disease claimed a high

Table 6. An outbreak of EPEC gastroenteritis in a maternity hospital (1982) – Ward A.

Onset (day)	Infant	Sex	Age	Stool frequency	pH	B.E.	WBC	Na/K
1	1	M	3	4	7.232	−13.3	4,100	131/4.2
	2	M	6	3	7.273	−14.2	10,700	130/5.7
	3	F	4	7	7.243	−12.4	8,250	139/3.9
	4	M	6	10	7.273	−10.4	7,800	139/4.7
	5	F	5	20	7.178	−19.2	11,600	128/4.0
2	6	M	4	5	7.31	−3.7	11,800	138/5.4
	7	F	6	8	7.27	−15.1	7,100	135/4.2
	8	M	4	7	7.316	−11.0	6,200	145/5.5
	9	F	3	10	7.31	−5.6	9,150	140/6.1
	10	M	3	6	–	–	10,900	140/5.6
	11	M	3	4	7.44	−4.2	8,500	142/4.7
	12	M	9	6	7.155	−21.2	12,400	132/3.8
3	13	F	5	4	7.544	−1.9	8,100	140/4.7
	14	F	2	10	7.310	−9.6	16,900	144/4.3
	15	M	2	4	7.354	−2.7	9,000	134/5.7
	16	F	2	3	7.454	−3.7	14,500	147/5.8
5	17	M	11	6	6.943	−30.1	29,200	120/5.1

EPEC 0126 present in Cases 1, 2, 3, 4, 5, 6, 7, 8, 9, 10, 13.
Fever in cases 2 & 7. Blood & mucus in case 15.

Table 7. Summary of an outbreak of EPEC gastroenteritis in a maternity hospital (EPEC 0126).

Ward	Infants (diarrhoea)	Spreading period (days)	Positive cultures	Neomycin prophylaxis*	
				Commenced (date)	Duration (days)
A+	17/44 (4)	4	11/17	2	10
B	2/66 (7)	6	0/2	4	9
C	1/64 (12)	3	0/1	3	12
N	3/61	7	1/3	3	12
P	1/25 (5)	7	0/1	3	12

Legend: A, B, C, = Post-natal wards, on level 2; N = Special Care Nursery, P = P.N wards, on level 4; + Ward closed for 2 weeks; ( ) = Breast feeding; * Neomycin 15 mg 8 hourly × 5 days to all infants.

mortality, tended to the much more protracted in the clinical course; it was associated with much higher incidence of severe sepsis and other complications. Recently, as we are seeing more viral infections among our children, we are also seeing a significant increase in the total number of diarrhoeal children as well. The disease however has become much less lethal than before. There are also relatively less young infants under 3 months affected by the condition compared to 12 years ago. The proportion of infants developing protracted diarrhoea has also been substantially reduced.

There is no indication as to the contribution of breast feeding to the development of gastroenteritis in this study, due to the lack of genuine statistics. The trend of breast feeding practices has been decreasing over the past 15 years. If this indirect information was correct, then reduced breast feeding was positively associated with increased number of gastroenteritis admissions but not associated with increased number of infants less than 3 months requiring hospitalization for such. As most of the protective effect against enteropathogens are derived from colostrum and early milk [11], the present finding of having less infants under 3 months with diarrhoea in 1981/82 provides indirect evidence contrary to the usual belief of the protective effect of breast feeding against infantile gastroenteritis. What is even more distressing was the finding of high mortality rate in the 1971/72 series when the incidence of breast feeding was believed to be much higher than what it was in 1981/82. To draw conclusions from these observations that the change of mortality and incidence of diarrhoea was the result of a change in the incidence of breast feeding is therefore not only highly dangerous but scientifically incorrect. There are multiple factors resulting in the change of disease pattern and improved survivals in our community, much more than a mere change of infant feeding practices.

Improvement in social economic status, educational level, and other public health measures together with comparable advances of standard of health care deliverance are all contributary to the improved survival of gastroenteritis seen in the past few years. In this regard, Hong Kong has joined other developed countries for not deriving significant benefit from breast feeding in regard to protection of young infants from developing severe and potentially fatal infective diarrhoea [12].

References

1. Bull WHO: 58:183—198, 1980.
2. Black RE, Brown KH, Becker S, Yunus M: Mortality and morbidity of gastro-enteritis in developing countries. Am J Epidemiol 115:305, 1982.
3. Gall DG, Hamilton JR: Infectious diarrhoea in infants and children. Clin Gastroenterol 6:431, 1977.
4. Cunningham AS: Morbidity in breast-fed and artificially fed infants. J Pediatr 90:726, 1977.
5. Bullen CL, Willis AT: Resistance of the breast-fed infant to gastroenteritis. BMJ 3:338, 1971.

6. Rosenstein BJ: Salmonellosis in infants and children. Epidemiologic and therapeutic considerations. J Pediatr 70:1, 1967.
7. Szeto M, Yeung CY: Camybobacteriosis in Hong Kong (in press).
8. Yeung CY, Lam BCC, Lam J: Unpublished, 1983.
9. Rodriguez WJ et al.: Clinical features of acute gastroenteritis associated with human reovirus-like agent in infant and young children. J Pediatr 91:188, 1977.
10. Yeung CY: Annual report of Paediatric B Unit, Queen Elizabeth Hospital, Hong Kong, 1971.
11. Welsh JK, May JT: Anti-infective properties of breast milk. J Pediatr 94:1, 1979.
12. Cushing AH, Anderson L: Diarrhoea in breast-fed and non-breast fed infants. J Pediatr 70:921, 1982.

Diarrhoeal diseases in children and oral rehydration in Nigeria

T.C. OKEAHIALAM

Summary

Diarrhoeal diseases are responsible for high mortality and morbidity in infancy and early childhood in tropical countries. Oral rehydration therapy, which is simple and cheap, has been found to be effective in most parts of the world. This is confirmed also in a study carried out in Nigeria. For immediate intervention, it is important that all health workers are conversant with its use; the long term measure will depend on efforts made by various governments to implement effectively their national programmes for control of diarrhoeal diseases.

Introduction

Diarrhoeal diseases are major causes of infant and early childhood mortality and morbidity in tropical countries. It is estimated that over five to ten million children die annually in these parts of the world from diarrhoeal dehydration. The high incidence is related to poor social and environmental factors – inadequate sanitation, overcrowding, lack of clean pipe borne water, malnutrition, poverty and ignorance. Within the past three decades, the unfortunate decline in breast feeding and the popularity of bottle feeding even among the rural communities of third world countries are also responsible for the increase in episodes of diarrhoea and its complications. The efficacy of breast milk in the prevention of diarrhoeal diseases is well documented [1–3].

One important social factor which has heightened the problems of diarrhoeal diseases in tropical countries is rural–urban migration, particularly within the past two decades. Social, economic and political changes have suddenly transformed little towns into cities without adequate infrastructural facilities. Peri- and intra-urban slums made up of shanty houses are characteristic features of most of these cities. The young illiterate population from the villages in search of regular wage-earning employment arrive and find accommodation in these parts of the city only to swell the number of the urban poor. Many children seen in the urban hospitals and clinics with diarrhoea come from this population. A recent study we have carried out indicates that children from these periurban slums experience more episodes of diarrhoea than those in the rural areas.

Diarrhoea in children occurs worldwide and the global challenge posed has led to several studies and advancement of knowledge on the epidemiology, aetiology, pathogenesis, better methods of treatment and possible prevention. Routine microbiological studies identify bacterial causative organisms in less than 25% of cases [4–6]. More elaborate investigations have incriminated viruses notably the rotavirus in diarrhoeal diseases of children [7–9]. Bacteriae isolated from stools include various pathogenic strains of E. coli – enterotoxigenic (ETEC), enteroinvasive (EIEC), and enteropathogenic (EPEC). Others include Yersinia enterocolitics, campylobacter jejuni/coli, staphyloccus aureus, pseudomonas aeruginosa, vibrio, clostridium and brucella.

In tropical countries, diarrhoea is also a commonly associated clinical feature of systemic diseases of infancy and childhood such as measles, malaria, kwashiorkor otitis media and pneumonia. Iatrogenic causes include the effect of potent traditional medicines, regular administration of aperients by parents and side effects of drugs particularly antibiotics often used indiscriminately.

Pathophysiology

In recent years, there has been a better understanding of production of diarrhoeal stool. Some bacteria directly invade and damage the villi of the intestinal mucosa, and others produce enterotoxins which affect the gut. A study of the cholera toxin shows that it activates adenyl cyclase in the cell membrane of the mucosal cells of the gut. This leads to an increase in the production of cyclic adenosine monophosphate (c-Amp). This paralyses the normal function of absorption of sodium and chloride and stimulates the secretion of these electrolytes by the crypt cells. It is likely that specific enterotoxins produced by other bacteria cause diarrhoea by this mechanism; however, the action of the rotavirus is not clear. In these cases, the mechanism of absorption of the gut is not disturbed. The consequence of these infections is loss of water and electrolytes in large quantities from the extracellular and later the intracellular compartment. The marked reduction of body fluid volume may lead to shock, decrease in renal blood flow and oliguria. These changes may take place rapidly and, if treatment is not promptly instituted, may lead to death or to irreversible changes particularly in the central nervous system.

It is becoming clear that recurrent episodes of diarrhoea within the first year of life are important precipitating factors of nutritional marasmus which is on the increase in tropical countries. The outlook of an infant with marasmus in terms of growth and development is not encouraging [10, 11]. There is need therefore for the adoption of simple methods of immediate intervention in the management of diarrhoeal diseases apart from the long-term programmes of prevention related to socio-economic changes.

Oral rehydration therapy

The efficacy of oral rehydration therapy (ORT) for the correction of electrolytes and water losses in diarrhoeal diseases has been established [12, 13]. The experiences obtained from the treatment of cholera with oral electrolyte solutions have heightened the enthusiasm of several workers on the use of this simple, cheap and effective method of therapy [14–16]. These have been applied to other forms of diarrhoeal diseases in children in many parts of the world [17, 18]. The effectiveness of salt-sugar solution (SSS) is based on the principle that glucose is a 'carrier' and one sodium ion is reabsorbed from the lumen of the gut into the mucosal cells along with one molecule of glucose. Thus the coupling of sodium and glucose is mandatory for this process to take place [19].

Oral electrolyte solutions can be prepared at home from salt and sugar. In our environment, mothers are instructed to use a quarter of a teaspoon of salt and 4 cubes of sugar dissolved in a pint of water. Some workers have pointed out mistakes that may occur in the measurement of salt used [20, 21]. To overcome this, special spoons have been recommended and found to be effective [22, 23]. Furthermore, the World Health Organisation has introduced prepacketed oral rehydration salts which can be made up into a solution with a litre of water. Each packet contains:

Sodium chloride	3.5 g
Potassium chloride	1.5 g
Sodium bicarbonate	2.5 g
Glucose	20 g

The prepared solution is isotonic and contains (mEq/l), sodium 90, potassium 20, bicarbonate 30, chloride 80. This solution has been tried in many parts of the world and found to be suitable. However, there has been debates on the possible risk of hypernatraemia as a result of the level of sodium content, especially among paediatricians in Europe and North America. Some have recommended three ORT solutions of varying compositions and expressed the view that the WHO solutions should be recommended only 'for developing areas of the world'. Experience has however shown that as long as breast feeding is continued during oral rehydration and adequate water is given, WHO ORT solution is safe [24–27).

ORT study in Nigeria

A multicentered study has been carried out to determine the effectiveness and acceptability of WHO ORT solution. This is a brief report of the results of part of this study in Enugu.

Two-hundred-and-twelve children with diarrhoea were seen at the Paediatric Clinic of the University of Nigeria Teaching Hospital and in four peripheral health centres. They comprised 94 males and 118 females. Their ages ranged from less than six months to two years, but the majority were between 12 and 18 months (Figure 1).

The clinical features on admission are shown in Table 1. One-hundred-and-forty-nine children (70%) presented with watery stools 4 to 6 times a day and dehydration was mild in 143 (67.5%) children and seven in 11 (5.2%). Drugs had been given at home in 79 cases (37%), and these consisted of various anti-diarrhoeal mixtures containing kaolin, pectin, and antibiotics, chloroquine, paracetamol, aspirin, phenergan, and plasil (metoclopramide). Traditional medicines were used in 6.5% of cases (Table 2).

Most of the children came from young families (Table 3) of the low income group. Pipe borne water was available to only 91 (43%) families involved in this study. There was rapid decline in breast feeding practice among the mothers (Table 4). Only 61 (28.7%) children were fully immunised. The response to ORT

Table 1. Clinical presentation on admission.

A.	Stool frequency	No. of patients (%)
	4–6 stools/day	149 (70)
	7–10 stools/day	17 (8)
B.	Other associated features	No. of patients (%)
	Fever	51 (24)
	Blood in stool	16 (7.5)
	Cough	35 (16.5)
	Convulsion	3 (1.4)
	Rashes	5 (2.4)

Table 2. Treatment given at home before attendance.

79 children (37%) given treatment

Anti-diarrhoeal mixtures containing antibiotics, pectin, kaolin

Chloroquine
Paracetamol, aspirin, phenergan
Plasil (metoclopramide)

Traditional medicines

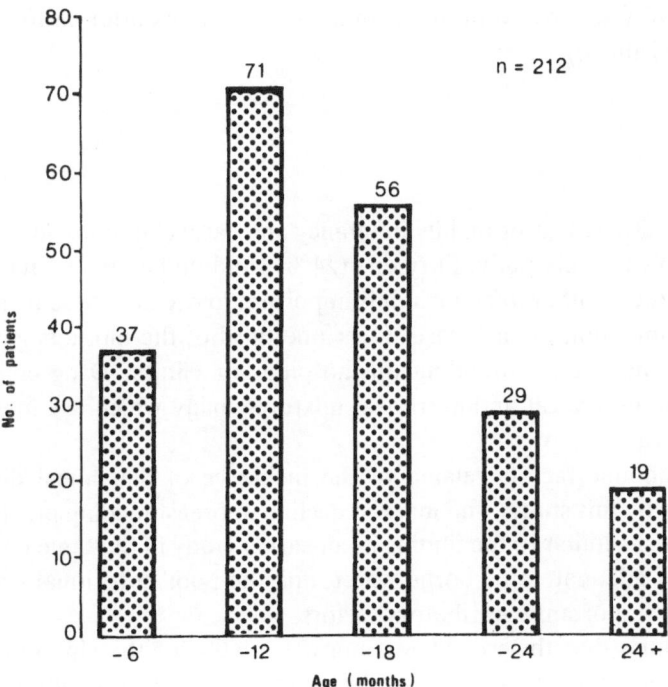

Figure 1. Age distribution of children with diarrhoeal disease.

was assessed by the frequency of the stool and the state of rehydration of each child (Table 5). The stools decreased in frequency or stopped within three of five days of therapy. Although 46 children presented with vomiting on admission, it was possible to treat 28 with ORT; the rest received intravenous fluids. Accept-

Table 3. Size of family.

No. of children per family	No. of families (%)
1–3	157 (74)
4–6	47–22
7+	8 (4)

Table 4. Children with diarrhoeal diseases and breast feeding.

Ages (months)	No. of patients	No of children still breast feeding
0–6	37	21 (56.7%)
7–12	71	28 (39.4%)
12+	104	11 (10.7%)

ability of ORT was based on the comments of mothers after 48 to 72 hours of treatment (Table 6).

Discussion

Diarrhoeal diseases occur mainly in infancy and early childhood in our environment as shown in this study. Fifty-one (24%) children had fever, and this could have been due to other infections; it is important to exclude these by a thorough clinical examination in each case. Over one third of the mothers gave various drugs at home before attending the hospitals or clinics. Drug companies in Nigeria market several antidiarrhoeal mixtures many which are ineffective or even dangerous.

Socio-economic factors related to the incidence of diarrhoeal diseases are brought out by this study. The marked decline in breast feeding practice among these mothers, similar to the finding of an earlier study in the same environment [28], lack of adequate pipe borne water, and the poor nutritional status of the children are important contributory factors.

It was found that the weight was normal in 60% of the children below six months (Table 7); above 18 months, the weight of half of the children was below the 50th percentile of the Nigerian standard [29]. The estimation of the amount of fluid required for mildly-dehydrated children based on weight may be unreliable; however, a clinical assessment is also necessary. Over two-thirds of the children were mildly dehydrated and these responded quickly to ORT. At the end of 72 hours, 162 (76.4%) were rehydrated and the frequency of the stool was significantly reduced in 151 (71.2%) children. Nineteen (9%) children who had per-

Table 5. Response to oral rehydration therapy.

Duration of treatment (h)	No of children (%) as shown by	
	Rehydration	Decreased stool
24	71 (33.5)	54 (25.5)
48	108 (50.9)	119 (56)
72	162 (76.4)	151 (71.2)

Table 6. Acceptability of oral rehydration therapy – response by mothers.

Found it useful	Found it easy to prepare	Will recommend to friends	Will give ORT again if child has diarrhoea
143 (67.4%)	196 (92.5%)	156 (73.6%)	155 (73%)

sistent vomiting and were severely dehydrated were placed on intravenous therapy after 48 hours, three of these died, and the mortality in this study was 1.4%.

Oral rehydration therapy is effective provided it is instituted early at the onset of diarrhoea and the mothers well instructed on its use. Mothers found the solution useful and easy to make at home. One basic problem one encounters with ORT is the lack of standard measures in many homes especially in the rural area. In Nigeria, the empty beer bottle which measures approximately two-thirds of a litre is found in most homes except in strict muslim families. It is therefore important to adopt a measure preferably a plastic container which is universally acceptable to the population of each country, for the preparation of oral rehydration solutions. Health education is very important for the success of ORT and it should emphasize the essential need of continuing with breast feeding during treatment. The need for immunisation should be stressed; in this study, only 61 (28.7%) were fully immunised.

It is important that doctors, nurses and other health workers are conversant with the use of ORT; it should form an integral part of maternal and child health in a national primary health programme, particularly in tropical countries. However, the long-term solution requires the political will of the various governments in Tropical Africa to implement their national programmes for diarrhoeal disease control and to give priority to the improvement of environmental sanitation, provision of good water supply and promotion of child health services. [30] Along these lines, it is hoped that the Government in Nigeria will initiate a programme for the local production of pre-packed ORT powder which will be available at a cheap price in most homes throughout the country. This will reduce not only the use of intravenous therapy which is expensive and could be dangerous, but also the high mortality and morbidity associated with the paediatric problem of diarrhoeal diseases.

Table 7. Weight of children on admission.

Ages (months)	0–6	7–12	13–18	19–24	25+
No. of patients	37	71	56	29	19
Centiles					
above 50th	24 (65%)	38 (53.5%)	21 (37.5%)	15 (51.7%)	10 (52.6%)
below 50th	13	33	35	14	9

88

References

1. Jelliffe DB, Jelliffe EFP: The uniqueness of human milk. W Ind Med J 20:190–195, 1971.
2. Mata L: Breast feeding: Main promoter of infant health. Am J Clin Nutr 33:2365–2371, 1980.
3. Ebrahim GJ: Breast feeding – The biological option. Macmillan, London, 1978.
4. Rowland HAK: The pathogens of diarrhoea. Trans R Soc Med Hyg 72:289–301, 1978.
5. Wamola IA: Bacterial stool pathogens in Kenyatta National Hospital. E Afr Med J 57:867–871, 1980.
6. Okeahialam TC: Gastroenteritis in children. Nig Med Prac 3:11–13, 1983.
7. Bishop RF, Davidson GP, Holmes IH, Ruck BJ: Virus particles in epithelial cells of duodenal mucosa from children with acute nonbacterial gastroenteritis. Lancet 2:1281–1283, 1973.
8. Walker-Smith S: Rotavirus gastroenteritis. Arch Dis Child 53:355–362, 1978.
9. Steinhoff MC: Rotavirus: the first five years. J Paediatr 96:611–622, 1980.
10. Stoch MB, Smythe PM: A 15-year developmental study on effects of severe undernutrition during infancy on subsequent growth and intellectual functioning. Arch Dis Child 51:327–336, 1976.
11. Okeahialam TC: Growth of Nigerian children with marasmus after hospital treatment. J Natl Med Assoc 75:75–80, 1983.
12. Darrow DC et al.: Water and electrolytes in infantile diarrhoea. Pediatric 129–156, 1949.
13. Harrison HE: The treatment of diarrhoea in infancy. Ped Clin N Am 1:335–348, 1954.
14. Phillips RA: Water and electrolyte losses in cholera. Fed Proc 23:705–712, 1964.
15. Nalin DR: Oral nasogastric maintenance therapy in paediatric cholera patients. Trop Ped 78:355–358, 1971.
16. Sack RB, Cassells J, Mitra R et al.: The use of oral replacement solutions in the treatment of cholera and other severe ciarrhoeal disorders. Bull. WHO 43:351–360, 1970.
17. Barker WH: Perspectives on acute enteric disease: epidemiology and control. PAHO Bull 9:148–156, 1975.
18. International Study Group: Beneficial effects of oral electrolyte-sugar solutions in the treatment of children's diarrhoea (Parts 1 and 2). J Trop Ped 27:62–67; 136–139, 1981.
19. Cutting WAM, Langmuir AD: Oral rehydration in diarrhoea: applied pathophysiology. Trans R Soc Trop Med Hyg 74:30–35, 1980.
20. Ransome-Kuti O, Bamisaiye A: Oral therapy in infant diarrhoea (letter). Lancet 2:471, 1978.
21. Harland PSEG, Cox DL, Lyew M, Lindo F: Composition of oral solutions prepared by Jamaican mothers for treatment of diarrhoea. Lancet 1:600–601, 1981.
22. Hendrata L: Spoons for making glucose-salt solution. Lancet 1:612, 1978.
23. Morley D, King M: Spoons for making glucose-salt solution (letter). Lancet 1:53–54, 1978.
24. Finberg L: The role of oral glucose solutions in hydration for children – international and domestic aspects. J Pediatr 96:51–54, 1980.
25. Hutchins P, Wilson C, Manly JA, Walker-Smith JA: Oral solutions for infantile gastroenteritis – variations in composition. Arch Dis Child 55:616–618, 1980.
26. Woodward WE: Oral rehydration for diarrhoea (letter). J Pediatr 97:515–516, 1980.
27. Finberg L, Harper PA, Harrison HE, Sack RB: Oral rehydration for diarrhoea (Editorial). J Pediatr 101:497–499, 1982.
28. Okeahialam TC: Breast feeding practices among Nigerian Igbo mothers. J Trop Ped (in press).
29. Janes MD, MacFarlane SBJ, Moody JB: Height and weight growth standards for Nigerian children. Ann Trop Pediatr 1: 27–37, 1981.
30. Bennett FJ: Diarrhoeal disease control (Editorial). E Afr Med J 57: 293–298, 1980.

Diarrhoeal diseases in Pakistani children

S.R. KHAN

Diarrhoeal diseases constitute a very important threat to child life and health in Pakistan. Some health statistics of the country relevant to the problem are given in Table 1.

Diarrhoea is the single most important disease of children in the country. It is responsible for 40–50% admissions and 25–30% of deaths of children in hospital. In the Pediatric Ward of Mayo Hospital, Lahore, in 1982 out of the 8760 admissions 4735 and out of 836 deaths, 206 were due to diarrhoea. This disease is also a cause of high morbidity and mortality in the community.

Doctors and other health workers in clinics and dispensaries see a third of their children patients suffering from this disease, and children constitute half of their work load.

Gordan et al. reported an incidence of 100 to 200 episodes per 100 children in Indian Punjab in 1963. Our socio-economic conditions are similar and working on a moderate rate of one episode per child per year, about *13 million episodes of diarrhoea occur every year among preschool children in the country with about a hundred thousand deaths.*

A nation wide survey is now being conducted to collect accurate incidence and mortality data which are expected to become available by the end of this year.

It is truly an infantile disease in Pakistan at least among hospitalised cases. 73% of 4735 cases admitted to the Pediatric Diarrhoea Ward of Mayo Hospital Lahore in 1982 were below one year of age. Similarly amongst hospital cases co-existant malnutrition is the rule. 88% of these had weights below the 10th percentile of the American standard, whereas in the community in general only 30% infants fall within that weight. According to the 1976 National Nutrition Survey, 16.7% of preschool children in the country are moderate to severely malnourished using waterlow's classification. Diarrhoea and poor and unhygienic feeding and weaning are considered to be the main causes of childhood malnutrition in the country.

Breast feeding generally considered an insurance against diarrhoea and malnutrition at least in the first six months of life does not seem to provide that cover on casual examination. The national survey of 1976 shows that breast feeding is a common practice both in rural and urban setting.

However diarrhoea and malnutrition are both very common at this age. The chief reason for this is that cow's milk (fresh or dried) is also being given to babies. 10% of infants receive additional cow's milk on the day of birth and 30% at 1 month of age. Nearly every woman brings with her a feeding bottle and a tin of milk when coming to hospital for delivery.

Another distinctive feature of infant rearing in Pakistan is the habit of giving water to them either pure or with herbs, etc. This begins the day of birth. These two practices – supplementary bottle and water feeding – greatly mitigate the safety of breast milk. In fact, some of us have launched a crusade against giving anything to infants other than their mothers' milk.

Soothers are very commonly used. The infant's environment is generally contaminated in low socioeconomic homes. There is a dearth of toilets and clean water. Personal hygiene is poor, and habit of frequent hand washing with soap is also not common. Abundant flies in summer complete the usual scenario of a developing country where diarrhoea thrives.

Etiology. There are hospital reports on the isolation of various pathogens (Table 4, 5).

Rota virus, EPEC, ETEC, Shigella, Vibrio Cholera and Salmonella have been isolated and reported from various centres in the country. However very little is

Table 1. Some relevant health statics of Pakistan 1982.

Total population	85 million
No. of children 0–4 years	13 million
Mortality of children 0–4 years	210/1000
Infant mortality	100/1000
Crude death rate	13/1000
Crude birth rate	43/1000
Population growth rate	30/1000

Table 2. Diarrhoea in children (0–4 years) in Lahore.

775 studied for 5 years
40% infantile mortality due to diarrhoea
25% ill with diarrhoea for more than 50 days in a year

Table 3. Ages of stoppage of breast feeding in infants.

6 months	7.4%
12 months	20.8%
24 months	72.0%

known of their relative frequencies in the patients and controls in the community. A multicentre study assisted by the WHO is now under way and will be completed by the middle of 1985. Studies on different aspects of diarrhoea pathogens are also being conducted at Lahore and 2 other centres.

The mortality pattern of hospital cases is presented in Table 6.

It was interesting to note that no death occurred in any case who did not have dehydration plus one or more of the above conditions and that in one death the patient had shock without dehydration.

Table 4. Isolates from the cases of infantile gastroenteritis (Khan et al.).

Organisms	Number
Rota virus	26
E. coli (EEC)* OK Poly A	05
OK Poly B	16
Pseudomonas aeruginosa	03
Rota virus + E. coli OK Poly A	01
Rota virus + E. coli OK Poly B	06
Rota virus + pseudomonas aeruginosa	01
Entamoeba histolytica	01
Negative	41
Total	100

* Enteropathogenic Each-coli.

Table 5. Causative organisms of gastroenteritis (Khan et al.).

Organisms	No. isolated
E. coli (EPEC) OK Poly A	29 (12.1%)
OK Poly B	36 (15%)
OK Poly C	7 (2.9%)
Proteus morganii	11 (4.7%)
Shigella boydii	2 (0.8%)
Shigella flexeneri	2 (0.8%)
Shigella dysenteriae	1 (0.4%)
Pseudomonas aeruginosa	4 (1.6%)
Salmonella stanley	2 (0.8%)
Salmonella typhi	2 (0.8%)
Giardia intestinalis	3 (1.3%)
Negative	141 (58.8%)
Total	240

Control measures. Considering its great importance the federal and provincial governments have launched control of Diarrhoea programmes since 1982.

Strategies adopted in Pakistan for control of diarrhoeal diseases.

---

1. Case management	ORS supply, training of health workers, education of community
2. Epidemic control	Chiefly based on returns from ORS outlets
3. M.C.H. practices	Breast feeding education/promotion
4. Environmental health	Water, excreta, flies

In this connection the province of Punjab, to which I belong, has organized the following activities.

ORS supply. Six million packets of ORS in 1983 are being procured from local manufactures and distributed free from 4000 outlets. Proper logistics for this has been worked out and depots, subdepots, vans and jeeps have been provided.

Training. One regional training centre of the World Health Organization, Eastern Mediterranean Region has been functioning at King Edward Medical College, Lahore, since December, 1980, and has trained 468 doctors and 370 paramedicals from all over the country in case management, diarrhoea control and programme management. Some of these participants came from other Middle Eastern countries.

8 subcentres of training have also been established at other institutions in the province; 2000 doctors and paramedicals are to be trained from these centres in 4-day courses by the end of 1984. Teaching material for mothers, community health workers and paramedicals have been prepared and are being distributed.

Health education. Health education of the community is being undertaken in the

Table 6. Mortality pattern in pediatric diarrhoea amongst hospital cases in Pakistan. Incidence of complications and associated illnesses in 106 deaths occurring in the Pediatric Diarrhoea Ward of Mayo Hospital, Lahore, 1980.

	No.	Percent
Dehydration	105	99
Acidosis	81	76
Bronchopneumonia	62	58
Marasmus	55	52
Shock	47	44
Distension	40	38
Meningitis	9	8
Convulsions	7	7
Prematurity	7	7

use of oral rehydration in diarrhoea, adoption of proper breast feeding, hand washing, use of clean water and proper excreta disposal.

In this connection booklets, posters and pamphlets have been prepared, and radio, TV and press, etc. and being used extensively.

References

1. Health and health related statistics of Pakistan planning commission. Government of Pakistan, Islamabad, 1975.
2. Pakistan Year Book, 1977 Planning Division, Government of Pakistan.
3. Gordon JE, Chitkara ID, Wyon JB: Weaning diarrhoea. Am J Med Sci 245:345–377, 1963.
4. Micro-Nutritient Survey of Pakistan, 1976–77: Nutrition cell, planning and development division. Government of Pakistan, Islamabad.
5. Khan MMA, Khan MA, Burney MI, Ghafoor A: Aetiology of infantile gastroenteritis. Pak J Med Res 21 (1), 1982.
6. Khan MMA, Ghafoor A, Burney MIJ: Pak Med Assoc 31, 1981.

Diarrhoeal diseases and mortality in infants and children

SUHARYONO

1. Introduction

1.1. Diarrhoeal diseases: 'a major health problem'

In developing countries, diarrhoea still ranks among the leading causes of death, and mortality rates continue to be as high as those of the industrial nations in 1900. In industrial nations, mortality due to diarrhoea declined from 4000 per 100,000 infants in 1900 to 35–45 in 1960; the corresponding decline for children 1–4 years old was from 200–400 to about 2.5 per 100,000 [1].

From 30 to 60% of all deaths in preschool children in developing countries are associated with diarrhoea. Incidence figures projected for children of 0–4 years of age etimate that there have been 457 million episodes of diarrhoea from 1975 in Asia, Africa and Latin America [2].

In some developing countries, attacks of acute diarrhoea may occur as often as once a month during a child's 2nd year [3]. An infant will have at least one diarrhoeal episode per year, between 1 and 2 years old will experience 2 episodes [4]. Longitudinal studies in a semirural community in Ujung Pandang (Indonesia) in 1976 revealed that the incidence or the episodes of diarrhoea was more than 400 per 1000 population per year, most (70–80%) occurring in children under 5 years of age.

1.2. Recent knowledge

Some recent research on the aetiology and pathogenesis of the common diarrhoea and advances in techniques to correct dehydration in a simple, effective and relatively inexpensive manner have brought optimism and enthusiasm to the area of health planning, particularly as applied to poor rural areas, to the extent that control of the effects of diarrhoea is now a real possibility [5, 6].

1.3. Chronic and other diarrhoeal diseases (e.g. acute diarrhoea with accompanying diseases in surgical cases): 'a major hospital problem'

1.3.1. Mucosal lesions in acute diarrhoea often diminish digestion and absorption of carbohydrates. Ingestion of lactose under such circumstances increases the diarrhoea and prolongs its course. Prolonged diarrhoea and repeated episodes of diarrhoea can lead to malnutrition and malabsorption [7].

Diarrhoea in malnourished children often is recurrent, particularly during the first two years of life. Each attack lasts for a few days or one week but its effects on nutrition may extend over a longer period. Malabsorption persists for days, and frequently for weeks or months. Therefore, diarrhoea is an important cause of malnutrition, growth retardation, and permanent stunting of children of developing nations.

1.3.2. In our hospital in Jakarta, the infant and child mortality rate of ('pure') acute diarrhoea has indeed been decreased to a minimum, but what later turns out to be chronic diarrhoea, and/or which goes with other accompanying diseases, is still relatively high. Therefore, it is now 'a major hospital problem'. The four main causes of infant and child mortality due to acute diarrhoea, which goes with other accompanying diseases, are: encephalitis, bronchopneumonia, sepsis and protein energy malnutrition.

1.3.3. Diarrhoea in surgical cases such as Hirschsprung's disease, causing CSBS or contaminated small bowel syndrome, post ilectomy in intussusception ileocoecal case, causing cholerrhoeic diarrhoea or bile acid malabsorption, and others are also a difficult and major hospital problem, since there are still many nosocomial infections in the wards of developing countries besides the difficulty of searching for the unknown determinants in these cases.

2. A national (Indonesia) diarrhoeal diseases control (DDC) programme (1974–1983)

2.1. Background information

Indonesia is an archipelago comprising more than 13,000 islands. It is a tropical country with a population of about 150 million which is distributed unevenly. The birth rate is approximately 44 per 1000 population, the crude death rate is 18% and infant mortality is 98 per 1000 live births according to the 1980 census.

The main health problems are communicable diseases and poor nutrition. The important causes of diseases and deaths are upper respiratory tract infections, diarrhoeal diseases and protein energy malnutrition (PEM). The low socioeconomic status and poor environmental health are important determining factors of the health condition of the majority of the people. Diarrhoeal disease belongs to the important public health problem in Indonesia. It is one of the leading causes of disease and death, especially before 1974.

2.2. Diarrhoeal diseases control programme

2.2.1. *Action and constraints*. Long- and short-term control programmes have been carried out since 1974. Oral rehydration using Oralit is one of the most important strategies in the programme. Although it is difficult to reduce the morbidity of diarrhoea, it revealed that deaths from diarrhoea could be reduced by oral rehydration.

Many constraints are faced by the programme, i.e. its management, technical and social constraints. The implementation of the programme can not rely exclusively on the existing health delivery care. The low coverage of the health delivery care system and the social constraints have pushed the government into a search of alternatives and oral rehydration should be a part of the social programme.

It has been proven that a solution of ordinary sugar and table salt, if measured properly, is capable of preventing dehydration if administered at an early stage of diarrhoea. Each household has sugar and salt; other kinds of sugars traditionally used were also found in most households. An easy method to prepare the sugar-salt solution is being done using a special spoon called 'blue-spoon'.

With simple but proper health education, the community can be taught how to prepare ORS (oral rehydration solution) from 'oralit' or salt and sugar using blue-spoon. The electrolyte composition is most accurate if the solution is prepared from 'oralit', the use of the blue-spoon was the next most accurate method of preparing the solution, while the less accurate method was preparing the solution using the ordinary tea spoon.

There are many old traditions and ways of treating diarrhoea. Some of these practices are of benefit to the patient with regard to rehydration, some are not and may even be harmful.

Methods which have a positive effect on rehydration should be encouraged or improved, while those people who practice methods which can be harmful should be taught that results would be much better if 'oralit' or sugar-salt solution were also given. At the first National Seminar on Rehydration in 1974, a motto was coined, i.e. 'No one should die from diarrhoea'. Rehydration with 'oralit' is without a doubt of paramount importance for preventing death of infants and children.

2.2.2. The estimate of morbidity of diarrhoeal diseases in 1983 dropped to 330 (1983) from 400 in 1976 per 1000 people.

2.2.3. The important enteropathogens are rotavirus (by electron microscopical method [8] and/or ELISA), E. coli (ETEC), Salmonella spp, Shigella, V. cholerae eltor, V.parahemolyticus, etc. There are numerous factors or other causes which induce diarrhoea.

2.2.4. A mortality study in 1976 revealed that 40% of all deaths in the first 2 years of life was due to diarrhoea. The CFR (case fatality rate) of diarrhoeal cases in hospitals in Indonesia, before the diarrhoeal diseases control program was launched, was 10–30% and at present, i.e. at the General Hospital Jakarta, was only 0.9%.

2.2.5. Malnutrition is one of the important contributory factors that may induce or increase the severity of diarrhoeal diseases in infants and children. Repeated bouts of acute diarrhoea can lead to undernutrition or PEM. Study in Indonesia revealed that about 30% of children under five suffer from undernutrition or PEM.

In some bigger cities the practice of breastfeeding has been on the decline since 1970. Although bottle feeding in Indonesia, especially in the rural area, is still less popular than in developed countries [9], it is nevertheless, posing a threat to the health of infants and children, i.e. causing diarrhoeal diseases and death in areas with a lack of proper drinking water and in unhygienic environmental conditions.

2.2.6. *Government's (health) target 'REPELITA IV' (1983–1988) include:*
1. Infant mortality 98/1000 → 74/1000
2. 'Under five'/'BALITA' mortality 48/1000 → 25/1000
3. Morbidity of diarrhoea 330/1000 → 250/1000
4. PEM 'under five' 30% → 22%
5. Clean and healthy water supply:
     rural 32% → 55%
     urban 60% → 65%
6. Latrine in rural area 25% → 42%
7. Life expectancy 56 years → 63 years.

3. Diarrhoeal diseases in hospital

3.1. The classification of diarrhoeal diseases

In the Paediatric Gastroenterology Ward at Dr. Cipto Mangunkusumo General Hospital, these diseases, are separated into 5 groups:
1. Acute diarrhoea (AD) or gastroenteritis
2. AD + complications (shock, acidosis, hypokalemi, etc.)
3. AD + accompanying diseases (encefalitis, bronchopneumoni, sepsis, PEM, etc.)
4. Chronic diarrhoea
5. Diarrhoea in paediatric (gastroenterology) surgical cases (CSBS, bile-acid or cholerrhoeic diarrhoea, etc.).

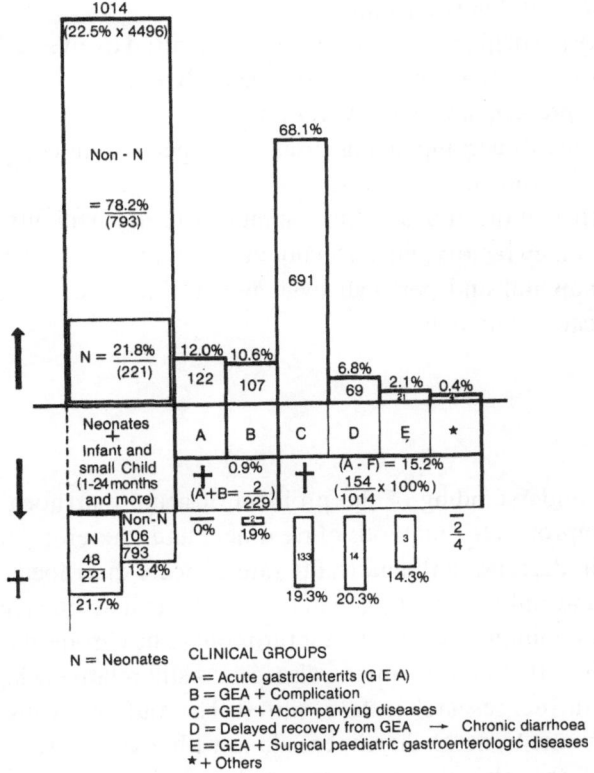

Figure 1. The prevalence of acute gastroenteritis (with or without complication and/or accompanying diseases) and the case fatality rate in the paediatric gastroenterology ward. Dr. Cipto Mangunkusumo Hospital Jakarta, 1980.

3.2. Morbidity and mortality

Figure 1 describes the 5 groups of infantile and childhood diarrhoeal diseases at Dr. Cipto Mangunkusumo General Hospital, Jakarta (1980).

3.3. Acute diarrhoea

This form of diarrhoea is still frequently found in the Department of Child Health at the Medical Faculty University of Indonesia/Dr. Cipto Mangunkusumo Hospital, Jakarta, but the prevalence of this disease is drastically decreasing as compared with previous years. This is partially due to the improved health programs.

However, of all cases which affect children hospitalized in the Paediatric Ward, acute diarrhoea is still the most encountered. Some of the more important factors contributing to acute diarrhoea are:

1. Community participation is not yet widely practised to give early treatment to acute diarrhoea patients by administering oralyte solutions at home by mothers so as to prevent severe dehydration.
2. There are many accompanying diseases (especially infection), which just severe the diarrhoea.
3. The incidence of diarrhoea in the community itself is still difficult to reduce, because of many factors which can not yet be improved or overcome, such as an environmental and personal hygiene, nutrition, socio-economic conditions, education and habit.

3.4. Mortality

An increased understanding of the problem of acute diarrhoea in infants and children has improved the methods of treatment and, therefore, has contributed considerably in decreasing the mortality rate of acute diarrhoea.

The infant and child mortality rate of ('pure') acute diarrhoea has indeed been decreased to a minimum, but what later turns out to be chronic diarrhoea, and/or which goes with other accompanying diseases, is still relatively high. Therefore, in this respect further research is still required. The four main causes of infant and child mortality due to acute diarrhoea, along with accompanying diseases, are: observation of convulsion and/or suspected encephalitis, bronchopneumonia, sepsis and aspiration pneumonia.

3.5. Efforts to reduce mortality

To decrease the mortality rate of acute diarrhoea in infants and children to a minimum, the following methods were applied:

1. to give the right and relevant treatment/medication;
2. to carry out 1., the problem faced should be clearly and correctly identified;
3. in certain cases, community participation (mothers of patients) should be an additional factor.

The ROSE system (R standing for rehydration with Ringer's lactate, O for oralyte, S for simultaneous and E for education) has been successful in the treatment of acute diarrhoea caused by cholera in infants and children.

Community participation is indispensible in the treatment of acute diarrhoea, be it within the ROSE system or through an early treatment which starts at home. It is manifested by administering a successful oralyte solution. Oral rehydration with oralyte, which begins at home, can be carried out by community members (housewives) themselves, even by those with poor socio-economic background.

By applying new technology, rotavirus, campylobacter and enterotoxigenic

Escherichia coli were discovered to be the aetiology of acute diarrhoea in a patient hospitalized in the Paediatric Gastroenterology Wards, Dr. Cipto Mangunkusumo Hospital/Medical Faculty University of Indonesia, Jakarta. Therefore, the treatment of acute diarrhoea in infants and children has been improved and reduces the mortality. The administration of oral antibiotics does not affect the recovery of acute diarrhoea very much, whereas oralyte solution proves to be more effective.

The realimentation method has been improved due to the discovery of malabsorption of sugar, fat and protein. Special formula for milk or porridge is required to realiment acute diarrhoea patients, who also suffer from malabsorption syndrome, without discarding the importance of breast milk and the provision of personal health counseling.

3.6. The study of 1014 hospitalized diarrhoeal cases at Dr. Cipto Mangunkusumo General Hospital, Jakarta, 1980.

3.6.1. There was a decrease in the number of acute diarrhoea cases in infants and children hospitalized in the Paediatric Gastroenterology Ward of the Dr. Cipto Mangunkusumo Hospital/Medical Faculty, University of Indonesia, Jakarta, from 37.2% (2085 cases out of 5606) in 1967 to 22.5% (1014 cases out of 4496) in 1980.

Classification into five clinical groups of acute diarrhoea cases has facilitated the detection of problems of each patient, leading to better management. The prevalence of neonates with acute diarrhoea was 21.8% (221 out of 1014) and almost half of them (41.5%, or 92 out of 221) is classified as low birth weight ones whereas the prevalence of infants with acute diarrhoea is 78.2% (793 out of 1014), and the majority (61.9% or 627 out of 1014) falls within the 5–12 months age group.

3.6.2. The nutritional state of the 1014 diarrhoea patients hospitalized in the Paediatric Gastroenterology Ward of Dr. Cipto Mangunkusumo Hospital/Medical Faculty, University of Indonesia (1980), were generally satisfactory. Apart from this, there were 75 out of 1014 infants (7.4%) with protein energy malnutrition (PEM), 16 of whom were kwashiorkor, 49 marasmus and 10 marasmic kwashiorkor.

3.6.3. The majority of the patients (68.1%, or 691 out of 1014) falls under group C (acute gastroenteritis with accompanying diseases). For group A and B (acute gastroenteritis with and without complications) the figure is 22.6% (229 out of 1014). The mortality rate for ('pure') acute diarrhoea was 0% (0 out of 122) whereas for group A + B (acute diarrhoea with and without complications) was 0.9% (2 out of 229). However, most of the cases who died were found in group C (acute gastroenteritis with accompanying diseases), i.e. 19.3% (133 out of 691). The three main diseases which cause death were suspected encephalitis/observation of convulsion, bronchopneumonia and sepsis. Acute diarrhoea complications, which were often found, were metabolic acidosis (85.1% or 91 out of 107) and hypokalaemia (30.8% or 33 out of 107 cases).

3.6.4. Electrolyte disturbance in PEM patients with acute diarrhoea was more serious than acute diarrhoea: 59.5% (31 out of 52) vs. 46.5% (33 out of 71) for hypokalaemia; 19.2% (10 out of 52) vs. 14.1% (10 out of 71) for hyponatremia; and 38.4% (20 out of 52) vs. 16.9% (12 out of 71) for hypochloraemia. Azotaemia was found in 57.5% (23 out of 40) of patients examined with acute diarrhoea.

3.6.5. The time required to reach rehydration in acute gastroenteritis cases without complications and accompanying diseases was less than 12 hours for almost half of the cases (42.3% or 44 out of 104), and half a day to one day for 53.9% (56 out of 104), whereas hospitalization was from 3 to 5 days for more than half of the patients (79.6%, or 97 out of 122) cases.

3.6.6. Patients with intractable diarrhoea and those who were hospitalized for more than 14 days (chronic diarrhoea) had, among others, the following backgrounds: malabsorption syndrome, severe PEM and accompanying diseases which were difficult to cure. Besides, there was suspicion that immuno-deficiency and/or gastrointestinal allergy especially cow's milk protein sensitive enteropathy (CMPSE) might also be the causes. However, this requires further research.

3.6.7. A significant number of acute diarrhoea cases accompanied by malabsorption syndrome was found in infants and children, i.e. 52.8% (452 out of 856) sugar intolerance, mostly lactose intolerance, and 57.0% fat malabsorption (194 out of 331). For low birth weight (LBW) and PEM infants, the figures were much higher, i.e. 89.5% (68 out of 76) and 67.2% (60 out of 89). Protein maldigestion was also found in severe PEM patients suffering from diarrhoea.

In PEM patients with diarrhoea, there was plenty of 'overgrowth' bacteria in the duodenum juice, e.g. 30.0% (6 out of 20) anaerob bacteria, which were thought to have some link with the cause of fal malabsorption besides that of the dysfunction of the pancreas, liver and intestine in PEM. The secretion of gastric acid (64.3%, 9 out of 14) decreased in PEM, and this was probably the reason for the plenty 'overgrowth' bacteria found in the upper part of the small intestine. Small intestinal biopsy revealed villous atrophy of second and third degree at 56.3% (9 out of 16), and of fourth, fifth and sixth degree at 43.7% (7 out of 16) in PEM and diarrhoea cases.

3.6.8. Based on humoral immunity research, immunological abnormality in PEM and diarrhoea (enteric infection) patients, showed a high degree of intestinal immunoglobulin. This immunoglobulinal increase was also found in patients with normal nutritional status (eutrofic) suffering from diarrhoea (enteric infection) as compared with healthy children. It was assumed that enteric infection was more likely the cause of increase in intestinal immunoglobulin. Compared with the situation in 1976, i.e. before breast milk was promoted, there was an increase in 1980 in the number of patients who still practised breast feeding, from 42.1% (439 out of 1043) to 64.2% (651 out of 1014). More than half (56.9% or 126 out of

221) of the acute diarrhoeal patients hospitalized had been given bottle feeding before they reached the age of one month. The reasons for this practice were unknown. While in hospital, breast feeding was continously applied to patients with acute diarrhoea, from the first day they were hospitalized until they were discharged.

3.6.9. There was no significant seasonal variation in the prevalence of acute diarrhoea in infants and children.

3.6.10. By virtue of new developments in technology, 80% of the causes of acute diarrhoea had been found in the Paediatric Gastroenterology Ward of Dr. Cipto Mangunkusumo Hospital/Medical Faculty, University of Indonesia. This was just the opposite compared with previous decades, where 80% of acute diarrhoea was not known as to its aetiology. A change in the microorganismic spectrum of the causes of acute diarrhoea was found, as compared to previous years, besides the discovery of several new microbes. Rotavirus, detected for the first time in an Indonesian child in 1974, has been known as the main cause of acute diarrhoea in infants and children (47.4%, or 9 out of 19); whereas during the period of 1980–1981 we found 30.4% (120 out of 395 cases) detected by electron microscope, ELISA and RPHA method. Next to it was E. coli (63.2%, or 122 out of 197); 14.3% (7 out of 49. E. coli isolation) was ETEC (Enterotoxigenic Escherichia coli), 30.3% (220 out of 725) Candida fungus, 22.2% (117 out of 528) Salmonella paratyphi (mostly 48 out of 117 S.oranienburg), 5.8% (17 out of 291) Campylobacter, 1.2% (6 out of 489) Shigella, 1.2% (5 out of 426) Vibrio cholerae,

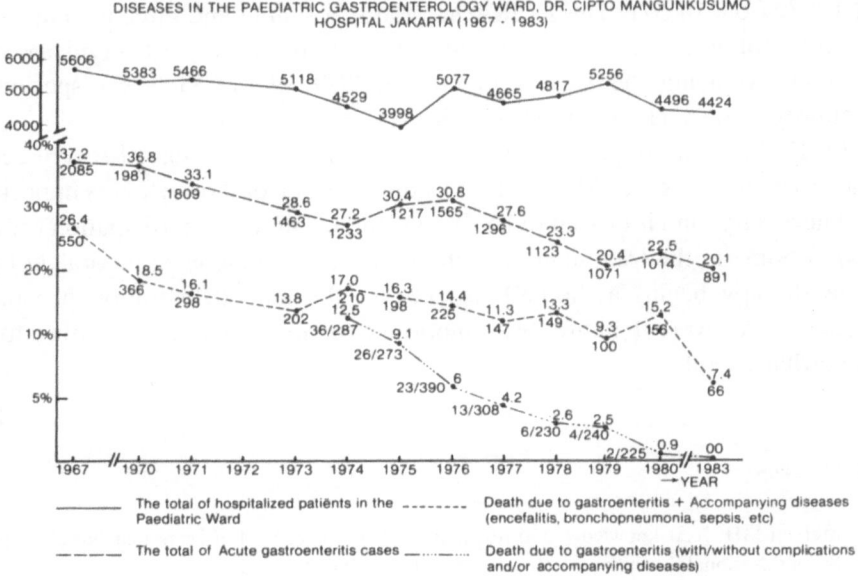

Figure 2. Decreased mortality of non-cholera diarrhoeal diseases (1967–1980).

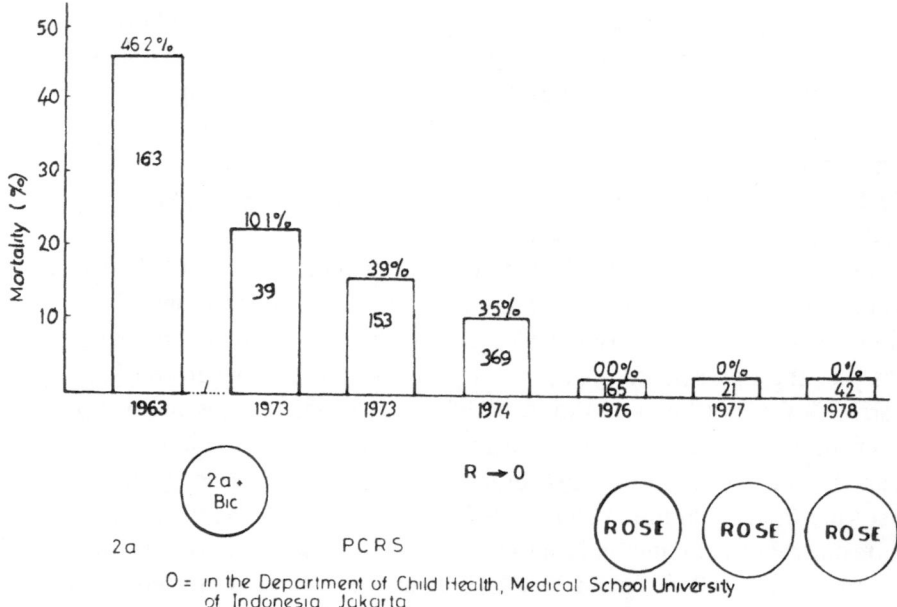

Figure 3. Decreased mortality of cholera diarrhoea and the use of ROSE system [10] (1963–1976, 1983).

0.3% (2 out of 725) amoeba, 0.1% (1 out of 725) giardia.

Some enterobacteriae were sensitive to colimycin (100%, or 57 out of 57), bactrim 89.5% (51 out of 57), gentamycin 77.2% (44 out of 57) and furadantin 42.1% (24 out of 57). The ELISA method is a simple and effective means to examine rotavirus without significant difference from the electron microscope method. Applying the ELISA method in 1979, of the 33 faeces specimens examined, 54.5% (18 out of 33) positive rotavirus was found.

3.6.11. Community participation (mothers) in the treatment of severe acute diarrhoea in clinics (ROSE system) by administering oral oralyte was important and necessary, and it proved to be very useful. Community participation (mothers) at home in the treatment of acute diarrhoea by administering oralyte ('oralyte therapy begins at home'), to prevent the mild dehydration becoming moderate or severe in nature, was important and necessary, and it proved to be somewhat useful.

References

1. Merson MH: New knowledge and research needs in the control of acute diarrhoeal diseases. Second National Seminar on Rehydration, Jakarta (Indonesia), 1978.
2. Rohde JE, Northrup RS: Taking science where the diarrhoea is. In: Elliot K, Knight J (eds) Acute diarrhoea in childhood. CIBA Foundation Symposium Ed. 2 (new series). Amsterdam, Elsevier-Excerpta Medica-North Holland, 1976, pp 339–358.

3. Mata LJ: Malnutrition: infection interaction in the tropics. Am J Trop Med Hyg 24:564, 1975.
4. Brotowasisto: Diarrhoeal diseases control programme in Indonesia. First National Seminar on Rehydration, August 26–30, 1974.
5. Sunoto: Diarrhoeal problem in Southeast Asia. In: proceedings of the 24th SEAMEO-TROPMED seminar on diarrhoeal diseases of children in S.E. Asia in the context of primary health care, Bangkok, 9–12 November 1981.
6. Tumbelaka WAFJ: Viewpoint from Indonesia. J Pediatr Gastroenterol:9–10, 1983.
7. Suharyono S, Aswitha B, Hentyanto H: Malabsorption syndrome in Indonesian children. Presented at the Vth World Congress of Gastroenterology, Ciudad de Mexico, 13–19 October 1974.
8. Thornhill TS, Wyatt RG, Kalica AR, Dolin R, Chanock RM, Kapikian AZ: Detection by immune electron microscopy of 26 to 27 nm virus-like particles associated with two family outbreaks of gastroenteritis. J Infect Dis 135:20, 1977.
9. Suharyono: Breastfeeding, supplementary feeding and the nutritional condition of infants/children in Jakarta. Workshop on the inter-relationship of maternal–infant nutrition, Surabaya, 26–27 April 1983.
10. Suharyono: Four principles of the treatment of diarrhoea (ROSE system). Presented at the 2nd Asian Congress of Paediatrics, Jakarta, August 3–6, 1976.

Acute diarrhea in the Dominican Republic

J.M. FERIS and H.R. MENDOZA

Introduction

As a necessary introduction to the topic of acute diarrhea in the Dominican Republic, it is necessary to remind you of the following data: The Dominican Republic is located in the Caribbean Sea, sharing the island of Hispaniola with Haiti, located between Puerto Rico and Cuba and separated from the Eastern coast of the United States by approximately 1200 km.

With a territorial extension of 48,442 km² and 5,648,000 inhabitants, we have a population density of 116 h/km² and a population growth rate of 3% [1].

The annual per capita income is US $483.00 [2] with an illiteracy index of 33% [3]. The climate is tropical, and the temperature oscillates between 18° C and 28° C.

The acute diarrhea as a national medical problem

Acute diarrhea is the principal cause of morbi-mortality in the Dominican Republic. Approximately 7% of the population reports to the state hospitals suffering from this illness, and the mortality rate is the highest at with 7% [4].

This illness, of course, is more frequent and severe at the pediatric age and, as shown by our statistics, which reveal that 16% of the deaths in children of a year of age or less, is caused by acute diarrhea as well as 15% of the deaths in children one to four years [5], taking into account that the infantile mortality rate is of about 80/1000 and the pre-school mortality rate is of 3.1/1000 [6].

Predisposing factors

The same environmental conditions that nurtured the high incidence of infantile diarrhea in the city of New York in 1900 [7] were present in the Dominican

Republic in 1983, i.e. lack of drinkable water. We should point out that in the urban area, drinkable water is available in 79% of the dwellings, and accessible to 14%, and in the rural zones it is present in 25% of the dwellings and accessible to 7% [8].

There is inadequate cleanliness, incredibly crowded quarters, lack of social and medical services; we have eight infirmary personnel available per 10,000 inhabitants, with only 0.9 graduate nurses in addition to one nurse per four doctors. There is malnutrition and a low level of personal hygiene. In a survey of an ample rural zone of the country, in which 34,000 homes were surveyed, it was detected that 4.5% of the homes surveyed had adequate means of proper removal of stools, i.e. latrines with sanitary specifications [1]. Families with many small children: 50.3% of the population is less that 18 years of age [1].

Furthermore, there is a decrease in breast feeding due to the poor orientation of the adolescents and young mothers as a consequence of the commercial advertisement for breast-milk substitutes [11].

Casual factors

The etiological agents related to diarrhea are: Rotavirus (20%), Campylobacter (15%), E. Coli Enteropathogenic (14%), E. Coli Enterotoxigenic (11%), Amebas (8%), Salmonellas (2%), and Shigellas (1%) [12–13].

Epidemiological pattern of the acute diarrhea

The epidemiological pattern of acute diarrhea has shown two frequency peaks related to climatological factors: one during the cold months (December to February) and another during the summer months (June to August). Rotavirus is more frequent during the cold months [12].

Evolutionary pathogenic and pathophysiological characteristics

Acute diarrhea is self-limiting. The majority of the deaths are due to dehydration along with occasional septicemia and malnutrition.

The pathogenic mechanisms currently accepted are the enterotoxicity and the microbic invasiveness.

The phenomenon of enterotoxicity is determined by the production of enterotoxins by the microorganisms (ETEC) which activate the adenylciclase within the intestinal cell, blocking the energetic ADP – ZTP mechanisms, resulting in the blockage of sodium and water absorbtion at the enterocytes level and influencing the secretion of sodium chloride and water at the enteroblast level.

The phenomenon of enteroinvasivity has effects that block the energetic mechanism which are not clearly understood.

Diarrhea by enterotoxicity are evidently the most dehydrating.

Prevention and treatment of dehydration caused by diarrhea

Since diarrhea is a self-limiting illness that leads to death by dehydration, to prevent or correct it is obviously the most important medical action. Moreover since dehydration due to diarrhea is known to be caused by the loss of water and sodium, to replenish these elements is obviously the correct therapeutic measure.

The discovery of the physiological mechanisms of sodium and water absorbtion by the enterocyte, and the determinant stimulatory factor of the energetic activity ADP-ATP of glucose, has made the oral administration of water, sodium and glucose the cornerstone in the prevention and correction of dehydration.

The oral administration of a solution of sodium and glucose is the most physiological, practical, economical and scientific mechanism for preventing and correcting dehydration.

The general acceptance of the oral rehydration therapy throughout the world, and its effectiveness in reducing mortality by diarrhea, is a deed that attests to its convenience and generalization in those countries, such as ours, where dehydration due to diarrhea is the principal cause of death.

At present, we are placing great emphasis on oral rehydration therapy, and we recommend the intensification of education and diffussion of oral rehydration therapy at all levels, doctors and communities, to develop a national campaign for the spread and generalization of the oral rehydration therapy, based on a program of sanitary education for the community along with the participation of the various incidental elements, such as medical educators, doctors, nurses, executors of health policy and the community, striving for the permanent government supply of the hydrating envelope at the health establishments of the Dominican government. Also, the search for effective means of obtaining the hydrating envelope for the people who most need it at the lowest possible price. It is necessary to point out that the envelope recommended by the WHO/UNICEF, the 'Rehydrate', costs US $ 0.90, a very high price for the population that needs it the most.

For this reason, and reasons of accessibility to the population, we recommend for oral rehydration therapy, the use of any solution with a scientific basis that contains glucose or carbohydrate, which is easily converted into glucose by the digestive processes (sucrose and starch), and common salt (NaCl). For this reason we recommended a solution of rice water and a teaspoon of salt per liter, or the home made solution of one liter of water, preferably boiled, adding six teaspoons of sugar and one teaspoon of salt, administered with a spoon instead of a bottle, to avoid the chance that mothers will relate any improvement in diarrhea with the bottle and continue to feed their children with hydrating solutions only. Furthermore, breast feeding should not be suspended in those cases where it is being received. These are the measures that we currently recommend, in addition to the 'Rehydrate envelope' and other commercial patents with the same price as or more expensive than the Rehydrate method.

Finally, a continuous evaluation of the conditioning factors of acute diarrhea, particularly its etiological factors, is of great importance in planning suitable strategies to erradicate this malady that is whipping humanity, above all, the infantile population.

In brief, if no improvement is made, acute diarrhea will continue to be the primary cause of morbi-mortality in our country. A list of important steps to be taken to control acute diarrhea is as follows:

1. promote breast feeding.
2. good hygiene in the preparation of foods and drinks.
3. provide the entire population with drinkable water.
4. proper elimination of feces.
5. promote hygienic habits.
6. improve general nutrition.
7. adequate control of insects and rodents.
8. adequate care of the sick.
9. adequate control of the carriers.

References

1. Secretariado Técnico de la Presidencia: Oficina Nacional de Estadística.: VI Censo Nacional de Población y Vivienda 1981, Enero, 1982, pp 1–2.
2. Secretariado Técnico de la Presidencia: Oficina Nacional de Estadísticas.: República Dominicana en cifras 1980, Vol IX. Santo Domingo, 1980, p 170.
3. Alvarez Del Real M: Almanaque mundial 1983. Editorial América, S.A. Panamá, 1983, p 299.
4. Rivera C: Gastroenteritis y Estadística. Seminario de Gastroenteritis y Rehidratación Oral. Mendoza H.R., Lebrón S.M. (Eds). Ediciones Médicas, Hospital de Niños 'Dr. Robert Reid Cabral', Santa Domingo, 1978, pp 145–184.
5. Martín J: Programa de Adiestramiento Médico y Paramédico en la Prevención y Tratamiento de las Enfermedades Diarreicas. In: Mendoza HR, Lebrón SM (eds) Seminario de Gastroenteritis y Rehidratación Oral. Ediciones Médicas, Hospital de Niños 'Dr. Robert Reid Cabral', Santo Domingo, 1978. pp 57–65.
6. Mendoza HR: Analisis sobre la Morbi-Mortalidad del Niño Dominicano, 1980. Arch Dom Ped 17:145–153, 1981.
7. Levine M: Relación entre Desnutrición, Mortalidad Infantil, Variables Demográficas y Diarrea Infantil. In: Mendoza HR, Lebrón SM (eds) Seminario de Gastroenteritis y Rehidratación Oral. Ediciones Médicas, Hospital de Niños 'Dr. Robert Reid Cabral', Santo Domingo, 1978, pp 15–21.
8. Mendoza HR: Morbi-Mortalidad, 1975. Folleto de la Cátedra de Pediatría, UASD.
9. Khoury S: Adiestramiento sobre Rehidratación Oral al Personal de Enfermería en la República Dominicana. In: Mendoza HR, Lebrón SA (eds) Seminario de Gastroenteritis y Rehidratación Oral. Ediciones Médicas, Hospital de Niños 'Dr. Robert Reid Cabral', Santo Domingo, 1978, pp 77–85.

10. Pichardo-Sardá ME: Contaminación Fecal en la República Dominicana. In: Mendoza HR, Lebrón SM (eds) Seminario de Gastroenteritis y Rehidratación Oral. Ediciones Médicas, Hospital de Niños 'Dr Robert Reid Cabral', Santo Domingo, 1978, pp 87–104.
11. Fernández Reid L: Lactar es Amar. Las Ventajas y Técnicas de la Lactancia Materna. Centro de Información Familiar, Santo Domingo, 1982, pp 2–4.
12. Mendoza HR, Levine MM, Kapikian A et al.: Factores Etiológicos de la Diarrea Aguda del Lactante en la República Dominicana. Arch Dom Ped 17:43–51, 1981.
13. Feris Iglesias J, Hernández A, Montás M et al.: Etiología Bacteriana de la Diarrea Aguda. Arch Dom Ped 17:125–133, 1981.

Effect of nutritional status of children on intake and absorption of nutrients

A. MOLLA, A.M. MOLLA and M. KHATUN

Introduction

Diarrhoeal disease is one of the most important causes for the mortality of children under 5 years in the developing countries [1–3]. Studies from Gambia and Guatemala showed that growth faltering and associated malnutrition are the direct consequence of diarrhoeal diseases [4–6]. Other infectious diseases were also found to cause a reduction in dietary intake due to anorexia and withdrawel of food [6]. Loss of nutrients due to vomiting and malabsorption could occur during enteric infections [7]. A child with fever may go into negative nitrogen balance due to increased rate of catabolism and even mild infections could result in a catabolic state with increased nitrogen loss [8]. Since diarrhoeal diseases adversely affect the child's growth [4, 6], the mechanism for this health hazard needs to be focused. Several of the following factors were considered to explain the mechanisms through which diarrhoeal diseases can affect children nutritionally:
1. reduced intake due to anorexia, withdrawel of food, as practiced by mothers to control diarrhoea, or feeding an altered diet for a prolonged period;
2. breakdown of body protein due to increased catabolism;
3. malabsorption of carbohydrates due to lactase deficiency [9].

All of these may lead to the supply of an inadequate quantity of nutrients, leading to malnutrition.

It was demonstrated in 1948 for the first time that , with three successive grades of the intake of calories (low, medium and high), absorption of nitrogen and fat in diarrhoeal children were proportional to the amount of intake [10]. In another investigation [11], it was further shown that duration of diarrhoea in a group of children was comparatively longer in the starved group compared to the group who were fed.

Hoyle and co-workers [12] studied preschool children with diarrhoea in Bangladesh and found that nutrient intake reduces to 50–70% compared to the controls of similar age group. In more recent metabolic studies in diarrhoeal children conducted in Bangladesh [13], it was observed that food intake was reduced from 15% to 36% compared to the intake at the recovery period. The exact estimation of calorie, fat, carbohydrate and nitrogen intake in acute diarrhoea due to cholera, rotavirus, E. coli and shigella were recently reported [14]. Absorption of nitrogen in children of 1 to 5 years with diarrhoea due to rotavirus or shigella was reduced (ranging from 25% to 40% of intake) during the acute stage of the illness [14]. Also, absorption of fat was significantly reduced to a range of 48% to 53% in acute diarrhoea due to rotavirus and shigella and less so in the case of diarrhoea caused by enterotoxigenic E. Coli and cholera [14]. Carbohydrate absorption was found to be least affected (77–91%) during acute diarrhoea caused by cholera, rotavirus, shigella and E. coli. All these absorption data obtained from the studies on diarrhoeal children appear to be reduced compared to the absorption of nutrients obtained in young American adults and children [15–17].

Although there is a belief that severe malnutrition does affect gut function, so far no attempt has been made to find out the impact of the nutritional status of children with diarrhoeal diseases on intake and absorption of nutrients. Data were reanalyzed from previous metabolic studies to focus mainly on three important aspects of feeding during diarrhoea. The aim of this paper is thus (1) to study the effect of the nutritional status of children on intake and co-efficient of absorption of nutrients during diarrhoea and 2 weeks after recovery (2) to find out the correlation co-efficient between the nutritional status of children and co-efficients of absorption of nutrients during acute diarrhoea and 2 weeks after recovery, and (3) to calculate the percentage of nutrient loss via faeces during feeding in diarrhoea and after recovery.

Patients and methods

The study was carried out in the metabolic study ward of the International Centre for Diarrhoeal Disease Research, Dhaka, Bangladesh (ICDDR,B). Sixty-seven children up to 5 years old with moderate to severe degree of dehydration were studied, and 28 were bound to have cholera, 17 rotavirus, 13 enterotoxigenic E. coli and 9 shigella. Most of the patients, nutritional status (based on Median Harvard standard for weight and age), ranged from mild to moderate degrees of malnutrition. However, patients with 3rd-degree malnutrition and without any complications were also studied. According to nutritional status, patients were divided into two groups, A and B. Group A consisted of children with normal, 1st and 2nd degree malnutrition and Group B consisted of 3rd degree malnutrition.

Prior approval of the human rights ethical committee of the ICDDR,B and informed consent from every guardian accompanying the patients were obtained. On admission, children were given standard intravenous rehydration therapy, the fluid composition of which is: Na^+ 133 mmol/l, K^+ 13 mmol/l, Cl^- 99 mmol/l,

HCO_3 (as acetate) 48 mmol/l. Usually after 4 to 5 hours of admission and subsequent rehydration, a familiar diet as previously reported [18], was offered ad libitum at regular intervals. Breast milk was allowed and the amount consumed was estimated by test weighing the child before and after breast feeding. Catheter stool samples were taken to determine the aetiologies for cholera, E. coli and shigella by stool culture [19]. E. coli isolates were tested for heat stable toxin (ST) by infant mouse assay and for heat labile toxin (LT) by Y_1 adrenal cell assay [20]. Rotavirus was detected by the enzyme-linked immunosorbent assay technique ELISA [21]. Xylose absorption test and a 72-hour metabolic study were carried out as previously described [14, 18]. All samples of study diet including breast milk, stool, urine and vomitus were analyzed for nitrogen content by micro-kjeldahl procedure [22], fat by the procedure of Van de Kamer et al. [23] and for calories by using adiabetic bomb calorimeter with benzoic acid as the standard. The co-efficient of nutrient absorption was calculated as before [18]. Patients were not given any antibiotic until the metabolic study was over.

Results

Table 1 shows the number, age, body weight and distribution of nutritional status of the study children. Patients with cholera were older compared to others, however the body weights were similar in all the groups of children. Nutritional status was poorer in the cholera group compared to the other children. In every aetiology of diarrhoea, second-degree malnutrition was most common. Results of xylose absorption are demonstrated in Table 2. A serum xylose level of less than 20 mg/dl was defined as xylose malabsorption. Xylose malabsorption was present in both the groups of A and B with acute rotavirus and ETEC diarrhoea. Children with acute cholera and shigella did not show any malabsorption of xylose during the acute stage. During recovery, serum xylose level of all patients were above 20 mg/dl.

Mean (± SD) intake of fat, nitrogen, carbohydrate and calories are presented

Table 1. Age, body weight (mean ± SD) and nutritional status of the study patients.

Aetiology	No.	Age (months)	Nutritional status (wt. for age)				
			Body wt (kg)	Normal (81%)	1st (76–80%)	2nd (61–75%)	3rd (60%)
Cholera	28	42.4 ± 12.9	9.5 ± 1.8	–	–	15	13
Rotavirus	17	24.8 ± 13.5	9.0 ± 2.2	5	1	7	4
Shigella	9	30.0 ± 18.5	9.2 ± 1.7	1	3	5	–
ETEC	13	33.0 ± 11.4	9.8 ± 1.9	3	1	8	1

in Tables 3, 4, 5 and 6, both during the acute stage and after recovery in every aetiology of diarrhoea. In general no difference in the intakes between Group A and B was obtained during the acute stage of all the aetiology of diarrhoea. However, in cholera and ETEC diarrhoea intake of calories and carbohydrates were higher in Group B than in Group A during the acute stage. During the recovery stage, the intake of nutrients was not different between the two groups (A and B) in any aetiology of diarrhoea.

Table 2. Effect of nutritional status on xylose absorption in children with acute diarrhoea and after recovery.

Aetiology	Serum xylose level (mg/dl)			
	Acute		Recovery	
	GR A	GR B	GR A	GR B
Cholera	20.3 ± 8.9	20.8 ± 8.2	27.3 ± 9.5	31.4 ± 6.8
Rotavirus	13.2 ± 5.4	17.3 ± 14.4	29.5 ± 6.7	23.9 ± 3.6
ETEC	17.5 ± 6.9	13.0 ± 2.8	25.6 ± 8.6	28.7 ± 10.2
Shigella	24.3 ± 13.4	*	30.1 ± 6.7	*

* Shigella with 3rd-degree malnutrition was not studied.

Table 3. Effect of nutritional status on intake of fat (mean ± SD) in acute diarrhoea, compared to recovery.

Aetiology	Intake (gm/kg/day)			
	Acute		Recovery	
	GR A	GR B	GR A	GR B
Cholera	1.7 ± 0.7	2.2 ± 1.2	2.6 ± 0.9	2.9 ± 1.3
Rotavirus	2.0 ± 0.6	1.5 ± 0.5	2.1 ± 0.7	2.5 ± 1.2
ETEC	3.4 ± 6.2	2.0 ± 1.3	2.1 ± 0.8	2.6 ± 0.9
Shigella	2.9 ± 2.9		2.3 ± 0.4	

Table 4. Effect of nutritional status on intake of nitrogen (mean ± SD) in acute diarrhoea, compared to recovery.

Aetiology	Intake (gm/kg/day)			
	Acute		Recovery	
	GR A	GR B	GR A	GR B
Cholera	0.3 ± 0.1	0.4 ± 0.2	0.5 ± 0.1	0.6 + 0.3
Rotavirus	0.3 ± 0.9	0.2 ± 0.5	0.4 ± 0.1	0.4 + 0.1
ETEC	0.27 ± 0.13	0.37 ± 0.3	0.4 ± 0.18	0.4 + 0.2
Shigella	0.3 ± 0.1		0.5 ± 0.1	

Percentages of loss of all the nutrients via faeces in the acute and recovery stages of diarrhoea were calculated and are shown in Table 7. Nitrogen loss was higher (range 39% to 53%) compared to other nutrients in acute diarrhoea of every aetiology studied. However, in acute rotavirus, loss of calories (30%) and fat (52%) were also higher than that obtained in other diarrhoea. During the recovery period, the percentage of loss of all nutrients was reduced, but in ETEC nitrogen loss was still as high as 42%.

Absorption of nutrients in healthy young American children and adults, eating

Table 5. Effect of nutritional status on intake of carbohydrate (mean ± SD) in acute diarrhoea compared to recovery.

Aetiology	Intake (gm/kg/day)			
	Acute		Recovery	
	GR A	GR B	GR A	GR B
Cholera	10.8 ± 5.0	13.5 ± 6.6	18.4 ± 5.8	17.9 ± 7.8
Rotavirus	10.7 ± 3.9	9.6 ± 3.2	14.3 ± 4.2	18.0 ± 5.5
ETEC	11.6 ± 5.7	15.1 ± 14.9	15.3 ± 5.4	15.2 ± 3.8
Shigella	11.0 ± 5.0		11.8 ± 4.9	

Table 6. Effect of nutritional status on intake of calories (mean ± SD) in acute diarrhoea, compared to recovery.

Aetiology	Intake (kcal/kg/day)			
	Acute		Recovery	
	GR A	GR B	GR A	GR B
Cholera	65.3 ± 28.9	83.7 ± 42.6	109.9 ± 30.8	113.3 ± 42.5
Rotavirus	72.5 ± 21.9	57.3 ± 15.7	84.9 ± 24.0	101.4 ± 31.5
ETEC	67.6 ± 30.7	87.7 ± 79.4	90.3 ± 31.0	94.3 ± 6.9
Shigella	67.7 ± 26.8		105.4 ± 25.7	

Table 7. Loss of nutrients (%) in acute and recovery stage of diarrhoea.

Aetiology	Acute (% of intakes)				Recovery (% of intakes)			
	Fat	N_2	CHO	Cal	Fat	N_2	CHO	Cal
Cholera	28	47	10	17	10	22	8	9
Rotavirus	52	46	18	30	17	27	8	12
ETEC	25	39	15	11	19	42	16	11
Shigella	28	53	20	26	13	26	16	16

an American diet, was found to be above 90%; however, with the Indians, the diet protein absorption was 80% (Table 8). In Table 9, effect of malnutrition on absorption of fat in acute and after recovery stages of diarrhoea are shown. Although children with third-degree malnutrition (Group B) tend to absorb more fat than those with better nutritional status (Gr A), this difference was not statistically significant. Fat absorption improved at the recovery stages of all diarrhoea.

Absorption of nitrogen (Table 10) was very low in the cholera Group A, Group B and in shigella Group A in the acute stage. In the recovery stage, nitrogen

Table 8. Absorption of nutrients in healthy American young children and adults, eating American and Indian diet.

	Co-efficient of absorption	
	American diet	Indian diet
Protein	91–92	80
Fat	93–97	93–97
Carbohydrate	97–99	97–99

Table 9. Effect of nutritional status on absorption of fat in acute diarrhoea, compared to recovery.

Aetiology	Co-efficient of absorption			
	Acute		Recovery	
	GR A	GR B	GR A	GR B
Cholera	60.7 ± 28.2	73.1 ± 19.9	88.5 ± 5	90.3 ± 9.0
Rotavirus	44.9 ± 25.0	64.5 ± 19.5	79.5 ± 20.7	88.3 ± 7.7
ETEC	74.0 ± 17.0	84.5 ± 1.2	75.4 ± 25.0	73.9 ± 30.8
Shigella	53.0 ± 59.0		86.7 ± 5.4	

Table 10. Effect of nutritional status on absorption of nitrogen in acute diarrhoea, compared to recovery.

Aetiology	Co-efficient of absorption			
	Acute		Recovery	
	GR A	GR B	GR A	GR B
Cholera	35.3 ± 32.3	50.6 ± 30.7	70.9 ± 8.9	79.1 ± 13.9
Rotavirus	57.2 ± 12.9	51.6 ± 8.3	72.3 ± 12.8	66.6 ± 16.9
ETEC	58.2 ± 18.6	65.4 ± 6.5	46.7 ± 34.2	67.1 ± 22.9
Shigella	25.0 ± 54.9		65.1 ± 15.9	

absorption improved significantly, although the improvement was less remarkable compared to the other nutrients. Effect of nutritional status of children with diarrhoea on absorption of carbohydrates and calories are presented in Tables 11 and 12. The lowest absorption of carbohydrate was noticed in the acute stage of Group B patients with ETEC diarrhoea, whereas in other acute diarrhoea carbohydrate absorption was least affected. In the recovery stage carbohydrate absorption was around 90% on an average. Calorie absorption was low in the acute diarrhoea due to rotavirus and shigella in the Group A patients. During recovery, absorption of calories improved (range 80% to 90%) in every aetiology of diarrhoea.

To correlate co-efficients of nutrient absorption (Table 13) with the nutritional status in the acute and recovery stages of diarrhoea, 32 'r' values were calculated from the correlation plots between nutritional status and absorption of fat, nitrogen, calories and carbohydrate in two different stages of diarrhoea. In the acute stage of rotavirus, a significant positive relationship was obtained between nitrogen absorption and nutritional status of children. Significantly negative correlation was obtained between nutritional status and all nutrients in the acute stage of shigella. Beside these, no positive correlation was seen between nutritional status and nutrient absorption in diarrhoea of any aetiology.

Table 11. Effect of nutritional status on absorption of carbohydrate in acute diarrhoea, compared to recovery.

Aetiology	Co-efficients of absorption			
	Acute		Recovery	
	GR A	GR B	GR A	GR B
Cholera	80.7 ± 26.6	91.9 ± 8.8	92.4 ± 3.5	93.0 ± 9.9
Rotavirus	82.1 ± 13.1	79.1 ± 27.2	91.3 ± 4.0	91.0 ± 6.4
ETEC	90.8 ± 6.0	55.4 ± 52.9	87.5 ± 9.9	90.5 ± 4.9
Shigella	76.5 ± 26.9		83.3 ± 18.0	

Table 12. Effect of nutritional status on absorption of calories in acute diarrhoea compared to recovery

Aetiology	Co-efficient of absorption			
	Acute		Recovery	
	GR A	GR B	GR A	GR B
Cholera	73.3 ± 9.9	83.6 ± 8.9	89.3 ± 4.3	92.7 ± 3.4
Rotavirus	69.3 ± 13.8	73.5 ± 22.8	86.7 ± 8.2	87.9 ± 6.8
ETEC	84.1 ± 8.5	88.4 ± 0.6	78.2 ± 17.5	85.2 ± 11.6
Shigella	66.9 ± 30.4		83.1 ± 11.9	

Table 13. Correlation co-efficients between nutritional status and absorption of nutrients in acute diarrhoea and 2 weeks after recovery.

Aetiology	Acute (r Values)				Recovery (r Values)			
	Fat	N_2	Cal	CHO	Fat	N_2	Cal	CHO
Cholera	− 0.09	− 0.07	− 0.02	− 0.21	− 0.06	− 0.19	− 0.27	− 0.05
Rotavirus	− 0.47+	0.47*	− 0.20	− 0.005	− 0.02	− 0.23	0.08	0.24
E. coli	− 0.20	0.44	0.15	0.32	− 0.24	− 0.15	− 0.04	− 0.01
Shigella	− 0.59+	− 0.59+	− 0.76+	− 0.79+	− 0.37	− 0.21	− 0.15	0.03

* Significantly correlated.
+ Significantly negatively correlated.

Discussion

Since the important work of Chung and Viscorova no comprehensive data have been available to demonstrate the value of continuing feeding during acute diarrhoea. From a recent study conducted in ICDDR,B [24], it was evident that enterotoxigenic Escherichia coli was the most common pathogen, followed shigella and rotavirus in rural Bangladesh. Although the duration of diarrhoea was longest in shigella, dehydration was more common in cholera and rotavirus. Since diarrhoea with these common pathogens is highly prevalent in this part of the world, it is likely to have significant impact on health and growth of children. The present study was designed to seek information about intake, loss and absorption of nutrients in diarrhoeal conditions and their relationship to the nutritional status of children. The overall objective was to interrupt the diarrhoea–malnutrition cycle and to give evidence to support the theory of continuing feeding in diarrhoeal diseases.

Previously [14, 18, 25], it was demonstrated that the gut transit time is independent of nutrient absorption in diarrhoeal diseases and that substantial absorption of nutrients does occur in all diarrhoeal aetiology and thus continuous feeding was encouraged to avoid the nutritional consequences of diarrhoea. How nutritional status may affect intake and absorption of nutrients in diarrhoeal diseases has not been examined before. The present results demonstrate some important information with regard to this question. However, we did not select diarrhoeal patients carefully from all nutritional status; thus, in our study, equal distribution of all nutritional status in every aetiology of diarrhoea is not evident.

Xylose absorption was lower in both Groups A and B in acute rotavirus and ETEC diarrhoea, but it has very little relation with nutrient absorption [25]. The poor absorption of nutrients in malnourished rotavirus children can be explained by two factors: (a) the children with rotavirus where younger and (b) virus particles may cause severe damage to the intestinal epithelial layer. During the recovery stage nutritional status seems not to affect the intake of nutrients. Rather a reverse trend, i.e. more intake of nutrients, were noticed in children with 3rd-degree malnutrition.

Loss of nitrogen was highest as was observed in the acute stage of every aetiology of diarrhoea perhaps due to the loss of faecal protein derived from intestinal secretions [26]. Also from a recent study, it was evident that in shigellosis serum protein was lost directly with the faeces through the gastrointestinal route [27]. The trend of higher absorption of nutrients in malnourished children might lead to the hypothesis that 3rd-degree malnutrition is probably not a limiting factor for intake and absorption of nutrients in acute diarrhoea. The study children were free from associated infections and thus probably intestinal lesion due to infections were minimal. Furthermore, in acute and recovery stages of diarrhoea, no positive correlation was obtained between the nutritional status and absorption of nutrients, except in acute rotavirus – a viral infection, absorption of nitrogen, was positively correlated with nutritional status. It is, however, surprising to find out that in acute shigella nutritional status is significantly negatively correlated with the absorption of all nutrients. This might be explained by the fact that it is the severity of the disease and not the nutritional status which determines the absorption of nutrients in diarrhoea. These results also suggest that children with 3rd-degree malnutrition tend to eat more and absorb more, once they are provided with sufficient amounts of food and as long as there is no mucosal lesion. Thus, in conclusion, feeding should be continued in all diarrhoeal children irrespective of their nutritional status. This measure will contribute immensely to the prevention of further malnutrition which already exists in the developing world.

Acknowledgements

This research was supported by the International Centre for Diarrhoeal Disease Research, Bangladesh (ICDDR,B). ICDDR,B is supported by countries and agencies which share its concern about the impact of diarrhoeal diseases on the developing world. Current donors giving assistance to ICDDR,B are: AG-FUND, Australia, Bangladesh, Japan, Saudi Arabia, Sweden, Switzerland, United Kingdom and USAID.

The authors gratefully acknowledge the help of Biochemistry and Statistical Branch for support; and nursing staff of the ICDDR,B Hospital.

References

1. Walsh JA, Warren KS: Selective primary health care: An interim strategy for disease control in developing countries. N Engl J Med 301:967–974, 1979.

2. Chen LC, Rahaman M, Sarder AM: Epidemiology and causes of death among children in a rural area of Bangladesh. Int J Epidemiol 9:25–33, 1980.

3. Puffer RR, Serrano CV: Patterns of mortality in childhood. Sci Public No. 262. Pan American Health Organization, Washington, DC, 1973.

4. Rowland MGM, Cole TJ, Whitehead RG: A quantitative study into the role of infection in determining nutritional status in Gambian Village Children. Br J Nutr 37:441–450, 1979.

5. Scrimshaw NS, Taylor CE, Gordon JE: Interactions of nutrition and infection. Geneva, World Health Organisation, 1968. WHO Monograph No. 57.

6. Martorell R, Habicht JP, Yarbrough C et al.: Acute morbidity and physical growth in rural Guatemalan children. Am J Dis Child 129:1296–1301, 1975.

7. Rosenberg IH, Solomons HW, Schneider RD: Malabsorption associated with diarrhoea and intestinal infections. Am J Clin Nutr 30:1248–1253, 1977.

8. Beisal WR, Sawyer WD, Ryll ED et al.: Metabolic effects of intracellular infections in man. Am Intern Med 67:744–779, 1976.

9. Brown KH, Parry L, Khatun M, Ahmed MG: Lactose malabsorption in Bangladeshi village children: relation with age, history of recent diarrhoea, nutritional status and breast feeding. Am J Clin Nutr 32:1962–1969, 1979.

10. Chung AW: The effect of oral feeding at different levels on the absorption of foodstuffs in infantile diarrhoea. J Paediatr 33:1–13, 1948.

11. Chung AW, Viscorova B: The effect of early oral feeding versus early oral starvation on the course of infantile diarrhoea. J Paediatr 33:14–22, 1948.

12. Hoyle B, Yunus M, Chen LC: Breast-feeding and food intake among children with acute diarrhoeal diseases. Am J Clin Nutr 33:2365–2371, 1980.

13. Molla AM, Molla Ayesha, Sarker SA, Raham MM: Food intake during and after recovery from diarrhoea in children. In: Chen LC, Scrimshaw NS (eds) Diarrhoea and malnutrition, interaction, mechanisms and interventions, 1983, pp 113–123.

14. Molla S, Molla AM, Sarker SA, Khatun M: Whole-gut transit time and its relationship to absorption of macronutrients during diarrhoea and recovery. Scan J Gastro 18(4):537–543, 1983.

15. Briscoe J: The quantitative effect of infection on the use of food by young children in poor countries. Am J Nutr 32:648–676, 1979.

16. Wollaeger EE, Comfort MW, Osterberg AE: Total solids, fat and nitrogen in the feces. III. A study of normal persons taking a test diet containing a moderate amount of fat; comparison with results obtained with normal persons taking a test diet containing a large amount of fat. Gastroenterology 9:272, 1948.

17. Stier LB, Taylor DD, Pace JK, Eisen JN: Metabolic patterns in preadolescent children IV. Fat intake and excretion. J Nutr 73:347, 1961.

18. Molla A, Molla AM, Rahim A, Sarker SA, Mozaffar Z, Rahaman MM: Intake and absorption of nutrients in children with cholera and rotavirus infection during acute diarrhoea and after recovery. Nutr Res 2:233, 1982.

19. Edwards PR, Edwin WH: Identification of Enterobacteriaceae. Burgen, Minneapolis, 1972.

20. Merson MH, Sack RB, Kibriya AKMG, SL Mahmood A, Ahmed QS, Huq I: The use of colony pools for diagnosis of enterotoxigenic Escherichia coli diarrhoea. J Clin Microbiol 9:493–497, 1979.

21. Yolken RH, Kim HW, Clem I Wyatt RG, Chanock RM, Kalica AR, Kapikian AZ: Enzyme linked immunosorbent assay (ELISA) for detection of human reovirus like agent of infantile gastroenteritis. Lancet ii:263–266, 1977.

22. Henry RJ: Clinical chemistry: principles and technics. Harper and Row, New York, 1964.

23. Vande Kamer JH, Ten Bokkel Huiniuk H, Wayers HA: Rapid method for determination of fat in feces. J Biol Chem 177:345–355, 1949.

24. Black RE, Brown KH, Becker S, Abdul Alim ARM, Huq I: Longitudinal studies of infectious diseases and physical growth of children in rural Bangladesh. Am J Med 115:315–324, 1982.

25. Molla A, Molla AM, Sarker SA, Khatun M, Rahaman MM: Effects of acute diarrhoea on absorption of macronutrients during disease and after recovery. In: Chen LC, Scrimshaw NS (eds) Diarrhoea and malnutrition, interactions, mechanisms and interventions. 1983, pp 143–154.
26. Holt LE, Courtney AM, Falls HL: The chemical composition of diarrhoea as compared with normal stools in infants. Am J Dis Child 9:231, 1915.
27. Rahaman MM, Wahed MA: Direct nutrient loss and diarrhoea. In: Chen LC, Scrimshaw NA (eds) Diarrhoea and malnutrition, interactions, mechanisms and interventions. 1983, pp 155–160.

Nutrition

CHAIRMAN: J.H.P. JONXIS

Methods for evaluating nutrition and health status

Y.N. MATHUR and D.H. RAO

Introduction

Malnutrition with its consequent effects on overall health is a major public health problem in most of the developing countries. There is a need to quantify the extent of malnutrition and health problems mainly from the view point of:
1. planning and implementing appropriate inter-sectoral strategies for the uplift-ment of the overall health and nutrition status of the population;
2. monitoring and surveillance of the nutrition and health status of communities for midcourse corrections;
3. assessing the effect and impact of the intervention programmes for necessary feed-back to the planning process.

In most of the developing countries, due to lack of resources and inadequacies in the infrastructural facilities, the available health records do not lend themselves to the above-mentioned requirements. While steps are being taken to improve the overall situation under the Primary Health Care approach, there is a need to review the available methodologies for evaluating the nutrition and health status of communities.

Clinical assessment detects extreme situations. Only severe forms of Protein Energy Malnutrition (PEM) in the form of Marasmus, Kwashiorkor or a combination of the two can be identified. Mild and moderate forms of PEM, which form the bulk of the problem in the community, are not detectable clinically.

This is clearly evident from our data base of the National Nutrition Monitoring Bureau of the Indian Council of Medical Research at Hyderabad [1]. Clinical forms of PEM were observed in only 2.7% of preschool children in a sample of 4025. Whereas 85.2% of the children (mild 47.9%, moderate 32.6% and severe 4.7%) were malnourished as judged by weight for age criteria and expressed as a percentage of well-to-do Indian preschool children [2]. It, therefore, indicates that for assessing the extent of undernutrition in a community, anthropometry is an important tool.

Use of anthropometry in nutritional assessment

Various anthropometric indicators are used for quantifying undernutrition. These are weight for age – Gomez's classification [3] – height for age, weight for height – Waterlow's classification [4] – and a combination of weight for age, height for age and weight for height – Seoane & Latham classification [5] – arm circumference [6] and fat fold at triceps.

While weight for age assesses the current nutritional status, height for age indicates undernutrition of long duration. The only constraint involved is correct assessment of age in rural illiterate communities. Parameters like height and weight which increase rapidly in the preschool age group can be easily and accurately measured. Use of indicators like weight for height have been shown to be quite useful in grading and quantifying malnutrition compared to the use of weight and height for age alone [7]. Use of the combination of weight for age, height for age, and weight for height has an advantage of indicating not only the extent of undernutrition but also the type of duration of undernutrition.

Arm circumference and fat fold at triceps do not increase much with age in the preschool age group [2, 8] and are, therefore, not very sensitive. Arm circumference, however, is useful in selecting communities for nutrition intervention on priority basis [9]. The extent of undernutrition in a community is quantified differently by various anthropometric criteria primarily due to different cutoff levels used [10].

The choice of anthropometric indicator depends on the objectives of the nutrition assessment. It has been shown that in cross-sectional studies weight for height is more valuable while in the longitudinal studies either weight for age or height for age is more useful [11].

Nutritional supplementation of populations

Extensive research carried out by the National Institute of Nutrition indicated that communities in India subsist on a cereal based diet which is predominantly deficit in calories and not in protein [12]. Based on this concept a number of supplementary feeding programmes are currently in operation. These large-scale feeding programmes attempt to bridge the calorie gap by using locally available, inexpensive and culturally-acceptable foods to the nutritionally vulnerable population. These groups which comprise nearly 40% of population include children of preschool and school ages and women who are pregnant or lactating. Under field conditions [13, 14] the nutritional supplementation has been shown to have a demonstrable biological effect.

Methodologies for evaluation of nutrition status of beneficiaries of feeding programmes

Ideally the beneficiaries should be assessed for their nutrition status before their inclusion under the programme and followed up periodically thereafter to observe the biological effect. Under the conditions of implementation of these programmes, this poses certain hurdles. Firstly, the baseline data on health and nutrition status of beneficiaries is not available. Secondly, the infrastructure does not lend itself to self monitoring and evaluation on a longitudinal basis. In such situations the nutritional status of the beneficiary group has to be compared with a similar non-beneficiary group. However, it is not always easy to select appropriate control groups. This is due to the reasons that environmental and socio-cultural situation, level of overall development and extent of utilization of health care services by the populations are difficult to match. Some studies which attempted to overcome this by taking controls from the same population group faced difficulties of getting 'real controls' as most of the non-beneficiary sibling children in the area were also sharing the food supplement at home.

These problems can be minimised by conducting a longitudinal study on a group of beneficiary and non-beneficiary children at an interval of at least one year. Within a population of 580 children in urban slums, it was observed that there was a significant improvement as per Gomez's classification [15].

However, this approach is time consuming and may not always be feasible for constraints of resources. An alternative method has been devised to overcome this in a cross-sectional study where children had been participating in the programme for varying periods of time [16]. Supervised feeding of about 300 calories on the spot for a year resulted in significant improvement of body weights of children [17]. Most of the programmes are not adequately supervised, to ensure on the spot feeding results in sharing by others. In view of this a period of 18 months of feeding was considered to be a desirable cutoff point. The results on about 21,700 preschool age children in urban slums and tribal areas revealed that children who had participated for more than 18 months had a better body weight for age status as compared to those who had participated for less than 18 months [16].

There is thus scope for extending these type of studies for knowing the duration

Table 1. Percent distribution of children of 1–5 years according to body weight status at two points of study.

Study	Normal	Grade-I	Grade-II	Grade-III	Total
Earlier	21.3	47.7	27.6	23.4	100
After one year	29.43	51.55	18.46	0.56	100

$\chi_2 = 22.460$; $P<0.001$; NIN – 1983.

of intervention under conditions of programme operation which are critical for demonstrating the biological effect on the growth status of children. Also such studies would indicate the period necessary to achieve the optimum growth potential through such interventions.

Assessment of health status

It is well known that some health disorders like diarrhoea, measles and infections of respiratory tract and skin adversely affect the nutrition and overall health status of children. It, therefore, becomes essential to collect information on these morbid situations. However, recall lapses hinder the accuracy of such data.

The availability of health care services, and its utilization by the communities, plays vital role in the outcome of overall health and nutrition status.

This also determines the outcome in terms of mortality in different age groups. Indicators like neonatal, infant and toddler mortality rates indicate the overall situation. However, the statistics available in most of the developing countries suffer from lack of adequate reporting, both quantitatively and qualitatively. In one of our recent community-based studies [18] covering a rural population of about 12,000 these inadequacies in vital statistics reporting have been highlighted.

Some comprehensive indicators like the physical quality of life index (P.Q.L.I.) which takes into account the life expectancy, infant mortality and literacy are more broad based indicators of community health.

It may thus be summerised that while evaluating the nutrition and health status of populations, data from various sources need to be collected, using appropriate methodologies for proper interpretation.

Table 2. Percentage distribution of children according to Gomez grading and duration of feeding.

Gomez grade	Age			
	Below 36 months		Above 36 months	
	Less than 18 months	More than 18 months	Less than 18 months	More than 18 months
Normal	25.9	41.7	30.1	38.3
I	37.8	37.9	41.1	39.7
II	24.4	16.1	22.4	17.3
III	11.9	4.3	6.4	4.7

NIN – 1983.

References

1. National Nutrition Monitoring Bureau: Report for the year 1980. National Institute of Nutrition, Indian Council of Medical Research, Hyderabad, 1981.
2. Hanumantha Rao D, Satyanarayana K, Gowrinath Sastry J: Growth of well-to-do Hyderabad preschool children. Ind J Med Res 64:629–638, 1976.
3. Gomez F, Ramos GR, Frenk S, Cravioto J, Chauez R, Vazquez J: Mortality in second and third degree malnutrition. J Trop Pediatr 2:77, 1956.
4. Waterlow JC: Classification and definition of protein-calorie malnutrition. Brit Med J 3:566, 1972.
5. Seoane N, Latham MC: Nutritional anthropometry in the identification of malnutrition in childhood. J Trop Pediatr Environ Child Health 17:98, 1971.
6. Shakir A, Morley DC: Measuring malnutrition. Lancet 1:758, 1974.
7. Gowrinath Sastry J, Vijayaraghavan K: Use of anthropometry in grading malnutrition in children. Ind J Med Res 61:1225–1232, 1970.
8. Pralhad Rao N, Darshan S, Swaminathan MC: Nutritional status of preschool children of rural communities near Hyderabad city. Ind J Med Res 57:2132–2146, 1969.
9. Vijayaraghavan K, Gowrinath Sastry J: The efficacy of arm circumference as a substitute for weight in assessment of protein-calorie malnutrition. Ann Hum Biol 3:229–233, 1976.
10. Gowrinath Sastry J, Srikantia SG: Using heights and weights how close are our estimates of undernutrition in a community. Ind J Med Res 64:193–198, 1976.
11. Nadamuni Naidu A, Hanumantha Rao D: Efficacy of various anthropometric indices in the evaluation of supplementary feeding programmes. In: Srinivasan K, Saxena PC, Kanitkar T (eds) Demographic socio-economic aspects of the child in India, 1979 (1st edn), pp 383–388.
12. Narasinga Rao BS, Visweswara Rao K, Nadamuni Naidu A: Calorie-protein adequacy of the dietaries of preschool children in India. J Nutr Diet 6:238–244, 1969.
13. Hanumantha Rao D, Satyanarayana K, Vijayaraghavan K, Gowrinath Sastry J, Nadamuni Naidu A, Swaminathan MC: Evaluation of the special nutrition programme in the tribal areas of Andhra Pradesh. Ind J Med Res 63:652–660, 1975.
14. Swaminathan MC, Hanumantha Rao D, Visweswara Rao K, Narasimham MVVL, Sinai Dumo N: An evaluation of supplementary feeding programme for preschool children in the rural area around Hyderahad city. Ind J Nutr Diet 7:342–350, 1970.
15. Gowrinath Sastry J, Hanumantha Rao D, Rameswara Sarma KV, Mathur YN, Swaminathan MC: Special nutrition pogramme – an evaluation study in Karnataka. Further studies in Bangalore slums. National Institute of Nutrition, Indian Council of Medical Research, Hyderabad, 1980.
16. Gowrinath Sastry J, Hanumantha Rao D, Rameswara Sarma KV, Mathur YN, Pralhad Rao N, Swaminathan MC: Special nutrition programme – an evaluation study in Karnataka. National Institute of Nutrition, Indian Council of Medical Research, Hyderabad, 1980.
17. Gopalan C, Swaminathan MC, Kumari Menon K, Hanumantha Rao D, Vijayaraghavan K: Effect of calorie supplementation on growth of undernourished children. Am J Clin Nutr 26:563–566, 1973.
18. Swaminathan MC, Vijayaraghavan K, Mathur YN, Radhaiah G, Rameshwar Sarma KV, Satyanarayana K: Bidar integrated rural development project – health and nutrition profile. National Institute of Nutrition, Indian Council of Medical Research, Hyderabad, 1980.

Assessing nutrition at village level

D. MORLEY

Abstract

Assessment can be considered an exploration and communication of values. In this paper emphasis will be particularly placed on how the values can be communicated at village level.

Introduction

All societies have nutritional problems. In terms of mortality, our problems in the north are perhaps not so different from those of the south except that the mortality arising from inappropriate nutrition comes in the later decades of life (Figure 1). The nutritional problems affecting children in the north were removed almost before we became medically conscious of their existence. Any attempts to assess adequate nutrition in communities in the north were only developed after most of the childhood nutrition problems had disappeared.

We now appreciate that most of the childhood nutritional problems in the south at the present time and in the north in the past were due to an energy deficit in small children. In the north, these energy deficits were overcome as high energy foods such as oils, fats and sucrose became widely available, and also with the development of specific weaning foods. The definition of good nutrition used here will be adequate growth, which at present in ignorance, we equate with maximum growth. We still do not know whether maximum growth is synonymous with a longer life and maximum mental and physical achievement. Even in Europe, a small proportion of children will show deficits in growth due to a variety of largely less common conditions. It is a sad reflection on the health care system in England that probably less than a quarter of children are weighed regularly and the health service still denies to the mother an ongoing record of her child's growth.

In this paper no attempt will be made to review all the methods of assessing

Nutrition and Life Styles: North and South TWO SIDES OF ONE COIN

Figue 1. Two sides of one coin. The nutritional poblems of the north and resulting mortality reflect a high energy density diet, high in salt content but low in dietary fibre. In the south, the low energy density diet with a low fat intake resuls in the child being deficient in energy intake.

nutritional status and only three types of anthropometric measurements will be considered. These are: weight for age, arm circumference, and weight for height.

In an important study from Bangladesh [1] over 2000 children aged 13–23 months were followed and mortality was related to anthropometric indices. Whatever indices were used severly malnourished children showed an increased mortality, unlike the normal, mild and moderately malnourished children all experienced the same risk. The best indicators were found to be weight-for-age, and arm circumference-for-age with 4-fold differentials. Height for age give 3-fold differentials and weight-for-height only a 2-fold differential.

Weight for age

Ever since I have worked with a public health nurse, Margaret Woodland, and the mothers of Imesi Ile in Western Nigeria, I have been convinced that of all measurements weight for age plotted on an appropriate growth chart is the most useful measure that we have to give guidance to mothers (Morley, 1979). Through this record we can help their children to achieve adequate growth and at the same time to take the necessary preventive measures including immunisation and spacing of births, which will also have a direct effect in improving the child's nutrition. Since the '70's, W.H.O. has also backed the use of such growth charts and in 1982 UNICEF also gave their support by emphasising monitoring growth as one of its priorities. A collection of over 280 charts held in the Institute of Child

Health from around the world suggest that there must be few countries where such growth charts are not used by some groups of health workers. In Indonesia and the Philippines many millions of colourful charts have been put into use. In Africa, they have been used widely. In Lesotho, Gambia, Malawi and Botswana probably three-quarters of all children have such charts and these countries probably have a better mother and child health service than other countries in Africa.

Understanding growth charts

The concept (Figure 2) is perhaps simple. Unfortunately, creating and understanding the meaning of a 'growth curve' involves the symbolism of charting. This symbolism is not taught in the 'Three Rs' of basic education and even in secondary and tertiary education, a proportion of individuals, including doctors, do not satisfactorily come to grips with the understanding of what a growth curve means. In the north with all the visual communication through the mass media a majority of people are becoming more 'picturate' and able to understand the appropriate symbolism. This is an area in which the south lags behind and there are many medical schools where the students will go through their course hardly ever seeing a projected aid such as a slide and have difficulty interpreting histograms.

When primary schools are more oriented to the needs of the environment in which children will grow up, emphasis may then be placed on the children understanding simple graphs. An understanding of the growth curves of their small brothers and sisters, and perhaps in the future of their own children, may then be achieved. The type of chart most appropriate is shown in Figure 3, in which the path of growth is replaced by a spectrum of colour, the more favoured colour in the upper part of the spectrum.

Arm circumference

The use of a coloured strip of plastic or old X-Ray film for assessing the nutrition of children between the age of one and five was first suggested by Shakir [3] in 1975.

This innovation spread quickly among health workers and was picked up by agriculturists and others as simple method of assessing the nutrition of the population for whom they were introducing additional agricultural inputs. The measurement of limb circumference has many advantages in the assessment of a child's nutritional state. The mid upper arm circumference is a measure of muscle, subcutaneous tissue and fat and these are all tissues that are dependent on the nutritional state of the individual. A recent analysis and bibliography of arm circumference [4] has confirmed this measurement as one of the more valuable in the rapid assessment of nutritional state.

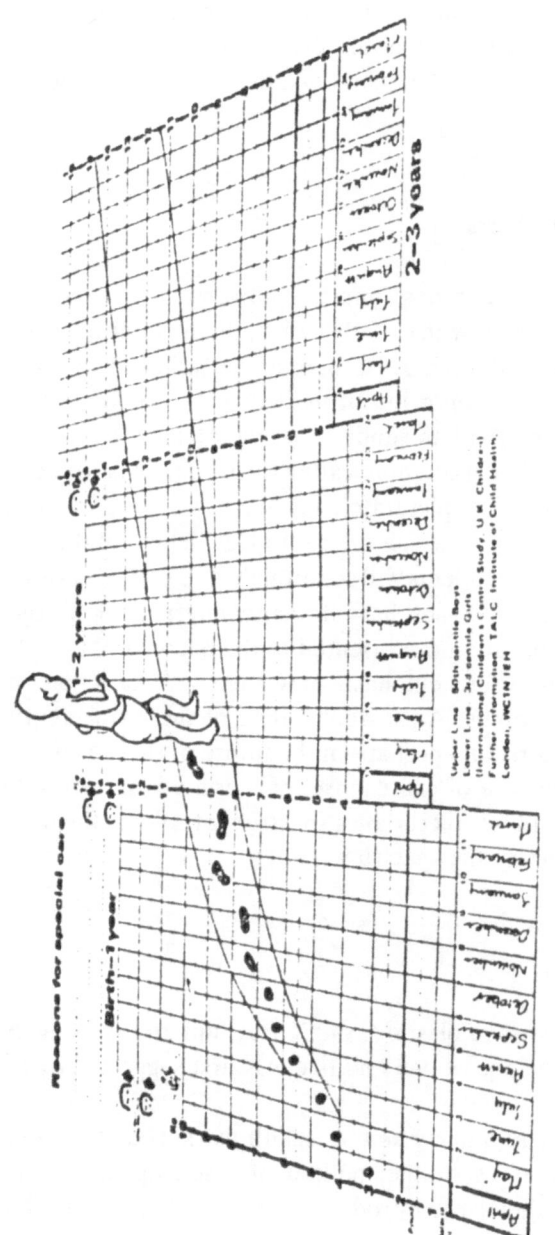

Figure 2. The concept is that of a child walking along the road of growth.

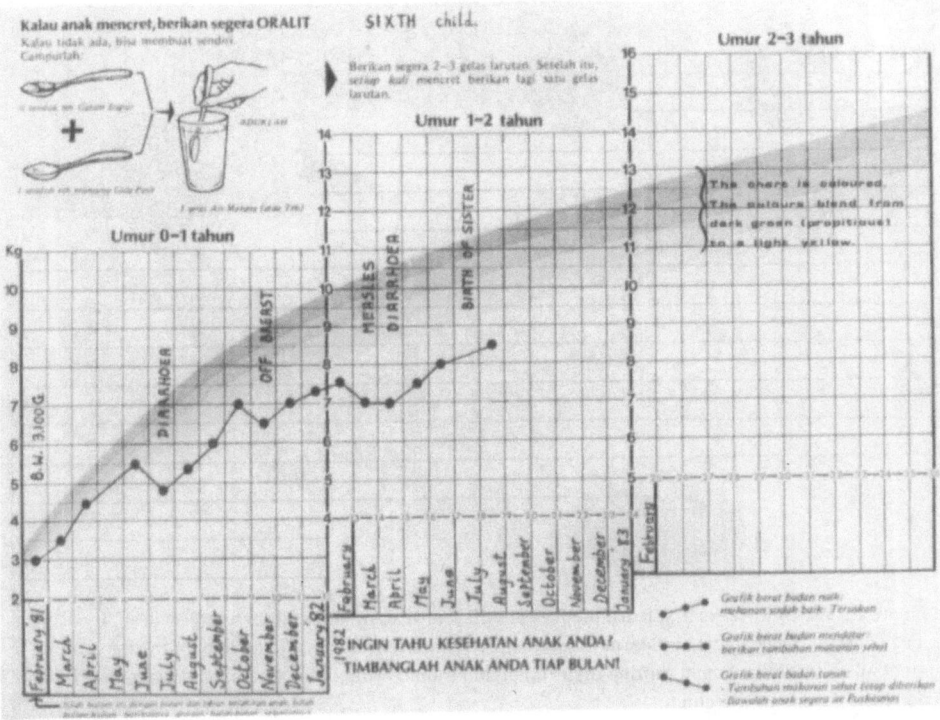

Figure 3. One of the more recently developed charts in which the path of the growth curve is coloured.

From a social and anthropological standpoint measuring the size of the arm can be recommended. In most hot climates where adults' arms are not covered people assess each other's state of nutrition perhaps more by the size of the arm than by the face, the latter is perhaps more used in temperate climates. Among the Ga tribe in Ghana mothers place a string of beads around the upper calf of their small children and are happy when this gets tight and they have to cut the string, but are worried if it starts to slip down the leg. Similarly, among one tribal group in South India, a metal band is placed round the upper calf and if this becomes loose the local tribal people say 'The devil is sucking the baby's juices . . .'

Weighing can also be a frightening experience for children, whereas measuring the arm circumference will rarely upset them. Perhaps, too, if we can train health workers to calibrate their own fingers and learn the feel of different sizes of arm, placing one's fingers around the arm of a child should be a routine clinical practice as well as a 'greeting' to the child (Figure 4).

138

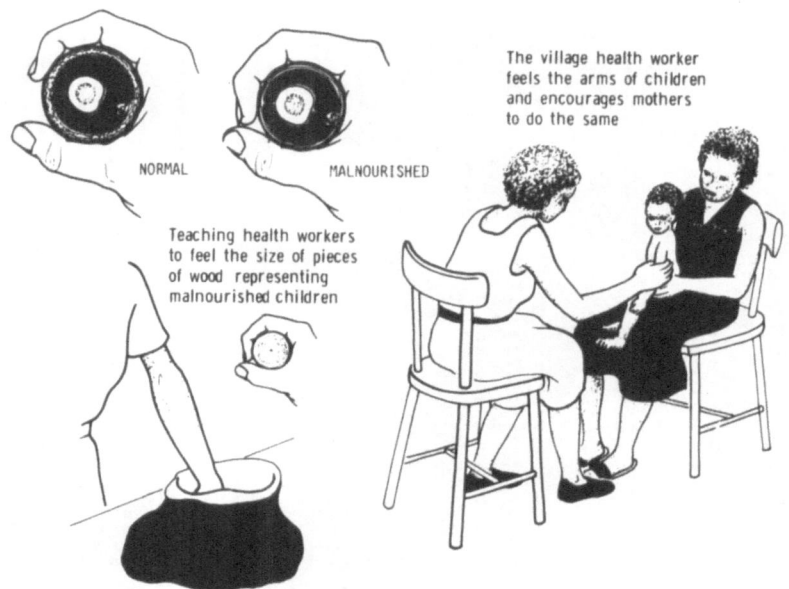

NORMAL

MALNOURISHED

Teaching health workers
to feel the size of pieces
of wood representing
malnourished children

The village health worker
feels the arms of children
and encourages mothers
to do the same

Figure 4. Health workers first learn the feel of different sizes of arm and then test their ability using a 'bag of arms'. Once they have learnt to assess the circumferences using finger and thumb they can then greet all children they meet putting their finger and thumb around the arm and assessing the size and nutritional state of the child.

The echeverri strip

The disadvantage of the Shakir strip is that it cannot be used until the child has reached the age of one and, therefore, it misses out on the vital early months. To overcome this a new plastic insertion tape has been developed which can be used from birth, and the reverse of which in the future may be used for measuring the enlarging uterus of the mother and perhaps her arm circumference.

Along with this tape there is a simple arm circumference growth chart which is so designed that the tape can be laid across it and the arm circumference marked. To make this simpler a cursor is placed on the plastic tape which travels along the tape as this is drawn tight. Instead of marking the child's weight every calendar month it may be simpler to do this at the new or full moon, a time that is easily recognised in most villages. A further development on these new charts is that drawings of syringes and dropper bottles are put for the various immunisations and those giving immunisations will pencil in the syringe so that it can be recognised at once what immunisations the child has or may need.

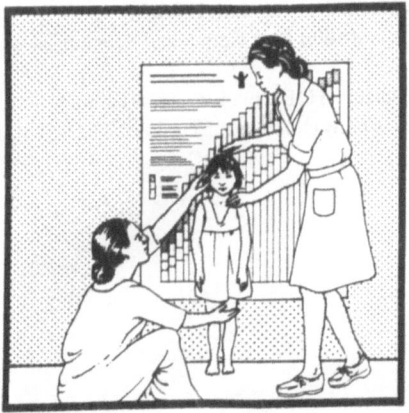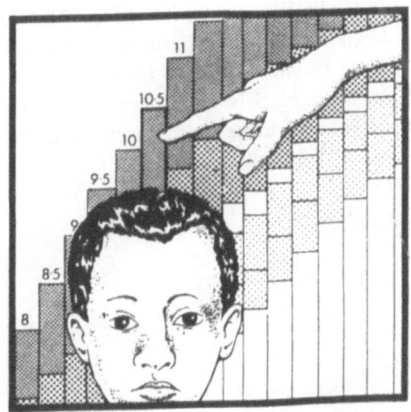

Figure 5. The Nabarro weight for height chart. This serves as a rapid method of relating weight to height. The charts are paticularly recommended for screening children to identify families requiring priority in feeding in a refugee camp.

Weight for height

Undoubtedly, for those undertaking scientific studies on growth, the measurement of length or height is the most valuable. Unfortunately, it is difficult to measure accurately in a clinic situation, may require quite expensive enquipment, and several months of training to achieve reliable results. For this reason, until recently the measurement of height in a clinic or emergency situation has not been attempted. However, thanks to developments in Nepal a simple wall chart has now been developed which rapidly relates the weight of the child to it's height. The child is weighed and then the column representing that weight is identified on the chart and the child stands in front of it (Figure 5).

If the child's head reaches into the green area, then the child's weight for height is likely to be satisfactory. If, however, the child's head reaches into a red area, then he is likely to be wasted and too thin for his height. This method is particularly suitable for use in refugee situations where the age of children is unlikely to be known and can be particularly useful in identifying wasted children who come from families who may need supplementary feeding. This chart can also be usefully used in the clinic in checking low-weight children to see whether they are either wasted or stunted.

References

1. Chen LD, Chowdhury A, Hoffman SL: Anthropometic assessment of energy protein malnutrition and subsequent mortality among pre-school children. Am J Clin Nutr 33:1836–1845, 1980.

2. Morley D, Woodland M: See How They Grow, Macmillan, London, 1979.
3. Shakir A: The surveillance of protein calorie malnutrition by a simple and economical means. J Trop Paediat Env Child Hlth 21:69, 1975.
4. Velzeboer M, Selwyn B, Sargent F II, Pollitt E, Delgado H: Evaluation of arm circumference as a public health index of protein energy malnutrition in early childhood. J Trop Ped 29:135–144, 1983.

A study of some aspects of marginal malnutrition amongst Egyptian infants and young children

R. SAKR, S. SAMUEL, D. FLEITA and A. ABDELWAHAB

Abstract

138 subjects aged 3 months to 4 years were chosen and classified into 3 groups: The first group comprised 45 normal controls, the second group consisted of 49 marginally malnourished patients and the third group included 44 patients who represented the 3 main varieties of PEM.

Final appraisal of nutritional status was based on clinical, anthropometric and laboratory data. A rather characteristic clinical picture for marginal malnutrition was presented. The anthropometric measurements that proved both practical and valuable were the mid-arm, mid-thigh circumferences and the weight/span ratio.

Estimation of serum total proteins, albumin, blood Hb, serum transferrin, ascorbic acid, creatinine and hydroxyproline was carried out and revealed: significant decrement in albumin, transferrin, Hb, hydroxyproline and hydroxyproline/creatinine ratio in MM and much more decrement in PEM patients. No significant difference was noted in vit C and creatinine levels in the whole material of study. Treatment of MM patients for 3 months revealed marked improvement. A scoring formula was deduced to assess individual nutritional status with a high degree of accuracy.

Abbreviations used

PEM	= protein energy malnutrition
MM	= marginal malnutrition
Wt	= weight
Ht	= height
MAC	= mid-arm circumference
MTC	= mid-thigh circumference
L	= length
KWO	= kwashiorkor
Hb	= hemoglobin

Introduction

Childhood malnutrition is a major health problem in developing countries where it has been estimated that 40% of children below 14 years are undernourished. Nutritional surveys of children under 5 years revealed that 34% of children in Asia, 31% in Africa, and 21% in South America were either severely or moderately malnourished [9].

Early detection of subclinical or MM is important; well-timed, appropriate management cuts short further deterioration in nutritional status and obviates serious sequelae.

The purpose of this communication is to highlight the problem and to provide the practitioner and nutritionist with some monitors that might help in evaluating the nutritional status of the young subject and in detecting the early stages of malnutrition.

Subjects and methods

Subjects of study comprised 138 infants and young children, 71 males and 67 females aged 3 months to 4 years. They were chosen from the poor or near poor attendants of the Outpatient Department of Children's Hospital of Cairo University, Egypt.

After detailed history and careful clinical examination the subjects were categorised into 3 groups. The first group included 45 healthy normal controls who were carefully selected to conform well with the median weights of well-to-do healthy age and sex matched Egyptians [1]. The second group consisted of 49 patients, 25 males and 24 females who were found to be at risk from malnutrition and were designated marginally malnourished. Diagnosis was made according to history, clinical presentation and Wt/Ht ratio percentage of more than 80% and less than 90% of the expected normal Wt/Ht ratio. The chief complaints and main signs of this group are summarised in Table 1. The third group included 44 overtly malnourished patients, 20 males and 24 females. All were below the 80% of expected Wt/Ht ratio of Egyptian 50th percentile. On clinical grounds, patients were divided into 36 marasmics who were further subdivided according to weight loss into 17 patients of second grade marasmus, and 19 of third grade (30–50% and more than 50% loss of weight respectively); 6 patients were diagnosed marasmic KWO and 2 patients severe KWO [2, 45].

The three groups of study were investigated as follows:

1. Anthropometric measurements (age dependent or independent) included: Wt, L or Ht, MAC, MTC, HC and span (Table 2). Ratios between different measurements included: Wt/Ht, HC/Ht MAC/Wt, MTC/Wt, $Wt/H^2 \times 100$, span/Ht and MAC/HC (Table 3).
2. Laboratory investigations: These included estimation of serum total proteins

Table 1. Main complaints and clinical data in the group of marginal malnutrition.

Chief complaints	No. of subjects	Percentage of total	Clinical examination	No. of subjects	Percentage of total
1. Failure to gain weight or weight loss	49	100	1. Wt/Ht (80–89% of Abbassy 50th percentile)	49	100
2. Anorexia	31	63	2. Pallor	44	89
3. Apathy	18	36	3. Apathy	28	57
4. Disturbed sleep	22	44	4. Vitamin deficiencies	32	65
5. Delayed walking	29	59	5. Rachitic manifestations	24	48
6. Delayed dentition	29	59	6. Conjunctivitis	12	24
7. Bouty diarrhoea	36	73	7. Stomatitis	14	28
8. Upper respiratory catarrh	40	81	8. Cheilosis	12	24
9. Wheezy chest	16	32	9. Otitis media	8	16
			10. Moon facies	36	73
			11. Oedema	–	–
			12. Liver enlargement	29	59

[26], albumin [12], blood hemoglobin percentage, serum transferrin level by single radio-immunodiffusion technique [28], serum ascorbic acid [8], serum creatinine [21, 34] and serum hydroxyproline [30].

The study also entailed clinical and laboratory follow-up of 9 MM patients for a period of 3 months during which they received appropriate therapy, and the results are shown in Tables 2, 3 and 4 and illustrated in Figures 1, 2 and 3. Figure 4 shows the Z-individual values in the different groups of study.

Discussion

The main concern of the study is to assist the practitioner to pick up subclinical or marginal forms of malnutrition at an optimal time by providing him with some useful indices whether these are clinical, anthropometric or laboratory.

On clinical grounds, subjects who were designated marginally malnourished

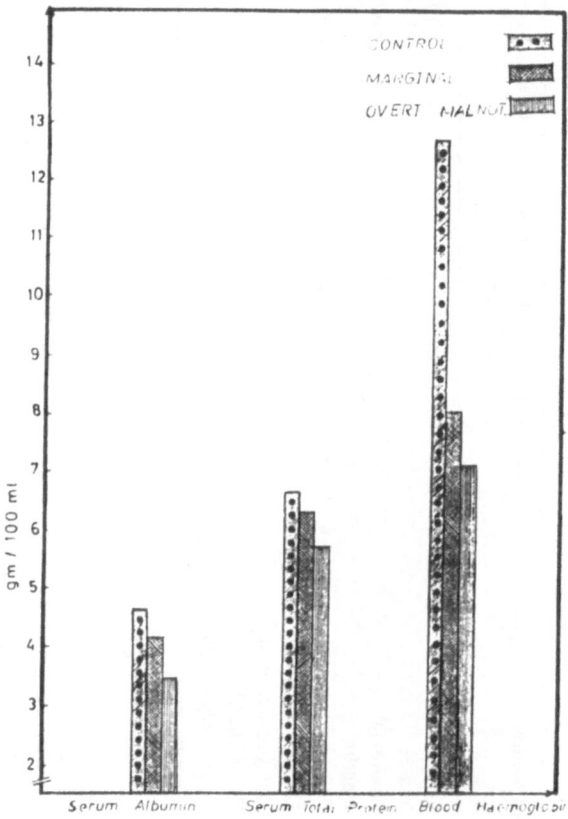

Figure 1. Serum albumin, total proteins and haemoglobin in the three groups of subjects.

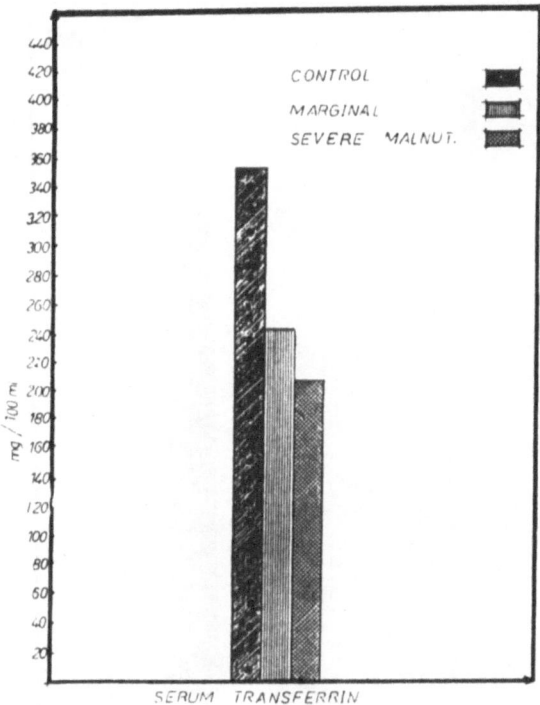

SERUM TRANSFERRIN

Figure 2. Serum transferrin in controls, marginally and overtly malnourished subjects.

were found to have common signs and symptoms which collectively compose a distinctive clinical picture that refers to under nutrition. The chief complaints, as shown in Table 1, were failure to gain weight or recent loss of weight, anorexia, apathy, disturbed sleep, excessive perspiration, delayed walking, delayed dentition, rhinitis, stomatitis, bouty diarrheal attacks, abdominal colics, upper respiratory catarrhs, otitis media and wheezy chest.

Their Wt/Ht ratio ranged between 80 to 89% of the standard value. Almost all patients looked pale with variable manifestations of vitamin deficiencies especially B, A and D. About 73% showed a characteristic unmistakable facies, the so called moon face appearance [22] with redundant hypotonic prominent cheeks; an appearance that is usually considered by parents and unaware practitioners as a sign of health and well being (Figure 5). Edema of any degree was absent in every member of the group of MM. The liver was enlarged in 59% of subjects – its consistency was always soft and it was not tender.

Age-independent anthropometric measurements have been widely appreciated for the detection of early cases of malnutrition, [21] especially in developing countries where the exact age of children may not be known to their parents.

In MM, the Ht and HC suffer least, while the MAC, MTC and body Wt are much more rapidly affected. Thus the MAC/Ht [6], the MAC/HC [25] and the

146

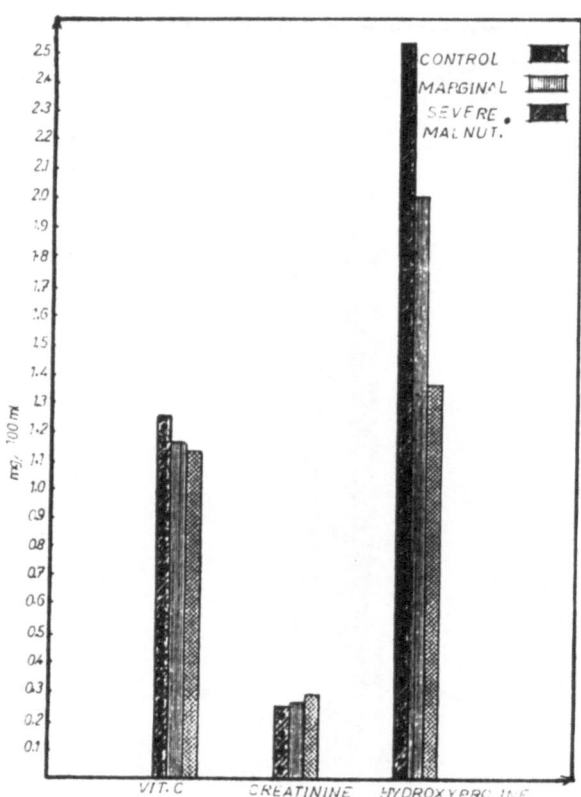

Figure 3. Serum vitamin C, creatinine and hydroxyproline in controls, marginally and overtly malnourished subjects.

Wt/Ht² × 100 ratios [15] have been suggested to gauge subclinical PEM in communities.

As regards Wt/Ht ratio in patients, a significant drop in its values was noted in the MM series as compared to controls and a more significant drop was obtained in the overtly malnourished series. This agrees with previous reports [25, 40, 44] which concluded that Wt/Ht ratio may be an adjuvant useful index in the detection of early malnutrition especially that of short duration.

Besides, a significant drop in MAC value was noticed in MM subjects as compared to controls. In the severely malnourished group more significant decrement was found. The results conform with those reported by other investigators [10, 16, 18, 36, 39] who stated that MAC varies more with nutrition than with age and thus recommended it as a useful measure especially when age is not exactly known. The same results were noted with MTC as the muscle represents a labile protein reserve. The mean values of MTC for controls, MM and PEM groups were 24.5, 20 and 15 cm respectively (Table 2). The thigh at its maximum circumference has the largest cross section of muscle mass. Thus muscle wasting

Table 2. Anthropometric measurement in the different groups of subjects.

Group of subjects		Age (months)	Weight (kg)	Length (cm)	H.C. (cm)	Span (cm)	M.A.C. (cm)	M.T.C. (cm)
Controls	Range	4–48	6–19.0	57.0–106.0	39.0–52.0	55–105	11.5–17.0	18.0–30.0
(45)	Mean	19.2	10.37	75.53	46.09	73.98	14.57	24.54
26 M	± S.D	14.8	3.75	14.84	4.68	15.51	1.46	3.44
19 F								
Marginal	Range	3–30	0–10.5	52.0–84.0	35.0–50.0	50–84	10.0–14.0	16.0–24.0
malnutrition	Mean	12.0	6.77	65.16	42.26	64.74	12.08	20.04
(49)	± S.D	7.2	1.70	8.20	3.21	5.96	1.14	2.66
25 M								
24 F								
Overt	Range	3–30	2.5–11.0	52.0–89.0	36.0–47.0	47.0–85.0	8.0–12.5	12.5–23.0
Malnutrition	Mean	10.6	5.45	64.80	41.29	61.45	9.67	15.02
(44)	± S.D	5.8	1.92	8.49	3.87	9.47	1.67	2.49
20 M								
24 F								

Legend: H.C. = head circumference; M.A.C. = mid arm circumference; M.T.C. = mid thigh circumference; ( ) = No. of cases; M = male; F = female.

whether in arm or thigh is a good indicator of protein depletion in malnutrition.

An insignificant difference was noted in the HC/Ht ratio between MM patients and parallel controls. Malnutrition of short duration has little or no marked effect on HC or Ht; thus the ratio HC/Ht is usually not appreciably affected by this type of malnutrition and is not recommended to substitute MA or MT values in the detection of MM. Even so in the severely malnourished patients, this ratio did not differ significantly from that of either the control or the MM series. It seems that even in the severe forms of malnutrition the HC and Ht may be affected simultaneously almost to the same extent so that the ratio may not reveal significant changes (Table 3).

Some workers [13, 25] suggested that if the Wt is divided by Ht^2 and multiplied by 100, the resulting ratio is independent of age. In the present study the $Wt/Ht^2 \times 100$ ratio showed highly significant lower values in MM when compared to those for controls and even a more significant drop in the ratio in the severely malnourished when compared to MM subjects. The results for controls ranged from 0.14 to 0.24 with a mean value of 0.17 ± 0.03, table [3]; the limit for good nutrition is a ratio of more than 0.15. These results agree with those obtained by other workers [10, 13, 15, 16, 18 25, 36, 40, 44] who concluded that this ratio is the most reliable index in the detection of MM in children of preschool age.

Concerning the MAC/HC ratio, a significant drop in its value was noticed in both the MM and the severely malnourished groups as compared to healthy parallel control values. These results agree with previous reports [15, 25]. It can be concluded that Ht and HC suffer least while the MAC and body Wt are much more readily affected in malnutrition and that MAC/HC ratio seems to be one of the useful tools in detecting MM. A ratio of 0.31 or more conforms with normal nutrition (Table 3).

As regards the values of the span/Ht ratio, a significant decrement in the values was obtained in both the MM and the severely malnourished groups as compared to the values obtained for the healthy controls. The span seems to be more affected than the Ht in malnutrition since in measuring the span, in addition to the chest, 4 long bones are included while 2 long bones only are included when measuring the Ht. So the span/Ht ratio can be used as a monitor to detect early or subclinical malnutrition. A ratio of 0.98 or more was obtained in healthy controls. The corresponding values for both the MM and PEM groups were 0.96 and 0.92 respectively (Table 3).

Concerning biochemical data the levels of serum albumin were significantly lower in MM than in controls and a marked decrement in serum total proteins and albumin was noticed in severely malnourished subjects (Table 4). These results are in agreement with those reported by other workers [18, 32, 38]. From the present study, serum albumin estimation when associated with suggestive clinical picture may be considered among the most reliable laboratory indicators of malnutrition.

Compared to controls, a significant drop in Hb levels was noticed in the MM

Table 3. Statistical parameters in the different groups of subjects.

Statistical parameter		Controls (45)	Marg. maln. (49)	Overt maln. (44)
Wt/Ht	Range	0.10–0.16	0.07–0.13	0.05–0.10
	Mean ± S.D	0.13 ± 0.02	0.10 ± 0.01	0.07 ± 0.01
	t		7.75	6.50
	p		<0.005**	<0.005**
M.A.C.	Range	11.50–17.0	10.0–14.0	8.0–12.5
	Mean ± S.D	14.57 ± 1.46	12.08 ± 1.14	9.67 ± 1.67
	t		9.22	10.04
	p		<0.001**	<0.001**
M.T.C.	Range	18.0–30.0	16.0–24.0	12.5–23.0
	Mean ± S.D	24.54 ± 3.44	20.04 ± 2.66	15.02 ± 2.49
	t		7.03	9.47
	p		<0.001**	<0.001**
H.C./Ht	Range	0.50–0.70	0.53–0.75	0.56–0.73
	Mean ± S.D	0.62 ± 0.08	0.63 ± 0.07	0.63 ± 0.03
	t		0.167	0.126
	p		>0.5 N.S	>0.5 N.S
$Wt/Ht^2 \times 100$	Range	0.14–0.24	0.12–0.16	0.08–0.14
	Mean ± S.D	0.17 ± 0.03	0.14 ± 0.02	0.11 ± 0.01
	t		6.36	6.67
	p		<0.001**	<0.001**
M.A.C./H.C.	Range	0.28–0.35	0.26–0.31	0.18–0.31
	Mean ± S.D	0.31 ± 0.01	0.28 ± 0.01	0.23 ± 0.02
	t		9.17	10.2
	p		<0.001**	<0.001**
Span/Ht	Range	0.77–1.05	0.82–1.01	0.78–1.02
	Mean ± S.D	0.98 ± 0.04	0.96 ± 0.05	0.92 ± 0.06
	t		2.09	2.61
	p		<0.025**	<0.01**

Legend: Wt = weight; Ht = height; M.A.C. = mid arm circumference; M.T.C. = mid thigh circumference; H.C. = Head circumference; ( ) = No. of cases; ** = highly significant.

Table 4. Comparative results in biochemical parameters estimated in different groups of subjects.

Biochemical test in serum		Controls (45)	Marg. maln. (49)	Overt. maln. (44)
Total proteins g%	Range	5.50–8.50	4.30–8.60	3.20–7.40
	Mean ± S.D	6.66 ± 0.80	6.34 ± 0.99	5.73 ± 1.19
	t		1.71	1.95
	p		>0.05 N.S.	>0.05 N.S.
Albumin g%	Range	3.80–5.50	3.00–5.50	2.40–4.30
	Mean ± S.D	4.65 ± 0.82	4.17 ± 1.02	3.47 ± 0.79
	t		2.30	3.30
	p		<0.025*	<0.005**
Blood hemoglobin g%	Range	12.0–14.0	7.10–9.40	6.00–8.20
	Mean ± S.D	12.8 ± 0.43	8.08 ± 0.62	7.11 ± 0.64
	t		2.44	7.45
	p		<0.001**	<0.001**
Transferrin mg%	Range	170.00–500.000	80.00–440.00	30.00–480.0
	Mean ± S.D	352.04 ± 133.21	242.83 ± 113.12	207.78 ± 108.
	t		3.97	4.52
	p		<0.001**	<0.001**
Ascorbic acid mg%	Range	0.46–2.60	0.20–2.83	0.45–2.00
	Mean ± S.D	1.24 ± 0.53	1.15 ± 0.55	1.12 ± 0.43
	t		0.761	0.333
	p		>0.25 N.S.	>0.4 N.S.
Creatinine mg%	Range	0.12–0.39	0.12–0.66	0.20–0.34
	Mean ± S.D	0.24 ± 0.05	0.25 ± 0.10	0.28 ± 0.04
	t		0.416	0.38
	p		>0.4 N.S.	>0.4 N.S.
Hydroxyproline µg/ml	Range	10.00–50.00	5.00–35.00	5.00–30.00
	Mean ± S.D	25.22 ± 9.52	19.48 ± 8.05	13.52 ± 8.48
	t		3.14	3.45
	p		<0.005**	<0.005**
Hydroxyproline/creatinine ratio	Range	2.58–25.00	2.50–26.42	1.47–10.71
	Mean ± S.D	11.50 ± 5.03	9.26 ± 6.41	4.83 ± 3.11
	t		1.99	4.31
	p		<0.05*	<0.005**

Legend: * = just significant; ** = highly significant; ( ) = No. of subjects.

patients and a more significant drop in the severely malnourished. Drop of Hb% in malnutrition has been attributed to protein deficiency [4, 5], deficiency of folic acid and iron [27], B 12 [23], vitamin C [42] or riboflavin [42]. Little has been written about Hb level in MM either in Egypt or abroad for comparison with the results of the study. In severely malnourished patients, the results obtained agree with previous reports [2, 3, 18, 37].

The values for serum transferrin in controls are in agreement with those reported in Egypt [3, 19, 37] and abroad. However the values were higher than those reported by others. This controversy may be partially attributed to differences in the clinical state, the subjects studied, variation of laboratory techniques as well as to differences in the composition of diet especially the protein content. The values of serum transferrin in the MM group were found to be reduced significantly when compared to those of controls and more significantly reduced in severe PEM subjects in agreement with the results obtained by other workers [3, 19, 37] (Table 4).

No significant difference was traced between values in plasma ascorbic acid concentrations obtained in the different groups studied. It was shown that vitamin C level depends on recent dietary intake [11] – and as the sources of vitamin C are usually cheap in Egypt, so it seems that malnourished subjects can get their requirements of the vitamin and hence the normal values achieved in the present study. No similar study was conducted in Egypt or abroad in MM. Only one work [14] reported low serum ascorbic acid in KWO in Nigeria. Such controversy may be partially attributed to a difference in dietary habits and method of estimation. Thus serum vitamin C cannot be utilised as a reliable indicator of the nutritional status of infants in areas where vitamin C sources are both cheap and adequate.

The serum creatinine level in MM showed no significant differences from control subjects. An insignificant increase was noticed in severely malnourished subjects as compared to either controls or MM groups. Serum creatinine concentration is related to muscle mass as well as to renal function and is largely unaffected by changes in diet, fluid intake or other factors apart from kidney diseases [37]. The slight degree of muscle wasting in MM as well as the preserved state of kidney function can explain the maintenance of a normal serum creatinine level in MM. This is in agreement with a previous report [43].

A significant decrement in serum hydroxyproline was noticed in MM as compared to controls. A higher significant decrease in serum hydroxyproline level was noticed in the severely malnourished patients compared to either controls or MM subjects (Table 4 and Figure 3). The amount of hydroxyproline in serum depends on the amount of total body collagen and the rate of its catabolism [33] and the kidney function and its ability to excrete hydroxyproline peptide. These findings agree with those of others [31] and show that determination of serum hydroxyproline is a reliable adjunct index for detection of MM.

As regards the serum hydroxyproline/creatinine ratio, the values obtained in MM were significantly lower than those obtained in controls. A significant reduction was obtained in severely malnourished patients compared to either controls or MM. Thus estimation of this ratio may be utilised as a monitor to assess the state of nutrition.

A 3-month treatment and follow up period of the 9 marginally malnourished patients revealed significant improvement in the values of Wt, MAC and MTC; the values were found to be approaching those of normal parallel controls. This supports our belief that rapid satisfactory improvement of the growth pattern in MM can be achieved when the syndrome is detected at an optimal time and is managed properly. With complete recovery all values are expected to be normalised.

Besides estimation of serum albumin, Hb, hydroxyproline and hydroxyproline/ creatinine ratio revealed almost normal values.

In order to consider the simultaneous effects of determination of different parameters, whether anthropometric or laboratory, in detecting malnutrition, multiple linear regression was chosen because it is a standard multivariate statistical approach for prediction.

A preliminary examination of the relation between pairs of variables, by calculating the correlation coefficient between every pair, was performed, including the nutritional status, using the data of the normal control group and that of the overtly malnourished one. Each normal control subject was considered as having nutritional status = 0, while those of classic malnutrition = 1. We concluded that MAC and Wt/Ht had the largest correlation coefficients. Serum total proteins, ascorbic acid and creatinine had the minimal correlation coefficients. A high coefficient was noticed between MAC and Wt/Ht ratio, also between serum hydroxyproline and hydroxyproline/creatinine ratio. Multiple linear regression analysis of the control and overtly malnourished subjects [42], was performed using a 'Wang' computer and taking into consideration the seven parameters that gave high correlation coefficients with the nutritional status. The regression models were calculated in the form:

$$Z = b_0 + b_1 x_{1i} + b_2 x_{2i} + \ldots b_k \times k_i,$$

where Z is the predicted nutritional status for subjects, the x are the values of particular parameters for patient i and the b's are calculated by conventional least quare methods. The optimal model is the higher the multiple correlation coefficient (approximating unity) [20]. The adequacy of a model containing a given set of factors for predicting the nutritional status is indicated by the correlation between the observed nutritional status and the predicted one. Correlation is measured by the multiple correlation coefficient R [41], this tends to increase when more variables are included, hence it is preferable to use the corrected correlation coefficient R which is adjusted for the number of variables [20]. The *Z value is calculated to be: 3–2.9 (Wt/Ht) − 0.1 (MAC) − 0.6 (Span/Ht) − 0.07 (Albumin g%) + 0.0002 (Transferrin mg %) + 0.006 (Hydroxyproline/μg/ml.) − 0.02 (Hydroxyproline/Creatinine). R for this equation is 0.914 and R' is 0.906. The*

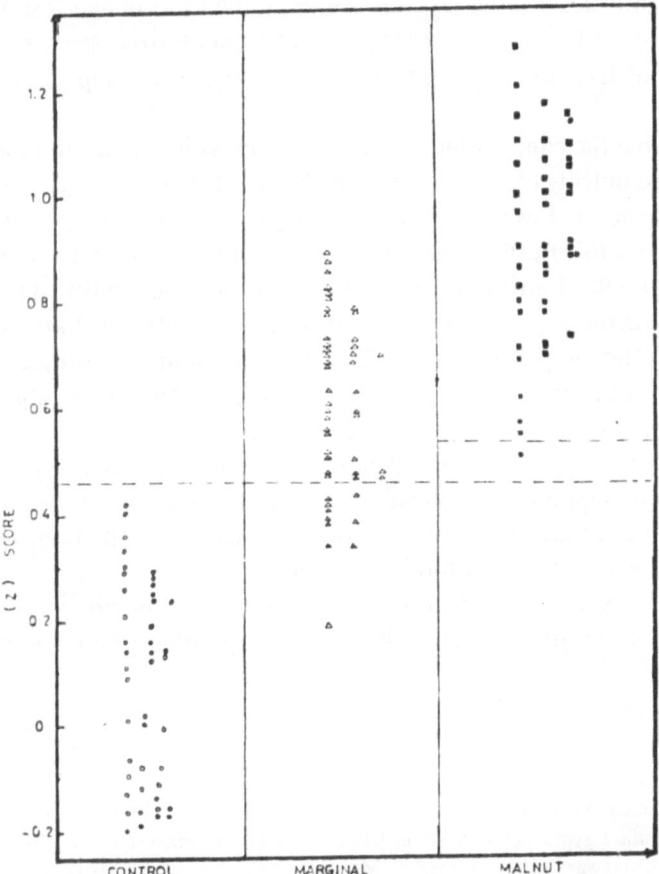

Figure 4. Z-individual values in different nutritional groups.

control group Z-score ranged from 0.21 to 0.42 with a mean of 0.08 and a S.D. of 0.19. So the upper limit of the 95% confidence level of the normal subjects (mean ± 2 S.D.) equals 0.46. The same Z-score of the overt malnourished subjects ranged between 0.51 and 1.27 with a mean of 0.92 ± 0.19, with a lower limit of 0.54. Figure 5 shows that there is no overlap between the 2 groups. By calculating the Z-score for each of the marginally malnourished subjects, it was found to range from 0.19 to 0.89 with a mean of 0.47 ± 0.18. Thirty-nine out of 49 (80%) of the MM subjects had scores above the upper limit of normal (0.46). This score gives a clear value for each subject suspected to be marginally malnourished.

In Egypt in poor sectors of population the prevalence of the overt forms of malnutrition in the preschool age period was found 10 years ago to vary from 1.3 to 15.4% with the highest prevalence in the age period 6 months to 3 years [39, 40]. One can confidently say that the state of affairs is better at present time. Yet it must be remembered that every patient of frank malnutrition represents about

10 play-mates suffering from less severe forms of the syndrome. Despite great advances in medical laboratory techniques and computerized science, clinical assessment – that has stood the test of time – remains the simplest and most rewarding.

Keeping in mind the clinical clues of MM together with few cut-off points that can be easily and quickly obtained, e.g. MAC below 14 cm in the age period 1–6 years, or Wt/Ht ratio below 90% of standard or blood Hb below 9 g%, will ease the recognition of MM. Besides, delineation of the child at risk from undernutrition from the normally nourished is of great value for the community. It improves the efficiency of screening programs for nutrition. Evidently paediatricians will be in a better position to pick up the subclinically undernourished subjects before the appearance of the classic signs of severe forms of PEM; thus morbidity and mortality are lessened and the financial burden is minimized.

Finally data obtained from history, dietetic survey, clinical and routine laboratory investigation all point to the value of some prophylactic measures namely:
1. Breast feeding, proper weaning (age of start, age of completion, mode of weaning and what articles of food to be offered).
2. Immunization especially against measles, pertussis and tuberculosis.
3. Eradication of parasites especially hook-worms, giardiasis and amoebiasis.

References

1. Abbassy AS, Hussein M, Hammed SA, Kassem AS, Aref M, Morsy MR, Araby JI: Growth and development of the Egyptian child from birth to 5 years. Dar El Maaref, Cairo, 1972.
2. Abdel-Aal A, El-Hawary MFS, El-Basousy MM, Khashaba AA, Hafez MI:GEPA 20(3):291, 1972.
3. Abdul Kader M, Rahman MA: Br J Nutr 28:191, 1972.
4. Adams EB, Scragg JN, Naidoo BT, Liljestrand SK, Cockram VI: Br Med J 3:451, 1967.
5. Allen DM, Dean RFA: Trans Roy Soc Trop Med Hyg 59:326, 1965.
6. Arnold RJ: Trop Pediat 15:243, 1969.
7. Awwaad S, Awny AY, Abdel Wahab EM, Abdel Fattah S: GEPA XIV (3.4):160, 1966.
8. Barker SB, Summerson WH: J Biol Chem 138:535, 1941.
9. Bengoa JM: In: Oslon RE (ed) Protein calorie malnut. Academic Press, New York, p 433, 1975.
10. Burgess HJL, Burgess AP: J Trop Pediat 15:189, 1969.
11. Cantarow A, Trumper T: Clinical biochemistry, 7th edn. Albert L. Latner, WB Saunders, Philadelphia, London, Toronto, 1975.
12. Doumas B, Bigg H: Standard methods of clinical chemistry, Vol 7. Academic Press, New York, p 175, 1972.
13. Dugdale AE: Am J Clin Nutr 24:174, 1971.
14. Edoxien JC: Nature 220:917, 1968.
15. El-Behairy F, Mostafa S, El-Mougi M, Osman NH, Saoudi F: GEPA 26(3&4):183, 1978.
16. El-Lozy M: Lancet 2:175, 1974.
17. Foy H, Kondi A, Mac Dougall L: Br Med J 1:97, 1961.
18. Fredrick L, Trowbridge MD: Am J Clin Nutr 32:758, 1979.
19. Gabr M, El-Hawary MFS, El-Dali MJ: Trop Med Hyp 74:216, 1971.
20. Haitovsky Y: Am Statis 23:20, 1969.

21. Hare RS: Proc Soc Exp Biol Med 2:95, 1950.
22. Hanson JDL, Buchaman N, Pettiefor IM: In: Mc Laren DS, Burman D (eds) Textbook of pediatric nutrition. Churchill, Livingstone, Edinburg, London, New York, 1976.
23. Herbert V: Megaloblastic anemia. Grune and Stratton, New York, 1959.
24. Jelliffe DB: Assessment of nutrition status of the community. WHO Monograph Series, No., 53, Geneva, 1966.
25. Kanawati AA, Haddad N, Mc Laren DS: J Trop Ped 15:233, 1970.
26. King EJ, Wooton IDP: Microanalysis, Medical Biochemistry, 3rd edn. Churchill, London, 1956.
27. Kondi A, Mac Dougall L, Foy H, Mehra S, Mabaya V: Arch Dis Child 38:267, 1963.
28. Macini G, Carbonara AO, Heremans JF: Immunochemistry 2:235, 1965.
29. Owen JA, Igg RJ: Biochem J 62:765, 1956.
30. Parekh A, Jung DH: Biochem Med 4:446, 1970.
31. Picon D, Alleyne GAO, Seakins A: Clin Sci 29:517, 1965.
32. Prasonna HA, Desai BLM, Rao MN: Br J Nutr 26:71, 1970.
33. Prockop DJ, Keiser HR, Sjoerdsma A: Lancet 2:527, 1962.
34. Ralston MJ: Clin Pathol 8:160, 1955.
35. Rao KV, Singh D: Am J Clin Nutr 23:83, 1970.
36. Rutishauser IHE, Whitehead RG: Br J Nutr 231:1969.
37. Said A, El-Hawayry MFS, Sakr R, Abdel Khalek MK, El-Shobaki FA, Noseir MB: GEPA 23(2):139, 1975.
38. Sakr R, Abdel-Khalek MK, Samuel S, El-Barbary M, El-Bishlawy A, El-Shobaki F. Abdin M: GEPA 26(3&4):167, 1978.
39. Shukry AS, Barakat MR, El-Gammal RA, Kamel LM: GEPA 20:151, 1972.
40. Shukry AS, Barakat MR, Kamel LM: GEPA 21:17, 1973.
41. Snedecor GW, Cochran WG: Iowa State University Press, Ames, Chap 13, 1972.
42. Velez H, Ghitis J, Pradilla A, Pud vitale JJ: Amer J Clin Nutr 12: 54, 1962.
43. Viteri FE, Alverodo J: Pediatrics 46:696, 1970.
44. Waterlow JC: Lancet 2:87, 1973.
45. Wellcome Trust Working Patry: Lancet 2:302, 1970.

Epidemiology and clinical assessment of vitamin deficiencies in Thai children

V. TANPHAICHITR

1. Introduction

Thailand is located in Southeast Asia. The recent census reveals a total population of 48.5 millions with 83% of the people living in rural areas. The children under 15 years of age constitute 38% of the total population. The economic foundation of the nation is rice farming.

Nutrition surveys carried out in different parts of Thailand indicate that malnutrition is one of the major problems affecting the life and well-being of the Thai population. The seven leading causes of malnutrition are protein-energy malnutrition, iron-deficiency anemia, beriberi, riboflavin deficiency, vitamin A deficiency, simple goiter, and pediatric bladder stone disease [1]. It is the objective of this paper to delineate the problem of the three vitamin malnutrition in Thai children, with the emphasis on thiamin deficiency.

2. Beriberi

Beriberi is caused by thiamin deficiency. It has been reported in almost every country but has never been endemic outside of Asia. Most of the occidental beriberi cases are confined to chronic alcoholics whereas most of the oriental beriberi cases are associated with the consumption of milled rice [2].

2.1. Clinical manifestations

The clinical manifestations of beriberi vary with age which is the basis of the classification of the disease into infantile beriberi and childhood, adolescent or adult beriberi [2, 3]. However, two major systems, the cardiovascular and nervous systems, are involved in both types of beriberi.

Infantile beriberi. This is a disease of the first year of life but is most commonly found between the age of two to three months [2, 3]. They may present as cardiac, aphonic, or pseudomeningitic form or as a combination of these three forms. Table 1 shows the common signs found in sixteen patients with infantile beriberi admitted at Ubol Provincial Hospital located in northeast Thailand [4]. They consisted of 8 males and 8 females, with the age ranging from one to eight months. Sixty-seven percent of these patients were in the age of one to two months.

Childhood or adolescent beriberi. Older children or adolescents suffering from thiamin deficiency manifest the same symptoms and signs as described in adults [2, 3]. They may present as dry (paralytic or nervous), wet, cerebral, or subclinical froms. Table 2 shows clinical data in sixteen patients with adolescent beriberi admitted at Ramathibodi and Siriraj Hospitals located in Bangkok [5, 6]. Seven patients were dry beriberi whereas nine patients were wet beriberi. Nine patients lived outside Bangkok.

The predominant feature in patients with dry beriberi is the presence of peripheral neuropathy with an insidious onset and chronic course. The neuropathy is characterized by a symmetrical impairment of sensory, motor, and reflex functions that affects the distal segments of limbs more severely than the proximal ones. Tenderness always appears at calf muscles. Muscular weakness in the early stage is demonstrated by the difficulty of the patients to rise from squatting position without assistance. Edema is absent in patients with dry beriberi.

Besides peripheral neuropathy, patients with wet beriberi also exhibit edema

Table 1. Physical signs present in sixteen patients with infantile beriberi.

Physical sign[a]	Percent of 16 patients
Cardiovascular system	
Dyspnea	87
Tachycardia[b]	81
Cardiomegaly[c]	73
Vomiting	63
Hepatomegaly	62
Edema	56
Cyanosis	19
Shock	6
Nervous system	
Decreased deep tendon reflexes	81
Aphonia	50
Convulsion	12
Ptosis	6

[a] More than one physical signs could be present in each patient.
[b] Heart rate was over 130 beats/minute.
[c] Confirmed by X-ray examination.

which is easily discernible over the lower extremities. Four out of nine patients with wet beriberi had a heart rate of over 100 beats per minute. The pulse pressure in seven patients was over 60 mmHg. All of the nine patients exhibited cardiomegaly evidenced by the roentgenologic examination. Congestive heart failure was also detected in six patients. The electrocardiogram in these six patients showed low or relatively low QRS complex voltages and definite ST-T abnormalities on admission. The increase of QRS complex voltage and the rapid reduction in heart size were observed concurrently with clinical improvement. These suggested that their transient low QRS complex voltage was most likely due to pericardial effusion [3, 7]. Hemodynamic data obtained from four adolescents with wet beriberi revealed that three patients had typical hemodynamic findings. These included high cardiac output failure and low peripheral and pulmonary vascular resistances [3, 8]. After thiamin therapy cardiac output was reduced and vascular resistance was increased. However, one patient exhibited low cardiac output which increased after thiamin administration. This may be due to myocardial damage caused by repeated episodes of thiamin deficiency. Thus low cardiac output in wet beriberi does not exclude the diagnosis. Our study has demonstrated that both nervous and cardiovascular systems were affected in patients with wet beriberi.

Table 2. Clinical data in sixteen patients with adolescent beriberi.

Patient	Age (yr)	Sex	Occupation	Residency
Dry beriberi				
1	17	M	Blacksmith	Bangkok
2	17	M	Jeweller	Bangkok
3	17	M	Farmer	Nonthaburi
4	18	M	Farmer	Chachoengsao
5	16	F	Trader	Samut Sakorn
6	20	M	Student	Bangkok
7	15	M	Watchrepairer	Nakhon Sawan
Wet beriberi				
8	21	M	Unemployed	Nakhon Pathom
9	18	M	Student	Samut Prakan
10	17	F	Factory worker	Bangkok
11	15	F	Factory worker	Bangkok
12	17	M	Student	Bangkok
13	15	M	Student	Ayuthaya
14	18	M	Carpenter	Bangkok
15	18	M	Student	Ang Thong
16	15	M	Student	Pichit

2.2. Diagnostic approach of beriberi

The diagnosis of beriberi can be made clinically by dietary history, physical examination, and therapeutic response to thiamin administration [3, 5, 6]. Clinical clues leading to the suspected diagnosis of infantile beriberi are as follows: the infant is breast-fed and has evidence of cardiac failure and/or aphonia whereas the nursing mother gives a history of food restriction and numbness and/or develops peripheral neuropathy. Adolescents usually give the history of excersive intake of carbohydrate derived mainly from milled rice, inadequate consumption of rich sources of thiamin, e.g. pork, beef and pulses. Some may consume foods containing antithiamin factors, e.g., raw fermented fish. These will cause inadequate thiamin status. A sudden increase in thiamin requirement due to strenuous physical exertion and/or fever will precipitate the clinical manifestations of beriberi.

Common suggestive signs in dry beriberi include glove and stocking hypesthesia of pain and touch sensations, loss of ankle or knee reflexes, tenderness at calf muscle, difficulty in rising from squatting position, and aphonia. However, other possible known causes of peripheral neuropathy must be carefully ruled out. Patients with wet beriberi exhibit both peripheral neuropathy and edema. Severe cases will have cardiac enlargement, wide pulse pressure, tachycardia and pulmonary congestion.

The response to thiamin treatment in infants or adolescents with cardiac beriberi is one of the most dramatic findings in medicine. Improvement can be observed within six hours after thiamin administration. This consists of less restlessness, disappearance of cyanosis, and reduction in heart rate and respiratory rate. Table 3 summarizes the outstanding changes following thiamin administration in nine adolescents with wet beriberi. These include diuresis evidenced by reduction in body weight, decrease in heart rate and pulse pressure. Reduction in cardiac size and clearing of the pulmonary congestion are also observed in patients with cardiomegaly. In dry beriberi, however, it is difficult to use the

Table 3. Clinical responses to thiamin treatment in nine adolescents with wet beriberi.

Parameter	Mean ± SEM	
	Before treatment	After treatment
Body weight, kg	51.6 ± 2.4	46.5 ± 1.0[a, c]
Heart rate, beats/min	97 ± 7	71 ± 6[b, d]
Pulse pressure, mmHg	57 ± 5	43 ± 4[a, d]

[a] Significant difference from before thiamin treatment: $P<0.02$.

[b] Significant difference from before thiamin treatment: $P<0.001$.

[c] Total weight loss of 5.1 ± 1.6 kg within 5.1 ± 0.5 days.

[d] 24 hr after thiamin treatment.

response to thiamin administration as a criterion for immediate diagnosis because more time elapses before improvement is observed [3, 5, 6]. Other possible known causes of peripheral neuropathy must be carefully ruled out.

2.3. Biochemical assessment

Various biochemical tests based on thiamin metabolism or the biochemical functions of thiamin pyrophosphate (TPP) have been developed to detect thiamin deficiency and establish thiamin adequacy in man [2, 9]. These include the measurement of blood thiamin, pyruvate, alpha-ketoglutarate, lactate and glyoxylate, urinary thiamin excretion, urinary thiamin metabolites, thiamin loading test and urinary methylglyoxal. At present the most reliable and feasible method to evaluate thiamin adequacy in man is the measurement of whole blood or erythrocyte transketolase activity (ETKA) and its percent enhancement resulting from the added TPP which is referred as thiamin pyrophosphate effect (TPPE) [2, 9]. Our studies have shown that biochemical diagnostic criteria for beriberi consist of low ETKA accompanied by high TPPE. Infants or adolescents with beriberi prior to thiamin treatment always have TPPE greater than 15%. Significant reduction in TPPE was observed within 24 hours in nine patients with infantile beriberi after receiving 50 to 100 mg of thiamin hydrochloride given parenterally (Table 4). The same finding was observed in their mothers (Table 4) and adolescents with dry or wet beriberi (Table 5).

Table 4. TPPE in nine patients with infantile beriberi and their mothers.

Subject		Mean ± SEM of TPPE, %	
Group	No.	Before treatment	After treatment
Infant	9	34 ± 6	7 ± 3[a]
Mother	9	24 ± 3	12 ± 4[b]

[a] Significant difference from before thiamin treatment: $P<0.005$.
[b] Significant difference from before thiamin treatment: $P<0.01$.

Table 5. TPPE in thirteen adolescents with beriberi.

Subject		Mean ± SEM of TPPE, %	
Group	No.	Before treatment	After treatment
Dry beriberi	6	36 ± 11	2 ± 1[a]
Wet beriberi	7	37 ± 9	6 ± 3[b]

[a] Significant difference from before thiamin treatment: $P<0.05$.
[b] Significant difference from before thiamin treatment: $P<0.02$.

2.4. Incidence

A comprehensive account of the incidence of beriberi in Thailand has been given [3]. The earliest reliable record of beriberi was made by Laurent in 1899. He described an epidemic of beriberi among Thai soldiers which promptly ceased when pork and fresh vegetables were introduced into the military ration. Subsequent report by Highet who collected statistics of the hospitals, the army, the navy, and the police, revealed that there were 22,670 cases of beriberi with 1063 deaths. In 1920, Hepburn et al. described 100 cases of beriberi. In 1956, Ramalingaswami reported that the incidence of peripheral neuropathy among adults and adolescents in Chiengrai, the province in northern Thailand, and Ubol province were approximately 24 and 12%, respectively. In 1959, Klerks and Bisolyaputra estimated the morbidity rate of beriberi for the whole population was 1 to 2 percents per year, including relapse. It was quoted in 1975 that beriberi had virtually disappeared from prosperous Asian countries such as Japan, Taiwan and Malaya, as well as in the big cities such as Hong Kong, Singapore, Manila, Bangkok, Rangoon and Jakarta and their surrounding countryside [10]. This, though, is not the case for Thailand because there are still reports of beriberi in children and adults from various parts of the country [4, 5, 11–14]. In September 1983, we had identified 24 cases of beriberi out of 164 adolescents living in Rayong, the province in eastern Thailand. Biochemical assessment revealed that 42% of these adolescents had TPPE greater than 15% (Table 6). Biochemical thiamin deficiency was also detected in Ubol children and adults (Table 7) (unpublished data).

2.5. Pathogenesis

TPP acts as a coenzyme required for the oxidative decarboxylation of alpha-keto acids which include pyruvate, alpha-keto glutarate, and keto analogues of leucine, isoleucine and valine, and the transketolase reaction in the pentose phosphate pathway. Circumstantial evidence also suggests that thiamin triphosphate (TTP) or TPP is the neurophysiologically active form which has a specific role in

Table 6. Prevalence of biochemical thiamin and riboflavin deficiencies in Rayong adolescents.

Sex	Age (yr)	No.	Percent of subjects with	
			TPPE >15%	AC ≥1.2
Male	10–20	144	40	37
Female	12–18	20	60	55
Both sexes	10–20	164	42	40

neural conduction independent of its coenzymatic function in general metabolism [2]. Inadequate thiamin status caused by impaired thiamin intake and/or increased thiamin requirement will deplete thiamin content of the tissues of the affected subject. Such event will lead to metabolic and neurophysiologic derangement and finally clinical manifestations will appear.

Dietary factors causing inadequate thiamin intake in adolescent beriberi include high consumption of milled rice, loss of thiamin due to methods of cooking, and lack of consumption of rich sources of thiamin, and/or regular consumption of antithiamin factors [3, 5, 6].

Dietary assessment in Ubol villagers revealed that 78% of their energy intake were derived from carbohydrate [15, 16]. Their staple diets were monotonous, consisting of glutinous rice and raw fermented fish. Some of the adult villagers habitually chewed betal nuts. Milled rice is a poor source of thiamin and about 85% of thiamin is lost by discarding the water after soaking the rice [2]. Vimokesant et al. [17] have shown that raw fermented fish contains the thermolabile thiaminase I whereas betal nut chew contains the thermostable antithiamin factor. These dietary habits explain the prevalence of biochemical thiamin deficiency in Ubol villagers (Table 7).

Most of lactating women residing in rural area eat only rice and salt during postpartum, with the restriction of nutritious foods. This dietary practice will lead to thiamin deficiency in the mothers whose breast milk contains low thiamin content [18]. This explains the occurrence of infantile beriberi in Thailand [4, 11, 14].

Conditions leading to increased thiamin requirement also play an important role in precipitating the clinical manifestations of beriberi. Fever caused by diarrhea or respiratory tract infection was observed in 12 out of 16 infants with beriberi on admission [4]. Out of 16 adolescents with beriberi, 6 had respiratory tract infection, one had urinary tract infection and one had skin infection [3, 5, 6]. Eight out of 9 patients with wet beriberi also gave the history of increased physical

Table 7. Prevalence of biochemical thiamin and riboflavin deficiencies in Ubol villagers.

Subject		Percent of subjects with	
Age group (yr)	No.	TPPE >15%	AC ≥1.2
6–12	50	18	38
13–16	7	43	14
17–59	82	40	28
60–70	9	33	11
Total	148	33	29
Male	61	33	34
Female	87	32	26

exertion before the development of beriberi. This factor was also observed in 24 Rayong adolescents with beriberi.

2.6. Treatment

A thiamin allowance for infants, children, adolescents and adults of 0.5 mg per 1000 kcal and for pregnant or lactating women of 0.6 mg per 1000 kcal is recommended [19]. Whenever beriberi is diagnosed or suspected prompt therapeutic dose of thiamin should be administered. The daily dosage usually ranges from 50 to 100 mg given intravenously or intramuscularly for 7 to 14 days, after which 10 mg per day can be administered orally until the patients fully recover. Since other water-soluble vitamin deficiencies may coexist with thiamin deficiency they should also be given in therapeutic dose. Nutrition advice must be done to change dietary habits of the patients. Such approach will prevent the recurrence of beriberi.

3. Riboflavin deficiency

Angular stomatitis is one of the common nutritional signs found in Thai villagers and is assumed to be caused by riboflavin deficiency [1]. Our study has shown that riboflavin and/or pyridoxine supplementation have reduced the lesion of angular stomatitis in Ubol children significantly [20]. This indicates that angular stomatitis can be due to riboflavin and/or pyridoxine deficiency. However, human riboflavin status can be specifically assessed by the determination of erythrocyte glutathione reductase activity (EGRA) and its activity coefficient (AC) [9]. The latter parameter represents the degree of stimulation of EGRA resulting from the added flavin adenine dinucleotide in vitro. An AC value of 1.2 and above indicates inadequate riboflavin status. Our recent studies have shown the high prevalence of riboflavin deficiency in children and adolescents resided in Rayong and Ubol provinces (Tables 6 and 7) (unpublished data). The data also indicate that thiamin and riboflavin deficiencies usually coexist in the target population.

4. Vitamin A deficiency

Thanangkul and Whitaker [21] reported that 56% of children with protein-energy malnutrition had vitamin A deficiency. Ten percent of these children remained partially or totally blind even with prompt therapy.

A dietary survey carried out in Ubol preschool children revealed their low vitamin A intake, i.e. 30–50% of the recommended vitamin A allowance. Their fat intake was also low which would reduce the biovailability of vitamin A.

Biochemical assessment showed that 70 and 17% of 146 preschool children had serum vitamin A in the low (10–20 μg/dl) and deficient (less than 10 μg/dl) ranges, respectively [22]. These data indicate the existance of vitamin A deficiency in Thai children.

5. Conclusion

Three out of seven leading causes of undernutrition in Thailand are due to thiamin, riboflavin, and vitamin A deficiencies which affect morbidity and mortality of Thai children. To combat these vitamin malnutrition correct nutritional knowledge including principle of nutrition and the value of consuming nutritious foods should be provided to teachers, community leaders, and parents. The application of their knowledge in daily dietary practice will improve the nutritional status of the family and community. It is also necessary to explore local foods and their nutritive value at the village level so that recommendation can be made to the people on using readily available food sources of vitamins. Since rice is the staple food of Thai people the process of milling rice at various mills should be studied in order to reduce the loss of nutrients including vitamins in rice milling.

Acknowledgements

This work was supported by a grant from the Faculty of Medicine, Ramathibodi Hospital, and the Rockefeller Foundation.

References

1. Subcommittee on Food and Nutrition Planning: Technical information and base-line data for the formulation of national plan on food and nutrition development (1977–1981). Thailand, National Economic and Social Development Board, 1977.
2. Tanphaichitr V: Thiamin. In: Nutrition Reviews present knowledge in nutrition. New York, The Nutrition Foundation, 1976 (4th ed), pp 141–148.
3. Tanphaichitr V: Clinical and biochemical studies in beriberi. A thesis submitted in partial fulfilment of the requirements for the degree of master of science (medicine). Faculty of Graduate Studies, University of Medical Sciences, 1964.
4. Cheunchit L, Tanphaichitr V: Infantile beriberi Supasitprasong. Hosp Gaz 1:97–101, 1975.
5. Tanphaichitr V, Vimokesant SL, Dhanamitta S, Valyasevi A: Clinical and biochemical studies of adult beriberi. Am J Clin Nutr 23:1017–1026, 1970.
6. Tanphaichitr V, Lerdvuthisopon N, Boongird P: Clinical and nutrition studies of adult beriberi. In: Abstracts of papers at the 4th Asian and Oceanian Congress of Neurology. Bangkok, Sompong Press, 1975, p 151.
7. Sukumalchantra Y, Tanphaichitr V, Thongmitr V, Jumbala B: Electrocardiographic findings in

adult beriberi: changes in the QRS voltage. Mod Med Asia 11:6–7, 1975.

8. Sukumalchantra Y, Thongmitr V, Tanphaichitr V, Jumbala B: Variability of cardiac output in beriberi heart disease. Mod Med Asia 12:7–10, 1976.

9. Sauberlich HE, Skala JH, Dowdy RP: Laboratory tests for the assessment of nutritional status. Cleveland, CRC Press, 1974.

10. Davidson S, Passmore R, Brock JF, Truswell AS: Human nutrition and dietetics. London, Churchill Livingstone, 1975 (6th edn), p 336.

11. Thanangkul O, Whitaker JA: Childhood thiamine deficiency in northern Thailand. Am J Clin Nutr 18:275–277, 1966.

12. Pongpanich B, Srikrikkrich N, Dhanamitta S, Valyasevi A: Biochemical detection of thiamin deficiency in infants and children in Thailand. Am J Clin Nutr 27:1399–1402, 1974.

13. Varavithya W, Dhanamitta S, Valyasevi A: Bilateral ptosis as a sign of thiamine deficiency in childhood. Clin Ped 14:1063–1065, 1975.

14. Sintarat S, Pansuravet S: Infantile beriberi in Nakornpanom Hospital. J Nutr Assoc Thailand 14:184–195, 1980.

15. Valyasevi A, Halstead SB, Pantuwatana S, Tankayul C: IV. dietary habits, nutritional intake, and infant feeding practices among residents of a hypo-hyperendemic area. Am J Clin Nutr 20:1340–1351, 1967.

16. Tanphaichitr V, Lerdvuthisopon N, Dhanamitta S, Broquist HP: Carnitine status in Thai adults. Am J Clin Nutr 33:876–880, 1980.

17. Vimokesant S, Kunjara S, Rungruangsak K, Nakornchai S, Panijpan B: Beriberi caused by antithiamin factors in food and its prevention. Ann NY Acad Sci 378:123–136, 1982.

18. Valyasevi A, Vimokesant S, Dhanamitta S: Chemical composition of breast milk in different locations of Thailand. J Med Ass Thailand 51:348–354, 1968.

19. Committee on Dietary Allowances, Food and Nutrition Board: Recommended dietary allowances. Washington, D.C., National Academy of Sciences, 1980 (9th edn), pp 82–87.

20. Tanphaichitr V, Lerdvuthisopon N, Valyasevi A, Dhanamitta S: Riboflavin and pyridoxine status in northeast Thai school children. In: Abstracts of 3rd Asian Congress of Pediatrics. Bangkok, Bangkok Medical Publisher, 1979, p 107.

21. Thanangkul O, Whitaker JA: Relationship of vitamin A deficiency to blindness in north Thailand. Chiang Med Bull 8:237–250, 1969.

22. Dhanamitta S, Valyasevi A: Vitamin A deficiency. In: Varavithya W (ed) Nutritional diseases, vol 1. Bangkok, Ramathibodi Hospital, 1977, pp 49–70.

Some aspects of protein-energy malnutrition in the highlands of Central Africa

D. BRASSEUR, Ph. GOYENS and H.L. VIS

Introduction

The studies presented are part of the work of the CEMUBAC medical team in the highlands of Kivu (Zaïre) and in Rwanda. Two special aspects of the protein energy malnutrition (PEM) encountered will be developed in detail: lactose malabsorption and trace element (TE) status during and after recovery of PEM.

Geographical and socioeconomic situation

The Kivu lake, just south of the equator, at the border between Zaïre and Rwanda, is surrounded by highlands with a mean altitude of 1700 m above sea level. The climate is temperate and two seasons divide the year: (1) a long rain season from October to June, interrupted by a very short dry season (2 or 3 weeks at the end of January) which enables the principal harvest; (2) a dry season from June to September.

These seasons influence the harvest and the food intake of the population especially the agriculturists. Nutritional surveys [1] show clearly that food consumption is the lowest at the end of the dry season before the first harvest; the energy intake at this moment is well below the requirements (Figure 1). Due to the fact that this population is also dependent on the harvest for its protein supply, the protein needs at this time are not fulfilled (Figure 2).

The food availability in the cities is less dependent on the seasons due to the regulatory effect of the monetary economic system [2, 3]. Whatever the season, the pastoral tribes depend essentially on the milk production of their cattle for their food supply; the size of their herd is usually large enough to provide sufficient milk [1].

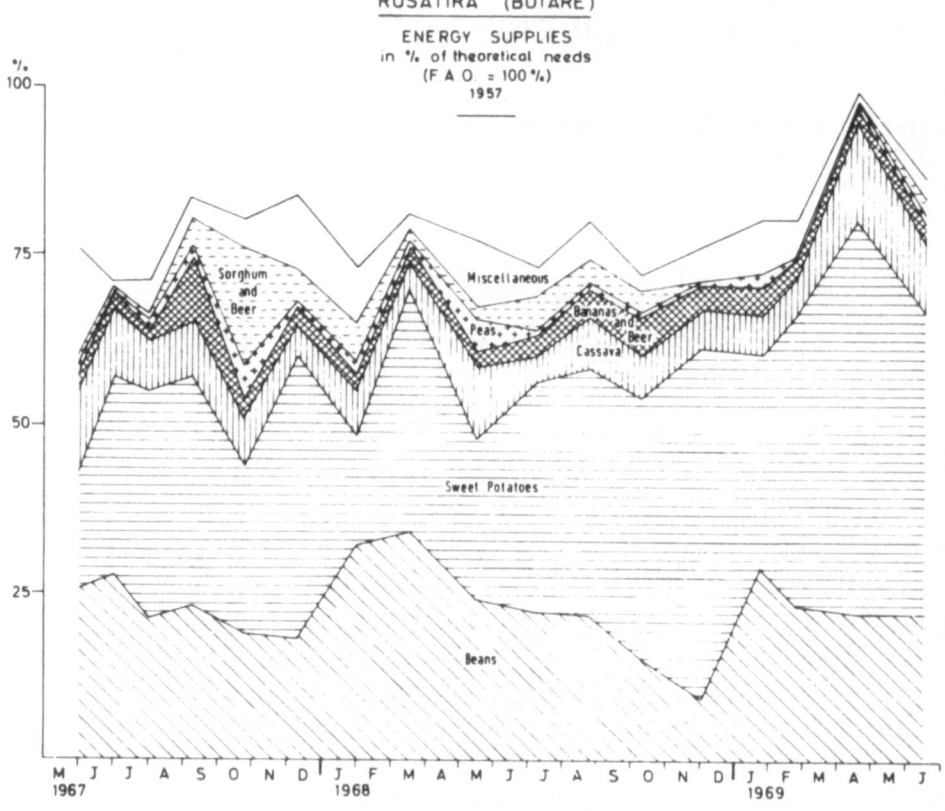

Figure 1.

Ethnic differences and nutritional habits

The Tutsi-Hima tribes originally lived in Rwanda, on the east coast of the Kivu lake and are cattlebreeders of nilotic origin. They are lactose tolerant and accustomed to drinking the milk of their cows [4]. Malnutrition as a rule does not occur with the Tutsi cattle breeders; however, some of them, for political reasons, lost their cattle and emigrated to Kivu in Zaïre and malnutrition prevails among these refugees.

The native Shi-Havu tribes are pure lactose-intolerant Bantus, living on the west shore of the Kivu lake in Zaïre. They are agriculturists. The women do nearly all of the work in the fields: they always take their youngest child with them so that prolonged breast-feeding prevails (usually more than 2 years) [4, 5]. Malnutrition is endemic. Overpopulation and soil erosion constantly reduce the arable surface, worsening the problem of insufficient food supply.

The Hutu tribes, native of Rwanda, have a mixed Bantu and nilotic origin. They are agriculturists, and lactose intolerance prevails among them, but at a lesser degree, when compared to pure Bantus (Table 1).

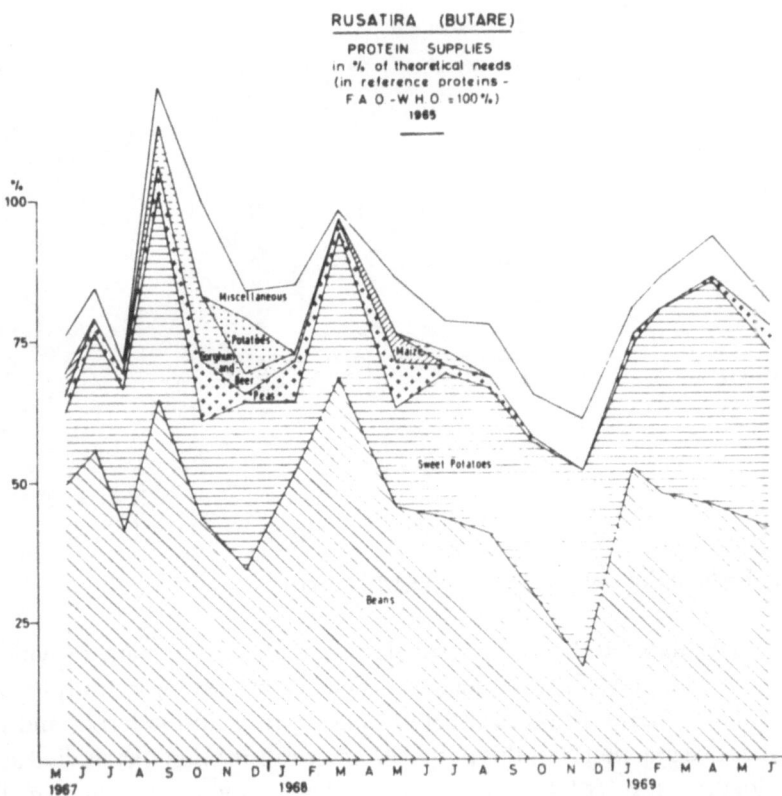

Figure 2.

In summary, the nutritional habits of the Tutsi-Hima, on one side, and of the Shi-Havu and Hutu, on the other side, are very different; lactose tolerance plays an important role in these habits. Cattle breeders have little problems of food supply; agriculturists and the refugees living among them have chronically low energy and protein intakes. The deprivation becomes particularly acute during a critical period in the year extending from October until February. Young weaned children, pregnant and lactating mothers are the most vulnerable.

Forms of malnutrition encountered

PEM is, for the reasons explained, endemic in the highlands of Kivu; edematous kwashiorkor is only encountered in cases of severe and pure protein deficiency. Most children develop marasmic kwashiorkor due to super added energy deprivation [6] (Figure 3). These two components have to be evaluated by two different parameters: the former by serum albumin levels; the latter by the weight for height ratio (after the child had lost his edema's), expressed as the percentage of the local standards defined by De Maeyer (unpublished data, 1959).

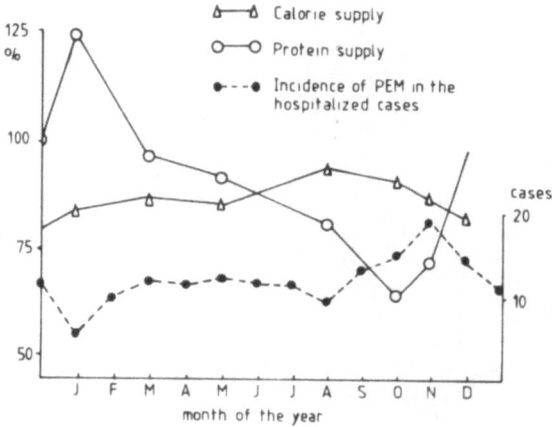

Figure 3.

Carbohydrate malabsorption during PEM in Kivu

It has been established that the intestinal sugar splitting enzymatic activities are depressed during PEM [7, 8]. It seemed particularly interesting to study them in a region where undernutrition is endemic and where lactose-tolerant and intolerant tribes live together. For this purpose, lactose absorption was studied using a lactose loading test (LLT) [9]. Disaccharidase activities (lactase, maltase, sucrase) were measured on a jejunal biopsy specimen using the method of Dahlqvist [10]. Histological sections of the mucosa were graded according to Welsh [11].

Table 1. Incidence of lactose malabsorption in the Shi-Havu, Tutsi, Hutu populations adults and children (aged from 2 to 5 years).

Subjects	Adults	Children
Traditional zone of non milking	97%	88%
Agriculturists Zaïre: Shi-Havu	(46/47)	(92/104)
Traditional zone of milking	23%	4%
Cattle breeders Rwanda: Tutsi	(3/13)	(1/26)
Mixed group originating from a traditional zone of non milking but living among cattle breeders	64%	88%
Agriculturists Rwanda: Hutu	(23/36)	(29/33)

Patients

Malnourished and recovered children (after at least 2 months of rehabilitation) were investigated: the Shi-Havu and Tutsi subjects in Zaïre (Children Hospital of Lwiro) and the Hutu subjects in Kigali (General Hospital of Kigali).

Lactose loading tests

197 Shi children were tested (Table 2), 98 were suffering from PEM. Among these, 95% were lactose malabsorbers. Still, 69% of the recovered children were lactose malabsorbers. The recovered children over five years of age showed an increased frequence of lactose malabsorption (Table 2) when compared to the younger subjects. 26 Tutsi children were tested (Table 3), 12 suffered from PEM and one of them had become lactose malabsorber. Moreover, the 14 healed Tutsi had a normal LLT. 33 Hutu children were tested (Table 3) – mixed group – the 14 malnourished subjects were lactose malabsorbers. 17 out of the 19 children healed from PEM remained lactose malabsorbers.

Mucosal histology and intestinal disaccharidase activities

This part of the investigation was only performed in the Shi-Havu children (Table 4). No child had a normal intestinal mucosa at light microscopy examination. Severe mucosal damage (Grade III, IV or V) was noticed in 80% of the cases in

Table 2. Incidence of lactose malabsorption in malnourished and recovered Shi-Havu children.

	2 to 5 years	5 to 15 years
Malnourished subjects	90% (n = 53)	100% (n = 45)
Recovered subjects	60% (n = 41)	73% (n = 58)

Table 3. Incidence of lactose malabsorption in malnourished and recovered Tutsi and Hutu children (aged from 2 to 5 years).

	Tutsi	Hutu
Malnourished subjects	8% (n = 12)	100% (n = 14)
Recovered subjects	0% (n = 14)	90% (n = 19)

both sick and recovered groups. Moreover very important lymphoïd tissue infiltration was also observed beyond the mucosal layer in both groups.

Among the sick children, lactase activity was severely depressed (from $16 \pm 6\%$ of the normal value) already when a moderate mucosal atrophy was described. This activity, however, did not recover after rehabilitation of PEM (Table 4). Maltase and sucrase activities were less severely depressed (from $34 \pm 9\%$ of the normal value for maltase and $65 \pm 19\%$ of the normal value for sucrase) and showed for the same histological grade some improvement after healing.

Discussion

The results of the LLT suggest that during PEM and after healing the lactose behaviour differs relatively to the tribe investigated. The Tutsi tribe seems to maintain lactose absorption and probably lactase activity: it is well known that these subjects never present adult-type hypolactasia [4]. The reason however for prolonged disappearance of the lactase activity among the Shi-Havu children remains questioned. We were surprised to see persistence of the mucosal injury even after 2 months of rehabilitation and after clinical recovery. It has been established that jejunal mucosal damage after a severe episode of PEM is very long to recover. Mucosal appearance is noted to remain unchanged even after one year [7]. This is thought to be due to environmental factors and clinical relapse as

Table 4. Histology and disaccharidase activity of the jejunal mucosa in malnourished Shi-Havu children (Serum albumin <2.5 g/dl) and in recovered children (Serum albumin >3.0 g/dl after two months rehabilitation) compared to the Belgian norms.

Shi-Havu subjects	Histology		Disaccharidase		
			Lactase	Maltase	Sucrase
Malnourished children	Grade I	0.0%	–	–	–
(n = 64)	II	3.1	7.4 U[a]	182 U	54 U
	III	15.6	5.3	130	49
	IV	50.0	2.7	120	34
	V	31.3	2.0	105	29
Recovered children	I	0.0	–	–	–
(n = 52)	II	7.7	8.2	223	65
	III	15.3	2.0	216	52
	IV	34.6	3.0	146	43
	V	42.4	3.3	108	33
Normal Belgian children	I	100%	32	421	64
(n = 88)					

[a] Enzymes are expressed in units (U) per gram of protein.

renourished children return to their family and their low socioeconomic conditions. As far as we know histological evaluation of the jejunal mucosa during the early stage of clinical recovery in parasite-free children has not yet been done.

The enzymatic and morphologic patterns of the intestinal mucosa in well-nourished Shi-Havu children is not better. In these conditions we are not allowed to conclude whether the anomalies observed in the studied children are due to their malnutrition or to environmental factors (e.g. parasitic infestation) or to hypothetical allergic mechanisms related to food consumption: the cow's milk proteins are usually used for the rehabilitation of severe PEM and might contain allergens.

Trace element status in PEM in Kivu

Numerous clinical and biological indices point to the fact that children with marasmic kwashiorkor in eastern Kivu suffer from associated trace element deficiencies (e.g. zinc deficiency). Indeed, hepatomegaly, hair and skin anomalies, diarrhea, increased susceptibility to infection, anemia, low levels of alkaline phosphatase and some behavioural changes are common to kwashiorkor and zinc deficiency.

Several studies [12–16] have already been conducted throughout the world on zinc status in malnutrition, demonstrating in most cases low serum zinc levels on admission, and a variable evolution of the serum zinc values after rehabilitation. Besides this, Golden and Golden in Jamaïca [17] were able to show that children recovering from PEM need zinc to gain weight. The same remark could be made for copper: bone x-rays of malnourished children are compatible with copper deficiency; tyrosinase responsible for the hair pigmentation is a cupro-enzyme. And effectively Cordano et al. [18] found in Peru low serum copper levels on admission in children with PEM. The same observation was made in a few other places in the world. In the case of selenium, it would also not be surprising to find some deficiencies, since it is known that this element is mostly associated with proteins in the diet. And once more, some authors found low serum or plasma levels in PEM, in Thaïland [19] and in Kivu [20]. However, in spite of the amount of research already done, we still have no clear insight in the patho-physiology of the TE deficiencies in malnutrition.

Patients

The patients studied were all children in severe malnutrition, mostly protein-energy malnutrition, but also pure kwashiorkor cases and a few cases of marasmus. They all live near the eastern border of Zaïre, in Kivu, in the highlands of Central Africa (predominantly members of the Shi-Havu tribe).

Activity of specific metallo-enzymes

The activity of some metallo-enzymes is reduced in experimental and pathological deficiencies of the metal in question; this methodology consequently permits an evaluation of the TE status. The activity of different metallo-enzymes was lowered in children with marasmic kwashiorkor in Kivu:

1. Serum alkaline phosphatase, a zinc enzyme (Table 5).
2. Erythrocyte superoxide dismutase, a zinc and copper containing enzyme, in which copper is much more specific than zinc; this activity returned to normal after recovery (Table 6) [20].
3. Erythrocyte glutathione peroxidase, a seleno-enzyme; this activity too returned to normal after rehabilitation (Table 7) [20].

This indicates anomalies in the intake or anomalies in the utilization of zinc, copper and selenium.

Table 5. Serum alkaline phosphatase activity (U/L) in PEM in Kivu (mean ± SD).

a)	Controls (n = 7)	112 ± 37
b)	On admission (n = 115)	79 ± 30
c)	Refed (n = 12)	120 ± 81
	a–b	p<0.01
	b–c	p<0.001

Table 6. Protein-energy malnutrition in Kivu. Erythrocyte superoxide dismutase activity (mg/g Hb; mean ± SD) (Fondu, 1977).

1.	On admission	0.26 ± 0.25 (n = 8)
2.	Refed	0.42 ± 0.23 (n = 7)
3.	Controls	0.42 ± 0.19 (n = 12)
	1–3	U = 17 p<0.05
	2–3	U = 42 N.S.

Table 7. Protein-energy malnutrition in Kivu. Erythrocyte glutathione peroxidase activity (μm/g Hb/min; mean ± SD) (Fondu, 1977).

1.	On admission	3.8 ± 0.9 (n = 9)
2.	Refed	4.1 ± 1.3 (n = 7)
3.	Controls	5.3 ± 1.8 (n = 12)
	1–3	U = 21 p<0.05
	2–3	U = 24 N.S.

Trace element determinations

Local controls had rather low serum zinc levels; children with PEM had very low serum zinc levels on admission (Table 8). The serum copper concentration was normal in local controls; values in PEM children on admission were significantly lower than those of the controls, although still within the limits of normal values (Table 8). Local controls had normal serum selenium levels; values in PEM children on admission were significantly lower; intra-erythrocytic selenium concentration on admission however was normal (Table 9) [20].

Supplementation trial

The previous observations seemed to indicate that children with PEM in Kivu suffer from zinc deficiency and perhaps from associated copper deficiency. It could therefore be supposed that, in order to reproduce the weight curves obtained by Golden and Golden in Jamaïca [17], children recovering from PEM in Kivu should receive zinc; therefore it was decided to give a peroral supplement of zinc and copper to some children during their rehabilitation, either zinc alone (1 mg/kg/day) or copper alone (0,3 mg/kg/day) or zinc and copper at the same time.

The supplementation of zinc and copper had no influence on the mortality rate which remained between 15 and 20%. There was no difference in mortality between the different groups. The zinc and copper supplementation did not influence the evolution of the serum albumin concentration. They have thus no influence on the evolution of the kwashiorkor component of PEM in Kivu (Table 10).

Table 8. Serum zinc and copper concentration (μg/dl) in PEM in Kivu (mean ± SD).

	Zinc	Copper
Controls	81 ± 24 (n = 39)	137 ± 27 (n = 43)
On admission	45 ± 22 (n = 157)	108 ± 35 (n = 157)
	p<0.001	p<0.001

Table 9. Serum and erythrocytic selenium levels (ng/ml) in PEM in Kivu (mean ± SD).

	Serum	Erythrocyte
Controls	59 ± 5 (n = 5)	102 ± 10 (n = 9)
On admission	42 ± 4 (n = 20)	112 ± 7 (n = 15)
	p<0.05	N.S.

By contrast it was noticed during the study that children receiving copper appeared healther than the others. This was true not only with regard to their behaviour but also with regard to their weight gain. Indeed, their complete recovery rate after 60 days of rehabilitation was slightly higher than in the other groups.

The percentage weight deviation calculated at the moment the child has completely lost his edemas gives a quantitative appraisal of the marasmic component of the PEM. The weight gain between the minimal weight and the weight after 70 days of rehabilitation, expressed in % weight deviation, was more important in the copper-supplemented than in the non copper supplemented group ($p < 0.01$) (Table 11).

Conclusions

A. 1) The trace elements zinc, copper and selenium interfere in the physio-pathology of PEM in Kivu.
   2) It seems that zinc and copper do not intervene in the recovery process of the kwashiorkor component of PEM in Kivu.
   3) On the contrary, and in spite of what could be expected from the serum concentrations of zinc and copper, which seemed to indicate a major

Table 10. Effect of zinc and copper supplementation on serum albumin concentration (g/dl) in PEM in Kivu (mean ± SD).

	n	albuminemia on admission	albuminemia after 45 days rehabilitation	p
Non supplemented	33	1.81 ± 0.43	2.78 ± 0.56	<0.001
+ Cu	28	1.90 ± 0.47	2.95 ± 0.51	<0.001
+ Zn	29	2.07 ± 0.43	2.79 ± 0.50	<0.001
+ Cu + Zn	28	1.90 ± 0.44	2.84 ± 0,38	<0.001
		N.S.	N.S.	

Table 11. Effect of copper supplementation on weight gain after 70 days of rehabilitation in PEM in Kivu (n = 13).

	Weight gain (% weight deviation)
Non supplemented	+ 5.0
Copper supplemented	+ 15.4
	(p<0.01)

problem of zinc homeostasis, copper supplementation influences the healing process of the marasmic component of PEM; zinc does not intervene.

B. 1) Furthermore, the present study gives once more evidence that transverse determinations of trace elements in biological fluids, especially plasma or serum, but also in erythrocytes are inadequate indicators of TE status. Plasma of serum levels of trace elements can change in a considerable manner with the circumstances of the blood puncture, the presence or not of carrier proteins, captation or release by different TE pools in the organism, stress situations and infection. They need therefore to be very cautiously interpreted.

2) The method which permits demonstration of a TE deficiency or dysutilization is:
   - either technically difficult to apply, as the balance technique;
   - or has to be rejected on an ethical basis, such as the isotopic technique;
   - or is very much time and energy consuming as therapeutic trials;
   - or are very rare and sometimes difficult to quantify, as metal-dependent physiologic functions (e.g. hypogeusia).

   An enlightened way to solve the problem is to determine the activity of specific metallo-enzymes through which perhaps the functionality of the TE in the organism at the level of the cellular metabolism can be evaluated. This might also be precisely the point where trace elements play a decisive part in the prognosis of PEM conditions, in terms of irreversible impairment, on the contrary, repair of TE dependent enzymatic activities which are essential for life is achieved.

C. Finally, this study shows very clearly that there is no overall point of comparison between children suffering from PEM in different parts of the world. They all suffer from generalized malnutrition, with deficient intakes of proteins and energy; but it is not known in most cases what their TE status is. It is clear, however, that the children described by Golden and Golden in Jamaïca [17] have a totally different zinc status from the children studied in Kivu, although the same diagnosis of marasmic kwashiorkor was made and low serum zinc concentrations were found in both cases.

References

1. Vis HL, Yourassowky C, Vanderborght H: A nutritional survey in the republic of Rwanda. Ann Mus Roy Afr Centr Sc Hum 87:192, 1975.
2. Hennart P, Vis HL: Breast-feeding and post partum amenorrhoea in Central Africa. I. Milk production in rural areas. Trop Pediatr 26:177–183, 1980.
3. Hennart P, Ruchababisha M, Vis HL: Breast-feeding and post partum amenorrhoea in Central Africa. 3. Milk production in an urban area. J Trop Pediatr 29:185–189, 1983.
4. Brasseur D, Mandelbaum I, Vis HL: Effects of an episode of severe malnutrition and age on

lactose absorption by recovered infants and children. Am J Clin Nutr 33:177–179, 1980.

5. Vis HL, Hennart P: Decline in breast-feeding (about some of its causes). Acta Paediatr Belg 31:195–206, 1978.

6. Vis HL: General and specific metabolic patterns of marasmic Kwashiorkor in the Kivu area. In: McCance RA, Widdowson EM (eds) Caloric deficiencies and protein deficiencies. Churchill Livingstone, London; 1968, pp. 119–134.

7. Cook GC, Lee FD: The jejunum after kwashiorkor. Lancet ii:1263–1267, 1966.

8. Barbezat GO, Bowie MD, Kaschula ROC, Hansen JDL: Studies on the small intestinal mucosa of children with protein-calorie malnutrition. S Afr Med J 41:1031–1036, 1967.

9. Gudmand-Høyer E, Jarnum S: The diagnosis of lactose malabsorption. Scand J Gastroenterol 3:129–139, 1963.

10. Dahlqvist A: Method for assay of intestinal disaccharidases. Anal Biochem 7:18–25, 1964.

11. Welsh JD, Zschiesche OM, Anderson J et al.: Intestinal disaccharidase activity in celiac sprue (gluten sensitive enteropathy). Arch Intern Med 123:33–38, 1969.

12. Sandstead HH, Shukry AS, Prasad AS, Gabr MK, Hefney AE, Mokhtar N, Darby WJ: Kwashiorkor in Egypt. I. Clinical and biochemical studies with special reference to plasma zinc and serum lactic dehydrogenase. Am J Clin Nutr 17:15–26, 1965.

13. Smit EM, Pretorius PJ: Studies in metabolism of zinc. Part 2. Serum zinc levels and urinary zinc excretion in South African Bantu kwashiorkor patients. J Trop Pediat 9:105–112, 1964.

14. Hansen JDL, Lehmann BH: Serum zinc and copper concentrations in children with protein-calorie malnutrition. S Afr Med J 43:1248–1251, 1969.

15. Kumar S, Rao KSJ: Plasma and erythrocyte zinc levels in protein-calorie malnutrition. Nutr Metab 15:364–371, 1973.

16. Golden MHN, Golden BE: Plasma zinc and the clinical features of malnutrition. Am J Clin Nutr 32:2490–2494, 1979.

17. Golden BE, Golden MHN: Effect of zinc supplementation on the dietary intake, rate of weight gain and the energy cost of tissue deposition in children recovering from severe malnutrition. Am J Clin Nutr 34:900–908, 1981.

18. Cordano A, Baertl JM, Graham GG: Copper deficiency in infancy. Pediatrics 34:324–336, 1964.

19. Levine RJ, Olson RE: Blood selenium in Thai children with protein-calorie malnutrition. Proc Soc Exp Biol Med 134:1030–1034, 1970.

20. Fondu P: Pathophysiology of the anemia of protein-energy malnutrition. Académie Royale des Sciences d'Outre-mer XX (3):80, 1983.

Perspectives on world malnutrition

J.M. BENGOA

Introduction

The world food problem, because of its amplitude, can be approached from many points of view. To try to cover the problem in all its dimensions would be almost impossible. For this reason, I will concentrate on four fundamental aspects. In the first place, the production and availability of food on a world level is still a very serious problem and has been made worse by the anomalies of international trade. In the second place, we will talk of poverty, both the poverty of men as well as the poverty of nations or countries, a problem that does not present a very encouraging view either. These two problems are the fundamental core of famine in the world.

We will not touch on the educational and health areas, which are also very important in determining malnutrition in the world, because in both these fields much more spectacular advances have been achieved than in those regarding production and poverty problems.

As a third point, we will discuss the quantification of the problem of world malnutrition, according to the different criteria used by international organizations.

Finally, without going into detail we will make a general review of food strategies and policies.

1. World agricultural production

1.1. The situation at the beginning of the eighties

According to the FAO in its latest publication on the state of Agriculture and Food, the world production of foodstuffs increased marginally in 1980 but was less than in 1979.

The instability of the present situation is such that the world now depends much more on the result of harvesting present food crops, especially cereals, than during any other year since 1973–74. The situation is alarming. The horizon is very serious for the developing countries but is especially critical in Africa where the annual increase of agricultural production from 1970 to 1980 was 1.8% while the population growth was almost 3%.

The situation in the Far East is somewhat better, with an agricultural production increase of 3.2%, and a population growth of 2.5%.

Latin America increased its agricultural production by 3.9%; that is to say, it almost reached the goal of 4% recommended by the FAO, while its population rose by 2.7%.

The total annual agricultural production of developing countries increased in the last decade by 3.2%, and the total of developed countries by 1.9%.

Although some countries reached the annual agricultural increase goal of 4%, no entire region has reached it in the last decade.

1.2. World food crisis in 1973

The 1973 crisis was probably the worst one within the last 40 years. In 1973 a series of facts were associated, though not all linked together, that caused an upheaval from which we have still not recovered.

In the first place, during the summer of 1972 the Soviet Union bought such a large amount of wheat from the United States that it caused an imbalance on the world market. At the time, no one realized what was happening. During that period the world price of a bushel (35.24 litres) of wheat and the price of a barrel of oil were almost the same, and fluctuated between $1.35 and a little over $2.00; at the end of 1973 – before the energy crisis – the price of wheat rose to more than $5.00. For a short period of time, a bushel of wheat could be exchanged for two barrels of oil.

Then suddenly, during Christmas of 1973, the price of oil rose over that of wheat, reaching $8.00 per barrel. The increase in the price of wheat, and at the same time that of rice and soya, therefore preceeded that of oil. Obviously, those countries that imported wheat and oil were the ones most affected.

But the crisis did not end here. Together with the problem of cereal and oil prices, in several areas of the world a series of natural disasters took place or became more acute, such as the drought in the Sahel and Ethiopia that needed international aid, particularly in the form of cereals; and in Pakistan the worst flood in history took place in which the entire wheat crop was lost.

In addition to this, during 1972 and 1973, Peru suffered its anchovy crisis. This country, which led the world in the fishing industry and whose main activity was the export of fish flour to the United States and Europe, was soon to see anchovies disappear from its coasts. This was a national disaster with serious international repercussions. Fodder for poultry and pigs had to be substituted by cereals.

As a result of all this, in 1973 the grain reserves dropped to critical limits. If in previous years reserves were equal to 95 or 100 days of consumption, which allowed a certain margin security, in 1973 they dropped to only 26 days. This figure was the lowest for the last 50 years.

1.3. Food availability patterns

As is well known, the availability of foods is collected from information on production plus the imports–exports of foods in each country. On an international level, the FAO periodically publishes national reports under the heading of 'Food Balance Sheets'. The latest edition is from 1980. In fact, these sheets include data on food supply on a national level and should not be confused with consumption data derived from other sources.

In previous publications the FAO offered information on calorie, protein and fat supply. In the latest publication, there is also information on the supply of minerals and vitamins. While in North America, western and eastern Europe, the energy food availability is more than 3300 calories per person/day (1977); in Africa and the Far East it is 2300 and 2000 in round figures respectively; Latin America and the Near East give intermediate figures; i.e., 2500 and 2600.

The supply of proteins also shows notable variations, North America having the highest with 106 g and the Far East the lowest with 49 g, or less than half. However, these differences can be seen most clearly in the supply of fats, which are almost four times less than in North America and in the Far East five times less. This explains without a doubt the enormous variations in caloric supply. It should also be pointed out that from the high availability of fats in North America, a large proportion is derived from animal fats, which compound this problem.

It has always been the motive of scientific and political questioning to find out what is the true world supply of foods for human consumption. Is there really sufficient food to feed the entire population on earth? Is there famine, when there is food enough for all?. The answer, though precarious, is affirmative, if we take as a model a moderate diet, sufficient for health and productivity; but, on the other hand, the answer is negative if adapted to the diet of North America or Europe. The energy supply would be 2571 calories per person/day, of which 83% would be from vegetable sources and 17% from animal sources. I must emphasize here that 50% of total calories comes from cereals.

1.4. Grain: the key to world nutrition

The term 'famine' – the hunger of countries – can be simplified and reduced to the problem of a shortage of grain. A large majority of developing countries live on grain, that is, on cereals and pulses. Some countries depend more on tubers and root vegetables, and certainly have more severe malnutrition problems than those which live on cereals.

In fact, international marketing politics plays with this exchange of grain. Today, wheat, corn, rice, soya and other products, form the most formidable strategic weapons that pose a threat to nations and continents. Never before in history has food been of such political importance. It is true that salt played an outstanding role in the social revolutions of the past, but it cannot be compared to the pressure exerted today by grain.

No nation can consider itself totally self sufficient if it does not have adequate grain production. American and Russian diplomats dedicate more time to the problem of cereal and soya exchange than to other activities, which are seemingly more pressing. Those countries that aspire to breed livestock sometimes tend to forget that it is difficult to produce meat, if there is not a surplus of grain.

Grain, therefore, cereals and pulses, are part of one of the most outstanding and obvious agricultural priorities. They simultaneously provide calories and proteins for man's direct food supply, and, moreover, though at a high cost, it is true, they guarantee animal production. For this reason, if we use the term hunger or famine in the world, we really mean that there is a grain crisis. Perhaps it was always so, but was overlooked as the real cause of vitamin deficiencies in the past.

Anyone following the drama of countries with famine, will have to follow the 'barometer' of the international grain trade. This is the key to the poverty and difficulties of an unequal world, subjected to the pressures exercised to feed its populations. What happened in 1973 was only a warning of what can happen in the future.

1.5. The international food trade

A little known fact is that the majority of grain sold by developed countries is acquired by other developed countries. If a line is drawn at the level of the GNP per capita above $ 3000, more than two-thirds of American exports of agricultural products were sent to well fed nations. Approximately only a fifth of grain produced in international trade goes to the less developed countries. This applies only to grain, because other foods and forrage on the world market move between the well-fed countries, and what is even more surprising, they move from the countries with famine to the rich ones. (George Kent). This same author adds: 'This is particularly noteworthy in relation to proteins, of which the well-fed countries have a net gain balance that surpasses one million tons.' The United States are the leading exporters of grain, but they are also the leading importers of meat in the world. This same country also imports even more fish than meat, in the form of animal food.

Of the foodstuffs that entered the international market (123,650 million dollars) in 1976, 11.9% went from the richest countries to the poorest, while 20.2% went from the poorest to the richest. The developed countries export four times more food to other developed countries than they do to developing countries. What is even more serious is that the developing countries export three times as much to developed countries as they do to other developing countries. Perhaps the responsibility of the richer countries lies not in giving more but in receiving less.

The Soviet Union absorbs a large proportion of the grain from the international market. The spectacular increase in meat consumption in Japan is based on growing imports, especially of grain, although from the United States. Therefore, there is not only a crisis in food production on a world scale, but an anomalous trade distribution that is detrimental to the developing countries.

1.6. The perspectives on a world level

According to FAO, in the year 2000, a world population of 6000 million will need an increase in agricultural production of 50–60% more than 1980. The demand for food and agricultural products in developing countries will double.

After these important production plans have been decided, the FAO estimates that it may take up to 20 years to implement them. The genetic improvement of plants, in order to substantially increase yields, requires at least 10 years of research and tests. It should not be forgotten – and the FAO emphasizes this – that agriculture is not merely a technical question but is the nucleus around which socially complex human cultures have developed.

It is possible that in the next decades agricultural production will double, which is an essential step to eradicate hunger, but, at the same time, it will not be sufficient, if we are not successful in overcoming poverty. This issue will be discussed further in the following section.

2. Poverty

We have already analyzed the syndrome of poverty past and present and its characteristics. In that analysis we pointed out that poverty was more serious than it is today in developing countries, but was less complex. It was an 'external' poverty, motivated by external factors, from which one could escape. Poverty today, especially in Latin America, is an 'internal' poverty, in which new elements are predicated and added to the social-economic factors, such as family instability, chronic parasitism and others.

The aspect of poverty in which we are now interested is that of knowing if there are universally accepted criteria to quantify poverty. In the first place, we must admit that for us, poverty – the fact of being poor – is something more profound than the simple fact of not reaching an adequate income level. Nevertheless, it is difficult to objectively establish criteria other than economic if we want to quantify poverty. It is worth emphasizing that some of the criteria by which poverty is measured are based on the cost of the family food basket, and this entails more responsibility by food and nutrition specialists.

The CEPAL considers that the 'poverty line' can be drawn when income is not more than double the cost of the food basket, and that of 'indigence' when income is not even sufficient to cover the cost of the food basket. According to this criteria, in 1980 in Latin America, 50% of the population lived in a state of poverty, and 26% in a state of indigence. Ten years later, 40% were still poor and 19% indigent. Although the proportion has decreased, it has really increased in absolute terms. This is now more evident and concentrated in the urban suburbs. In 1970, and according to the same criteria, Venezuela had 25% poor population and 10% indigents.

According to the CEPAL, poverty in Latin America in the seventies was basically restricted to rural areas; 62% of the rural population was poor against 26% of the urban population. Nevertheless, even if the percentages have changed recently, it should be pointed out that the characteristics of one or another type of poverty are different. Rural poverty is linked to a natural ecology and urban poverty to an anarchic and artificial way of life. However, urban population has the advantage of greater accessibility to services which a large part of the rural population lacks. This can be changed as will be shown in the discussion on poor countries.

The criteria used by the CEPAL cannot be applied to all countries, especially the developed ones. For example, the definition of poverty in the United States, although it is also based on the cost of the food basket, estimates that minimum income as rated above poverly level is four times that of the food basket. According to this criteria, 11.4% of the population was below this minimum in 1973 as against 45% in 1959. This means that if the United States of America's criteria were applied in Latin America, that is, multiplying the cost of the family food basket by four, almost the entire population would be defined as poor. But are all poor people equal? Can one compare solutions to the poverty of countries lacking coastlines with those of insular countries?

At present, four categories of underdeveloped countries, are distinguished:
1. the less developed countries (LDC);
2. the most seriously affected countries (SAC);
3. developing countries, lacking coastlines;
4. insular developing countries and territories.
Their characteristics are as follows.

2.1 The less developed countries (LDC)

In 1971, the General Assembly of the United Nations reached an agreement on the following criteria to be applied to characterize the LDC; an annual Gross Domestic Product per capita of 100 dollars or less – this amount was raised in 1975 to 125 dollars – participation of 10% or less of the manufacturing industries in the Gross Domestic Products and a literacy rate (proportion of literate persons over 15 years old) of 20% or less.

2.2. The most seriously affected countries (SAC)

These are developing countries which, in view of their low technological and developmental level, are considered as *most seriously affected by the present economic crisis due to the sudden increase in prices of essential imported goods*. Originally, 42 countries were chosen as the objective of the U.N.'s Special Fund created to help these most seriously affected countries. Since then, their number has increased to 45. Of these, 13 are countries without coastlines, five are insular countries, eight are in Sahel region and 25 are less-developed countries. The majority of the 45 SAC are included in the LDC group, and therefore are also characterized for having problems such as predominance of agriculture, low production per capita of food and agricultural goods, (usually very few), minimum production and industrial base and loss in terms of exchange.

2.3. Developing countries lacking coastlines

There are 20 nations which, with the exception of five (Bolivia, Paraguay, Swaziland, Zambia and Zimbabwe) also fall into the category of the LDC. Between 1970 and 1977, the growth rate of their real product per capita was, on average, only 1.2% per year in comparison with 3.1% for all the developing countries. Six of these countries had a negative growth rate.

2.4. Insular developing countries and territories

There are 60 nations and insular developing territories that have the following problems: a high incidence of natural disasters, such as volcanic eruptions, earthquakes, tidal waves and hurricanes. Low availability of resources, which make them dependent to a great extent on foreign imports, and a lack of variety in their agricultures. Their small surface area, combined with monoculture, makes them highly vulnerable to market fluctuations as well as to loss of crops.

An additional curb on their development is, paradoxically, their inability to exploit their own marine wealth. In spite of their close proximity to rich fishing grounds, many islands cannot improve their fishing fleet, nor compete with foreign fleets that exploit their resources to the maximum, and do not even protect them.

Both air and maritime transport is costly for insular developing countries; aid from the PNUD could help them to increase their national energy production in order to reduce these external costs.

In closing, it can be said that *homogenizing the problems* could be applied on a national level and in a specific manner to nutritional problems.

3. Quantification of world malnutrition

3.1. Clinical surveys in children under 5 years of age

Diverse criteria have been used to quantify the nutritional problems in the world. On one hand, in 1974 the WHO analyzed those surveys carried out in different countries on the basis of clinical and anthropometrical data. 101 surveys in 59 developing countries were analyzed. Some of these surveys covered only a small sample of the population, and this led to the decision to use only those surveys with more than 1000 children. The total number of children under 5 years of age who were clinically examined was approximately 175,000 in 17 developing countries.

The average figure for severe forms of malnutrition was 2.6% and for moderate cases 18.9% on a world level. In Africa, the average for severe forms was 4.4% and for moderate cases 26.5%. In Asia, it was 3.2% and 31.2% respectively, and in Latin America it was 1.6% and 18.9%.

If these surveys are extrapolated to the world population of developing countries (something which we hesitate to do), the total number of undernourished children in the world in 1974 was 10 million severe cases and 90 million moderate cases, making a total of 100 million. Using this figure, 19 million would correspond to Africa, 71 million to Asia and 10 million to Latin America. It would also be useful to carry out a new world analysis in 1983 or 1984 in order to observe the changes which have occurred during the last decade.

3.2. Low birth rate

The relationship between the standard of living, the nutritional state and the weight of newborn children is well known. A recent study carried out by the WHO offers an overall view according to continents. On the basis of 280 surveys carried out in 90 countries, it is estimated that out of 122 million live babies born in 1979, almost 21 million weighed less than 2500 g. This means that one child out of every 6 had a low birth weight; 90% of these children were born in developing countries.

Broken down into continents or regions, the percentage of low birth weight is as follows: Asia, 20%; Africa, 15%; Latin America, 11%; Europe, 8%; and North America, 7%. The average birth weight in Asia is 2900 g, in Africa, 3000 g, Latin America 3100 g and 3200 g in Europe and North America.

3.3. Caloric consumption

The FAO estimates the number of undernourished (or 'underfed') persons in terms of calorie consumption, per person per day. Data from the FAO are obtained from studies made on family budgets and from other surveys. According to the FAO, individuals who have a caloric intake represented on a Metabolic Base Rate (MBR) index of 1.2 as a critical limit would be 'undernourished', that is to say 20% more than the strict basal metabolism. For a 'small adult', MBR would be approximately 1520 calories. If we take a MBR of 1.5, as originally recommended, the caloric intake would be 1900 calories, and below this figure the small adult would be considered as undernourished. Based on this criteria, FAO estimates that 436 million people are seriously undernourished.

3.4. Towards an interpretation of chronic malnutrition

It is obvious that, except for severe forms of protein calorie malnutrition or specific mineral and vitamin deficiencies (anaemias, xerophthalmia, etc.), it is very difficult to evaluate the malnutrition level of the population; nevertheless, *chronic malnutrition is the fundamental problem of world malnutrition.*

Mortality from severe forms of protein–calorie malnutrition has decreased in the greater part of developing countries, probably due more to a decrease in infections and better medical care than to improvement in living conditions, although this should not be minimized. But the fact is that symptoms of Kwashiorkor (Plurideficiency Syndrome), so frequent in the forties, fifties and sixties, have decreased, especially in relation to mortality. However, there are still frequent forms of nutritional marasmus in children under 1 year of age.

What is most prevalent in the developing countries is chronic malnutrition, reflected in a short stature and distorted physical and functional development. These people are small or of short stature 'not because their (genetic) build determines it, but because they lack the building material to complete the project' (A. Chaves). This state of chronic malnutrition is the most serious problem Latin America faces, because, it is chiefly the result of an adaptation process that cannot be reversed in many of its parameters. Therefore, the prognosis is not very good for improving the present generation.

This adaptation is a self-defense phenomenon that is achieved through a reduction in the growth rate and a decrease of physical activity, which reduces nutritional requirements. Therefore, they are not physiologically 'normal' children or adults, but human beings adapted to conditions which the environment and social-economic factors impose on them.

Over 100 years ago, Europe was also in a similar situation. The stature of the European during that period was that of the Central American population today, and, although there are no references on what caused this biological underdevelopment of the European at that time, we suspect that it was simply a period of biological adaptation.

This adaptation phenomenon has been thoroughly studied by Ramón Galván who called it 'homeorhesis'. The adapted individual will never attain a normal height even with an improved diet and their performance will probably never increase in lineal proportion to an improvement in their feeding habits. Nevertheless, there will be changes in the body composition and functional development and social frustration will decrease to a large extent. An improvement in the diet of those adapted individuals will therefore be highly beneficial, but the results should not be evaluated in terms of an improvement in biological development (stature, etc.) but in the function of other parameters that are perhaps more important for the individual and for society.

Nevertheless, it is necessary to realize that the secular trend in stature is important not only in itself, but because stature is the best indicator of biological, harmonious, physical and functional development of human beings. The 'adapted' children and adults are more than ever today a serious problem – their case histories are even more serious – and we cannot accept them as 'normal' or even as 'apparently normal'. The problem is much more serious than one of simple underdevelopment. Short stature because of nutritional or social economic reasons hides a complete pathology of physical and functional development with repercussions on social development. Thus, an undernourished child who has reached the age of four, can be the same height as a three-year-old, can have a chest circumference of a two-year-old, a head circumference of a one-and-half-year-old, the speech capacity of a 14-month child and the weight and motor behaviour of a one-year-old.

A six-year-old child who at first sight looks like a three-year-old because of his physical development, obviously cannot be compared in his behaviour and learning capacity with a normal child of six years old neither with a child of three years old. He is a different human being, with his own biological and behavioural characteristics and an intersensory organization that is difficult to fit into a chronological age group.

Recent scientific publications have been using terms which, analyzed with a social sensibility, are overwhelming. They state, for example, that malnutrition, generally associated with repeated infections 'distorts the symmetry of the body; distorts development; causes inharmonious development; produces a disproportioned child; determines an unbalanced growth which can be cause of psycho-social disharmony and learning disorders'.

We are no longer dealing with mere growth retardation, which in itself could be important, but with distortion, perversion, disproportion, instability dishar-mony, disorder, etc., which are much more serious. This adaptation process that leads to chronic malnutrition explains the extremely low levels of caloric con-sumption reported by the FAO, and which results in nearly 500 million people in the world who can be considered as 'undernourished' or underfed.

I think this field is extremely important to physiologists, physicians, bioche-mists and specialists in public health care. More investigations are needed to explain the phenomenon of why so many millions of people can survive, carrying out a seemingly normal life, with a diet that hardly surpasses 20% of the Basal Metabolism.

3.5. Specific deficiencies

Apart from Protein-Calorie malnutrition, on a world level, xerophthalmia (lack of vitamin A) and nutritional anaemias are major problems. Regarding the first, it is estimated that in eastern Asia alone there are 250,000 cases of irreversible blindness. With regard to nutritional anaemias, on the other hand, Layrisse et al. estimated that in temperate zones, 10–15% of menstruating women and 20–30% of pregnant women can suffer from iron-deficient anaemias. In nursing children, the frequency of anaemia can be as high as 40% during the first year of life. In tropical regions, parasitic infection and the poor bio-availability of iron found in food, contributes to the high prevalence of iron deficient anaemias. The preva-lence is estimated in these regions between 20–40% in men and higher among women.

4. Conclusions

We will conclude this analysis of the world situation with some practical consider-ations for future action.

4.1. International institutional crisis

Over the past 40 years, the severity of the nutritional problem and the scant priority given to it by national and international political spheres has been reported. It is also true that the social communication media have been continu-ously on the alert about the magnitude of famine in the world with figures that do not always coincide with the true situation; but the fact is that the actions adopted and carried out have been timid, scattered, incoherent and lacking in clear and attainable objectives. This has resulted in a profound international institutional crisis on food and nutrition policy that has created a state of confusion on a national level.

The disappearance of the Interagency Project of the United Nations for Food and Nutrition policies in Latin America, (headquarters in Chile); of putting into effect the Food and Nutrition project of the SELA; the technical and administrative changes of the Nutrition Institute for Central America and Panama (INCAP); the deteroration of nutritional activities by some of the specialized agencies of U.N. and other examples, cannot be compensated by efforts of the World Bank and the University of United Nations that have involved themselves in food policies on a world level.

The international institutional crisis on food and nutrition is evident. Forty years ago ideas on how to tackle the nutritional problem were clearer than they are now. What we have won in depth we have lost in clarity. Forty years ago, when the conference on Food and Agriculture of the United Nations was held (Hot Spring 1943), ideas on what had to be done were quite clear. They dealt essentially with four interrelated measures:

(a) the necessity to increase agricultural production, taking into account, among other factors, the nutritional needs of the population;
(b) the struggle against poverty, so that the entire population would have access to basic foods;
(c) to raise the level of education of the population;
(d) health actions (especially against infections).

They were clear objectives, and it was insisted upon that effective coordination was essential in order to attain them. Today, things are somewhat more complex, due to the same complexity of society and its environment. In any case, it was not meant that a food and nutrition policy should cover or be responsible for the four areas mentioned, but rather that it was necessary *to present* the *definitions* and *strategies* of such policies.

Governments opted for another strategy. They considered that in the long run simple growth and social-economic development would resolve the problem, and that *meanwhile,* (I emphasize this because this has gone on for over forty years) free food would be supplied to the underpriveleged population (that is to say, the already damaged population). It has been forty years of interference and confusion, and while the complexity has increased, the efforts have diminished.

4.2. Levels of nutritional intervention

It would be convenient to arrange policies and actions on food and nutrition into two large complementary measures. On the one hand the macro-economic agricultural and social measures of a general nature, and, on the other hand, those that can be accurately developed into population groups with specific nutritional problems ('target or focal groups').

There is a strong tendency in some countries to carry out an excessively centralized nutritional policy, which probably will not solve the problems of the 'focal groups'. According to Bruce Stokes the cost of solving problems in a centralized manner has become prohibitive. This author adds that in this age of energy shortage and static economics, a new approach is necessary to solve these problems. René Dubois also said: 'Think globally but act locally'. And more than four centuries ago, Iñigo de Loyola warned us: 'Pray as if everything depends on God, but work and act as if everything depends on you' which, translated to modern day language, could be expressed as follows: 'ask as if everything depends on the Government, but work as if everything depends on you'.

The communities cannot expect that all solutions to their problems come from central powers, as if they were an Almighty being. An effort from the community itself is absolutely essential if it is to help in its own development. This is especially relevant when solving problems of 'focal groups'.

These considerations are also applicable in the international sphere. International organizations are too often made responsible for world crisis, when it is the countries themselves, through weakness or excessive power who are the cause of the crisis.

How can a world strategy for food production or a fight against poverty exist, if each country does not even have a strategy of its own? There does not seem to be any doubt that food production, directed towards the population's need, is a necessary but insufficient step to eliminate the risk of vulnerability and dependence on other countries. This point must be stressed and repeated a thousand times because the solution is not going to come from outside sources. I have said that the intensification of agricultural production is a necessary and urgent step, but it will not be sufficient if measures are not adopted that will allow the population to acquire the food produced. In other words, the eradication of poverty.

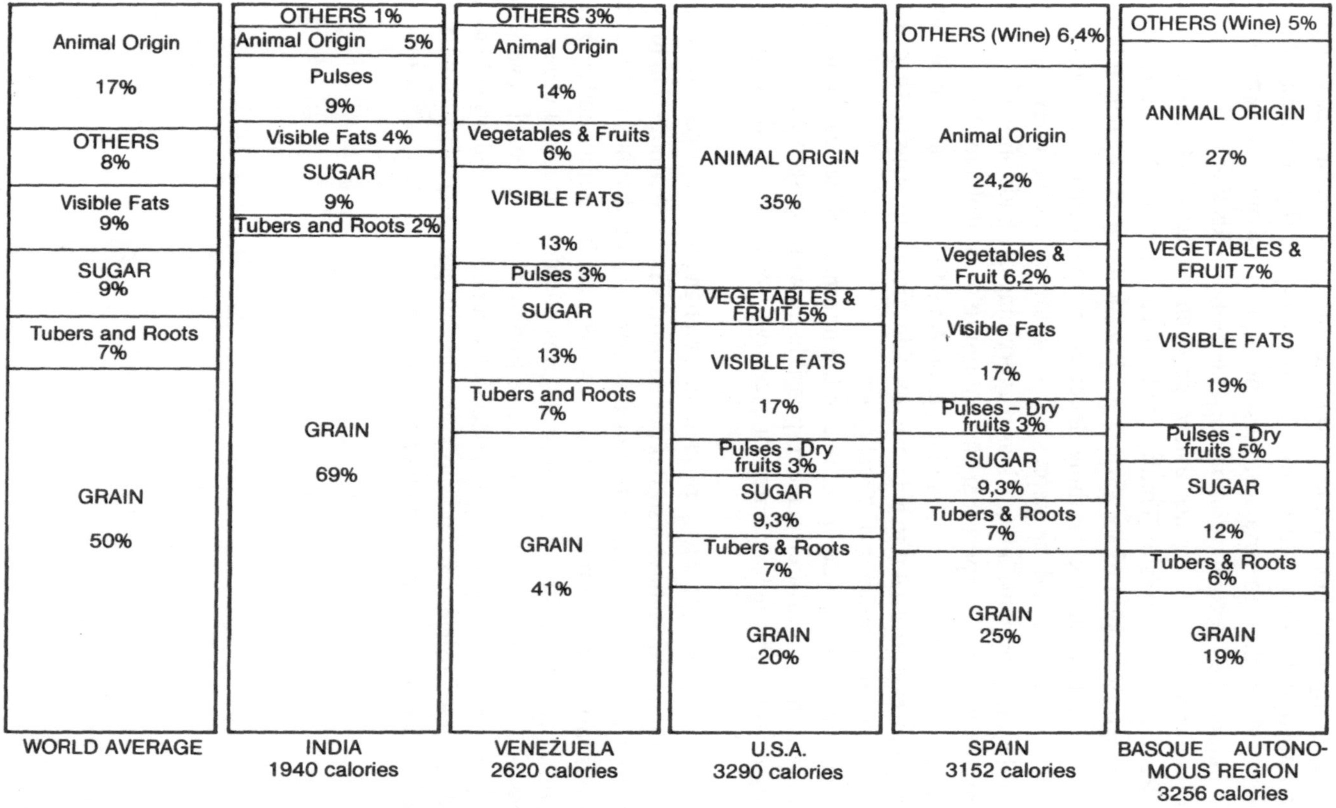

WORLD AVERAGE

- Animal Origin 17%
- OTHERS 8%
- Visible Fats 9%
- SUGAR 9%
- Tubers and Roots 7%
- GRAIN 50%

INDIA 1940 calories

- OTHERS 1%
- Animal Origin 5%
- Pulses 9%
- Visible Fats 4%
- SUGAR 9%
- Tubers and Roots 2%
- GRAIN 69%

VENEZUELA 2620 calories

- OTHERS 3%
- Animal Origin 14%
- Vegetables & Fruits 6%
- VISIBLE FATS 13%
- Pulses 3%
- SUGAR 13%
- Tubers and Roots 7%
- GRAIN 41%

U.S.A. 3290 calories

- ANIMAL ORIGIN 35%
- VEGETABLES & FRUIT 5%
- VISIBLE FATS 17%
- Pulses - Dry fruits 3%
- SUGAR 9,3%
- Tubers & Roots 7%
- GRAIN 20%

SPAIN 3152 calories

- OTHERS (Wine) 6,4%
- Animal Origin 24,2%
- Vegetables & Fruit 6,2%
- Visible Fats 17%
- Pulses – Dry fruits 3%
- SUGAR 9,3%
- Tubers & Roots 7%
- GRAIN 25%

BASQUE AUTONOMOUS REGION 3256 calories

- OTHERS (Wine) 5%
- ANIMAL ORIGIN 27%
- VEGETABLES & FRUIT 7%
- VISIBLE FATS 19%
- Pulses - Dry fruits 5%
- SUGAR 12%
- Tubers & Roots 6%
- GRAIN 19%

Figure 1. Food availability patterns in the world and in specific countries: percentage distribution of caloric supply (1970s).

Table 1. Two decades of economic development in poor* densely-populated countries.

Country	Population (millions) 1979	GNP per inhabitant Annual % growth rate 1960–1979	Life expectancy 1960–1978	
Bangladesh	88.9	0.1	43	49
Ethiopia	30.9	1.3	36	40
Burma	32.9	1.1	44	54
India	659.2	1.4	42	52
Vietnam	52.9	–	43	63
China	964.5	–	–	64
Pakistan	79.7	2.9	44	52
Tanzania	18.0	2.3	42	52
Zaire	27.5	0.7	40	47
Indonesia	142.9	4.1	39	53
Sudan	17.9	0.6	39	53
Egypt	38.9	3.4	46	57
Thailand	45.5	4.6	51	62
Philippines	46.7	2.6	51	62
Nigeria	82.6	3.7	39	49
Peru	17.1	1.7	48	58
Morocco	19.5	2.6	47	56
Colombia	26.1	3.0	53	63
Rep. Korea	17.5	3.5	54	63
Turkey	44.2	3.8	51	62
Rep. Korea	37.8	7.1	54	63
Algeria	18.2	2.4	47	56
Mexico	65.5	2.7	58	66
South Africa	28.5	2.3	53	61
Brasil	116.5	4.8	55	63
Rumania	22.1	9.2	65	71

* GNP per capita less than 2000 dollars in 1979.

Table 2. Supply per person (1977).

Country	Calories	Proteins	Fats
North America	3,557	105.9 g	164.4 g
			(1) v. 63.4
			a. 101.0
Latin America	2,557	65.5	57.5 g
			v. 25.6
			a. 31.9
Africa	2,310	59.0	44.5 g
			v. 32.9
			a. 11.1
Near East	2,620	73.5	51.6 g
			v. 34.0
			a. 17.6
Far East	2,029	48.7	30.3 g
(Developing countries)			v. 22.7
			a. 7.7
Western Europe	3,376	94.8	138.6 g
			v. 48.4
			a. 90.2
Eastern Europe and U.S.S.R.	3,481	103.3	106.8 g
			v. 29.5
			a. 77.3
Steady world average	2,571	68.8	62.2 g
			v. 28.7
			a. 33.5

Table 3. Summary of food availability according to large groups of countries.

	Calories	Proteins	Fats
Developed countries with market economy	3,353	97.0	134
Developing countries with market economy	2,203	54.9	38.6
Countries with centralized planning economies:			
Asian countries	2,380	62.5	37.9
Eastern Europe and USSR	3,481	103.3	106.8
All developed countries	3,395	99.1	125.3
All developing countries	2,260	57.3	38.4

Table 4. Percentage distribution of calories produced for human consumption on a world level (1977).

	Calories		%	
General total	2,571			
Vegetable products	2,136		83.08	
Animal products	435		16.92	
Grain	1,278		49.71	
– Wheat		465		36.38
– Rice		505		39.52
– Maize		146		11.42
– Millet and sorghum		102		7.98
Roots and tubers	161		6.26	
Sugar and honey	234		9.10	
Pulses	77		2.99	
Nuts and oleaginous seeds	48		1.87	
Vegetables	41		1.59	
Fruit	59		2.29	
Meat	205		7.98	
Eggs	21		0.83	
Fish	25		0.97	
Milk	116		4.51	
Oils and fats	225		8.75	
– Vegetable origin		159		70.67
– Animal origin		66		29.33
Others	81		3.15	
Total	2,571		100	

Sources: Food balance sheets. Average 1975–77.

Table 5. The rich, the poor and the poorest.

	The 31* least advanced countries	89 other developing countries	37 developed countries
Population (in million of inhabitants)	283	3,001	1,131
Infant death rate (per 1000 live births)	160	94	19
Life expectancy (in years)	45	60	72
Percentage of children born weighing over 2,500 g	70%	83%	93%
Supply of drinking water	31%	41%	100%
Literacy rate of adults	28%	55%	98%
GNP per inhabitant	$ 179	$ 520	$ 6,230
Public health costs per inhabitant	$ 1.7	$ 6.5	$ 244
Public health costs in percentage of the GNP	1.0%	1.2%	3.9%
Number of inhabitants per physician	17,000	2.700	520
Number of inhabitants per sick person	6,500	1,500	220
Number of inhabitants per health assistant of any rank	2,400	500	130

* The figures indicated are steady average ones, based on estimates corresponding to 1980 or to the last year when data was collected.
Source: World Health (WHO), Geneva. June 1982.

Table 6. Dispersal and averages of the prevalence of protein-calorie malnutrition in surveys carried out in communities (1963–1973).

Areas	Number of surveys	Number of children examined (thousands)	Severe forms		Moderate forms	
			Dispersal %	Average %	Dispersal %	Average %
Latin America	11	109	0.5– 6.3	1.6	3.5–32.0	18.9
Africa	7	25	1.7– 9.8	4.4	5.4–44.9	26.5
Asia	7	39	1.1–20.0	3.2	16.0–46.4	31.2
Total	25	173	0.5–20.0	2.6	3.5–46.4	18.9

Source: Bengoa, J.M. and Donoso, G. PAG Bulletin 1974.

Table 7. Estimated number of seriously undernourished persons in developing countries (according to the FAO).

Countries	1974–76 (millions)
86 developing countries	436
Africa	72
Far East	304
Near East	19
Latin America	41
Countries of medium income	87
Countries of low income	349

There is no information on 4 of the developing countries.
Source: Agricultural Horizon 2000 FAO. Rome. 1981.

Table 8. Consumption tendencies of calories per capita in developing countries.

Countries	1974–76	2,000
90 countries	2,180	2,370
Africa	2,180	2,305
Far East	2,025	2,200
Near East	2,560	2,845
Latin America	2,525	2,700
Medium income	2,485	2,690
Low income	2,010	2,175

Source: Agricultural Horizon 2000 FAO. Rome. 1981.

The newborn infant

Chairman: O.P. GHAI

Sources of excess low birth weight in developing countries

N. TAFARI

Introduction

The state of low birth weight (LBW) arises from adverse maternal and fetal factors that bring about shorter gestation or a slower rate of intrauterine growth, or both. Measurement of birth weight has been epidemiologically useful since the combined effects of maternal and fetal factors are manifested in a single quantifiable variable. Thus variations in LBW rate reflect variations in the frequency of abnormal maternal and fetal factors. It has been postulated that the LBW rate reflects not only the health status of the mother–fetus dyad but also the socio-economic conditions under which the particular reproduction has taken place [1].

According to the WHO [2], nearly one-fifth of the worlds births during 1979 were classified as LBW. Of these, 90% were born in developing countries where protein-energy and other forms of malnutrition, infections and parasitic infestations are common. There is a compelling body of evidence that undernutrition and infections during the perinatal period underlay most of the excess prevalence of premature termination of pregnancy and intrauterine growth retardation.

The role of nutrition

The role of nutrition on fetal growth and development has been the subject of continuous study over the last 70 years. There is consensus that maternal nutrition is a factor in fetal growth. The data are derived from observational studies, international comparisons and the 'natural' experimental data from the 'hunger-winter' of 1944–45 [3]. The reported pregnancy abnormalities associated with protein-energy undernutrition are summarized in Table 1.

If deficiencies in the home diet are factors in fetal growth, nutritional supplementation during pregnancy of mothers at risk of producing LBWs should produce large increases in birth weight. It appears that under normal living conditions in industrialized countries, such supplementation of the home diet of gravida at risk result in increase in birth weight of only 40 to 60 grams. Larger increases in birth weight are seen in gravida who were undernourished, and under conditions of acute food deprivation, such as during famine, in which the average increase in birth weight following food supplementation may be as high as 300 to 400 grams [3].

The study from Guatemala [4] was among the first to demonstrate that dietary deficiency in energy was more important than deficiency in protein. When the villagers in Guatemala who habitually consumed 1500 kcal/day, were given supplementary diets containing either energy alone, or energy with protein, significant increase in birth weight and decrease in the proportion of LBW did not occur until the supplement approached the energy cost of pregnancy. On the other hand protein supplementation was not only without effect on birth weight in undernourished gravida in Guatemala, it was associated with excess frequency of termination of pregnancy prior to 30 weeks in New York City where the gravida's home diet probably contained adequate amounts of the nutrient [3]. Although the importance of dietary protein may not be apparent from these studies, it cannot be entirely discounted since during normal pregnancy some 900 grams of new protein is synthesized in the fetus, placenta and maternal reproductive tissues [5]. The synthesis of this quantity of protein in the face of marginal dietary intake requires significant modification of the intermediary metabolism of amino acids [6]. There appears to be a physiologic suppression of amino acid catabolism in early pregnancy with protein storage followed by a catabolic phase in late pregnancy. The catabolic phase in the pregnant rat occurs irrespective of the level of protein intake, suggesting that the phenomenon is not under dietary control [7]. Naismith and colleagues, using the amino acid 3-methylhistidine, showed that muscle protein breakdown in apparently healthy gravida and in positive nitrogen balance, began at around 30 weeks of gestation and increased until birth [7].

Vitamins and micronutrients [8]

The role of specific nutrients, such as vitamins and trace elements, have been the subject of many studies. Studies on dietary vitamins, folate and vitamin B6, have not yielded positive correlation with fetal growth or pregnancy outcome. Studies

Table 1. Reported effects of protein-energy undernutrition on pregnancy outcome.

Fetal growth retardation [3, 4, 14, 18, 20]
Placental underperfusion [14, 18, 19]
Abruptio placentae [14]
Maternal hypotension [14, 21]
Maternal hypovolemia [14]

on 'routine' iron supplementation show no beneficial effect on the health of the mother/fetus pair. The role of micronutrients such as copper, chromium and iodine on fetal growth and pregnancy outcome await further evaluation.

Zinc deficiency and reproductive performance

The role of the micronutrient zinc in fetal growth and pregnancy outcome has received considerable attention. The possibility that zinc deficiency state may occur in association with low intake of animal protein [8] is of great public health importance since zinc deficiency may be coextensive with protein-energy under-nutrition.

Zinc is a constituent of many metalloenzymes, and is present in almost all human tissues. The metal is apparently essential in carbohydrate and fat metabolism for the synthesis of proteins and nucleic acids and for optimal function of the immunological and endocrine systems. The fetus accumulates most of the body zinc during the third trimester of pregnancy.

Recent animal experimental data and observations from humans indicate added risk for reproductive failures in association with apparent zinc deficiency states [8, 9]. The reported perinatal abnormalities are summarized in Table 2. Severe zinc deficiency in rats, and possibly also in humans, leads to gross congenital malformations of several organ systems [9]. In the pregnant rat [10] and rhesus monkey [11], dietary zinc restrictions lead to anorexia which may retard fetal growth without affecting the nutritional status of the mother. The conversion of arachidonic acid to '2 series' prostaglandins in the placenta is increased by 50–150% in the zinc deficient rat [12]. The cardiac output of such zinc deficient rats is also decreased to 50% of control values. The associated increase in prostaglandin E2 and F2-alpha decreases the proportion of the cardiac output reaching the placenta, uterus and adrenals [13]. Blood flow to these organs was also reduced. If these observations in the rat are true of humans, zinc may play a central role in the genesis of such common perinatal disorders as placental abruptions, prostaglandin mediated preterm labor and fetal growth retardation

Table 2. The reported effects of zinc deficiency on pregnancy outcome.

Fetal growth retardation [9, 14]
Congenital malformation [9, 14]
Maternal hypovolemia
Reduced cardiac output [13, 18, 19]
Reduced utero-placental blood flow [13]
Increased protaglandin synthesis [12]
Dystocia and postpartum bleeding [9]
Reduced antibacterial activity of amniotic fluid [14]

from reduced placental nutrient transfer and chronic fetal hypoxia [14].

Zinc deficiency has also been implicated in impaired antimicrobial activity of amniotic fluid [14]. The antibacterial activity of amniotic fluid resides in a polypeptide that requires the presence of zinc. The action of zinc in this system is counteracted by the presence of high concentrations of phosphorus in amniotic fluid. Some workers have suggested that a treshold ratio of 'phosphate'-to-zinc of 200 as the upper limit of antibacterial activity, while others have not found such a relationship. As Gibbs et al. [15] point out there are important differences between the various studies both in design and population. At the time of this writing the role of zinc and inorganic phosphorus in antibacterial activity of amniotic fluid during late gestation, and hence in the pathogenesis of intra-amniotic fluid infections, are not clearly defined.

Zinc supplementation of the diet has not produced added bacterial growth inhibitory activity on amniotic fluid [14]. One recent study from the United States [16] describes the effect of zinc supplementation in a double-blind experiment in 213 'free-living' Hispanic gravidas. This study showed that although the mean serum or hair zinc levels were not higher in the treatment group, the proportion of gravida with severely depressed zinc levels (<54 μg/dl) in late pregnancy was significantly reduced. The importance of this reduction to perinatal outcome is not stated. Extrinsic factors such as presence of phytic acid, dietary fiber, tin and iron reduce the bioavailability of zinc. The inhibitory effect of these extrinsic factors may be counteracted by intrinsic regulation of zinc absorption through intestinal adaptations, particularly when content of zinc in the diet is marginal [17]. Until these determinants of the bioavailabilty of zinc are better understood, it would be difficult to interpret the results of these dietary zinc supplementation studies.

The role of hemodynamic changes

Plasma volume expansion is recognized as one of the most important signs of successful adaptation to pregnancy. In normal pregnancy plasma volume expansion starts at 6 weeks gestation and continues until 24 to 34 weeks [5]. Expansion in plasma volume is accompanied by increase in heart rate at rest of about 15 beats/min. It is estimated that cardiac output in the healthy gravida increases from a mean of 4.5 l/min to 6.0 l/min. The increase in cardiac output follows the expansion of plasma volume, and is brought about by increase in heart rate and stroke volume. The systemic arterial pressure falls in the first trimester of pregnancy followed by a rise in the last trimester. The fall in diastolic blood pressure is greater than that in systolic pressure. The fall in systemic arterial pressure in the face of rising cardiac output implies a decrease in systemic peripheral resistance. Since cardiac output and plasma volume do not rise appreciably during the third trimester, the observed rise in blood pressure during the

third trimester must be due to increase in total peripheral resistance.

Several lines of evidence suggest associations between maternal protein-energy undernutrition and decreased pregnancy plasma volume, cardiac output, systemic arterial blood pressure, uterine and placental blood flow [18–21]. In the rat, when maternal diet is restricted to 50% of that given to controls, cardiac output is reduced [18, 19]. The reduction in cardiac output is accompanied by significant reduction in uterine blood placental blood flow in late gestation. Measurements of plasma volume in human pregnancies date back from the 1950s, but there has been no attempt to correlate the observed abnormalities with clinical outcome. Recent studies suggest that failure to expand plasma volume in response to pregnancy is associated with intrauterine fetal demise [22]. The associated uterine underperfusion is thought to underlie such disorders as abruptio placentae, placental infarctions and chronic fetal hypoxia [14].

A decline in the frequency of toxemia of pregnancy was noted in the original analysis of the data from the Dutch hungerwinter of 1944–45. Re-examination of the data by Robeiro et al. [21] showed that this decline was due to fall in blood pressure in communities exposed to severe food deprivation. The fall in blood pressure was best correlated with energy intakes below 1900 kcal/day. Higher blood pressures were associated with presence of dependent edema. Goodlin et al. [23] suggest several clinical and laboratory signs to identify the woman with inadequate plasma expansion in response to pregnancy. These signs include absence of dependent edema, failure to develop a fall in hematocrit, hypo-albuminemia and absent systolic flow murmur. Failure to increase systemic arterial pressure in late gestation is associated with decrease in birth weight [24]. The effect is compounded by maternal pregravid undernutrition.

The effects of protein-energy undernutrition on maternal hemodynamic adjustments is further augmented by maternal physical exercise. Studies on pregnancy hemodynamics in response to exercise show rise in cardiac output as a result of increase in heart rate and stroke volume [24]. The total peripheral resistance is lowered inducing further fall in blood pressure and redistribution of the cardiac output away from the utero-placental unit. With pre-exercise hypovolemia and hypotension, marked reductions in utero-placental blood flow may occur with heavy muscular work [14]. Figure 1 summarizes the possible interaction between protein-energy and zinc undernutrition, and hard physical work in the pathogenesis of LBW.

The role of infections [14]

Viruses, bacteria and protozoa reach the placenta and the fetus and bring about damage or death without causing clinically apparent infection in the mother. Infectious agents may produce LBWs by causing fetal growth retardation or by shortening the duration of gestation (Figure 2).

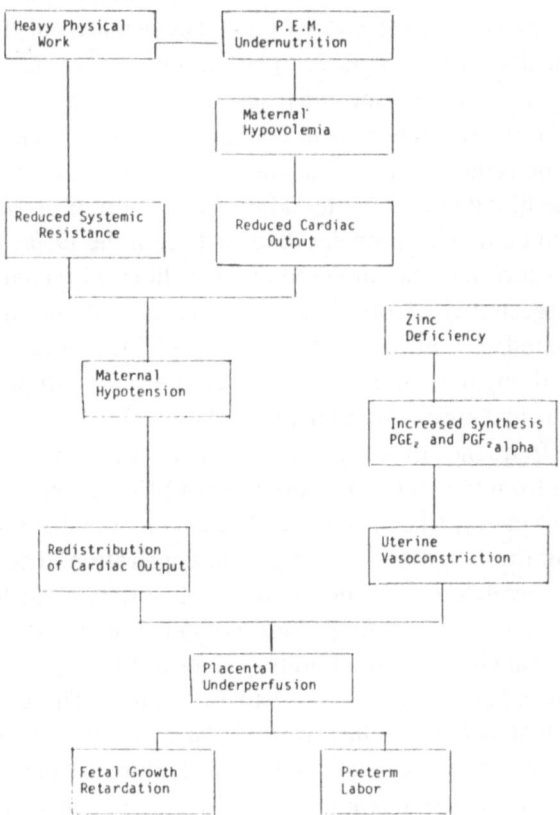

Figure 1. Combined effects of protein-energy undernutrition, heavy physical work and zinc deficiency on pregnancy outcome [3, 5, 12–14, 18, 19, 21].

Malaria is perhaps the most ubiquitous infection in developing countries. Malaria infections have been associated with fetal growth retardation. The mechanism of fetal growth retardation in malaria is due to fetal hypoxia due to extensive placentitis and maternal anemia [14]. There is very little known about the effect of the other tropical diseases on the prevalence of LBW. Maternal leprosy is associated with excess LBW delivery, but most gravida with this disorder live under conditions of extreme poverty so that it is not possible to separate the effects of nutritional and other environmental factors from those due to the infection. There is no information on the effect of the other common tropical parasitic infections such as schistosomiasis, trypanosomiasis, leishmaniasis and onchocerciasis.

The prevalence of perinatal rubella and cytomegalovirus infections in developing countries is not known. The occasional sero-epidemiologic surveys indicate that there is no excess in the proportion of women of the reproductive age group

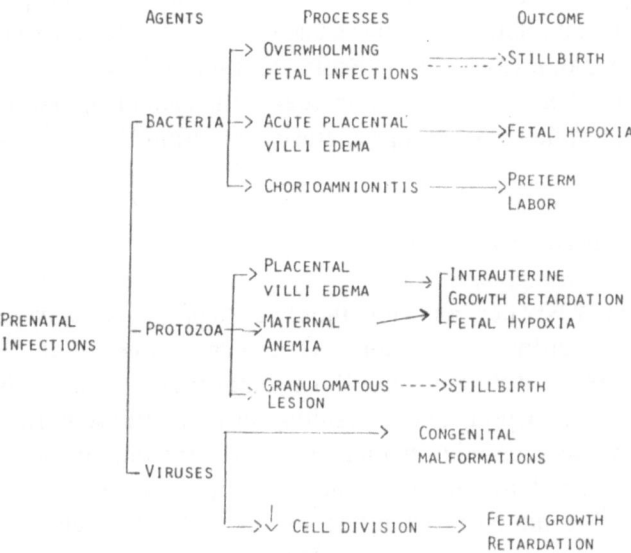

Figure 2. The role of infection in the pathogenesis of LBT [14, 26, 27].

at risk of developing the infections during pregnancy. It therefore appears that the excess LBW observed in developing countries cannot be explained by excess prevalence of fetal infections with these viruses.

Studies from the United States, Addis Ababa and Durban have shown that ascending, transcervical bacterial infections of the fetus as the leading cause of excess perinatal mortality [14]. The infections occur across intact membranes in the majority of cases. These infections are the result of complex interactions between maternal and pregnancy factors. The exact mechanism by which bacteria gain access to fetal membranes is not known. Dilatation of the cervical os that normally occurs in late gestation, coitus and the presence of semen may facilitate the entry of bacteria into the gravid uterine cavity. Infections of the fetal membranes are associated with diminished antimicrobial activity of amniotic fluid. As detailed above, the lack of amniotic fluid antimicrobial activity is associated with low levels of zinc.

These infections lead to intrauterine fetal demise following the development of intrauterine pneumonia and septicemia. Many of the bacteria recovered from the lungs of fatal cases of amniotic fluid infections are usually considered to be of such low virulence that they are seldom reported in perinatal infections [26]. Several of these organisms were recently shown to have an active phospholipase A2 system [27]. It is postulated that in chorioamnionitis due to these organisms phospholipase A2 is elaborated. Phospholipase A2 splits arachidonic acid from phospholipids normally present in fetal membranes. Arachidonic acid so formed enters into the synthesis of prostaglandin F2 alpha and E2 leading to premature labor.

If this hypothesis is upheld, most preterm labors should be prevented by controlling chrioamnionitis due to these bacteria. It is interesting to note that 20 years ago, a group of investigators in Boston [28] showed that a 6-week course of tetracyline in non-bacteriuric women increased the mean length of gestation by one week, representing a drop in prematurity rate from 15.2% to 5.4%.

Some clues to preventive measures

The separation of LBW newborns into those due to premature delivery and those due to intrauterine growth retardation has been clinically useful. It has, however, implied that there are different causes for two disorders. Examination of recent evidence suggests that pregnancies resulting in prematurely born and growth retarded infants have certain characteristics in common: previous fetal loss, hypotension or hypertension, and possibly also protein-energy and zinc under-nutrition. If such common mechanisms are operative it should be possible to demonstrate correlations between rates of fetal growth retardation and premature delivery. In a large population based study from the United States, Spiers and Wacholder [29] demonstrated significant correlation between intrauterine growth retardation at term and premature birth indicating common origins for the diseases leading to the two disorders (Figure 1).

Critical areas of intervention to reduce the prevalence of LBW must take into consideration the environmental, demographic and economic conditions under which reproduction takes place. Most gravid women in developing countries are undernourished, are often engaged in heavy physical work and suffer from recurrent infective disorders. Nutritional supplementation of the kind that were undertaken in the 60's and 70's cannot in themselves produce the desired effect. The introduction of labor-saving devices may have a higher biological and social value in that they do not induce dependency on the recipient. Zinc supplementation has the potential of reducing LBW rate through prevention of amniotic fluid infections, improving maternal appetite, and enhancing placental underperfusion. Reduction of chrioamnionitis is key to the reduction of premature labor.

The medical literature is surfeit with reports of recent decline in perinatal mortality as a result of advances in clinical obstetric and neonatal care. Two population based studies from the United States [30, 31] show that most of the decline in perinatal mortality during the 70's was due to reduction in birth weight-specific mortality rate as a result of improved intrapartum and neonatal care. As can be expected these measures had no effect on birth weight distribution so that despite enormous expenditures on perinatal health care, there has been no change in the proportion of LBW newborns in certain underprivileged populations. It is evident that the definitive solution to the problem of excessive perinatal mortality and longterm morbidity in the 'tropics' is the reduction of the variance around the optimal birth weight for a given population.

References

1. Sterky G, Millander L (eds): Birth weight distribution: an indicator of development, Swedish Agency for Research Cooperation with Developing Countries, Report No. 2, 1978.
2. WHO: The incidence of low birth weight, a critical review of available information. World Health Stat Quart 33:197–224, 1980.
3. Susser M: Prenatal nutrition, birthweight, and psychological development: an overview of experiments, quasi-experiments, and natural experiments in the past decade. Am J Clin Nutr 34:784–803, 1981.
4. Habicht JP, Yabrough C, Lechtig A, Klein RE: Relation of maternal supplementary feeding during pregnancy to birth weight and other sociobiological factors. In: Winick M (ed) Nutrition and fetal development. Proceedings of the Syposium on Nutrition and Fetal Development. Current Concepts in Nutrition, Vol 3. New York, John Wiley, pp 124–146, 1974.
5. Hytten FE, Leitch I: The physiology of human pregnancy. Oxford, Blackwell Scientific Publications, 1971 (2nd edn).
6. Naismith DJ, Morgan BLG: The biphasic nature of protein metabolism during pregnancy in the rat. Br J Nutr 36:563–566, 1976.
7. Naismith DJ: Maternal nutrition and the outcome of pregnancy – a critical appraisal. Proc Nutr Soc 39:1–11, 1980.
8. Michael AJ, Dreosti IE, Gibson GT: Maternal zinc status and pregnancy outcome: a prospective study. In: Clinical applications of recent advances in zinc metabolism. New York, Alan R Liss, pp. 53–66, 1982.
9. Jameson S: Effects of zinc deficiency in human reproduction. Acta Med Scand Supl 583:3–89, 1976.
10. Greeley S, Fosmire GJ, Sandstead HH: Nitrogen retention during late gestation in the rat in response to marginal zinc intake. Am J Physiol (Endocrinol Metab) 2:E113–E118, 1980.
11. Sandstead HH, Strobel DA, Logan GM Jr, Marks EO, Jacob RA: Zinc deficiency in pregnant rhesus monkeys: effects on behavior of infants. Am J Clin Nutr 31:844–849, 1978.
12. Cunnane SC: Zinc deficiency increases prostaglandin synthesis from arachidonic acid. Proc Nutr Soc 40:114A, 1981.
13. Cunnane SC, Majid E, Senior J et al.: Perinatal mortality in zinc deficient rats is associated with significantly reduced placental blood flow. Proc Nutr Soc 40:69A, 1982.
14. Naeye RL, Tafari N: Pregnancy risk factors and diseases of the embryo, fetus and neonate. Baltimore, Williams and Wilkins, 1983.
15. Gibbs RS, Blanco JD, Hnilica VS: Inorganic phosphorus and zinc concentrations in amniotic fluid: correlation with intra-amniotic infection and bacterial inhibitory activity. Am J Obstet Gynecol 143:163–166, 1982.
16. Hunt IF, Murphy NJ, Cleaver AE, Faraji BF, Swendseid ME, Coulson AH, Clark VA, Laine N, Davis CA, Cecil Smith J Jr: Zinc supplementation during pregnancy: zinc concentration of serum and hair from low-income women of Mexican descent. Am J Clin Nutr 37:572–582, 1983.
17. Solomons NW: Biological availibility of zinc in humans. Am J Clin Nutr 35:1048–1075, 1982.
18. Rosso P, Kava R: Effects of food restriction on cardiac output and blood flow to the uterus and placenta in the pregnant rat. J Nutr 110:2350–2354, 1980.
19. Ahokas RA, Anderson GD, Lipshitz J: Cardiac output and utero placental blood flow in diet-restricted and diet-depleted pregnant rats. Am J Obstet Gynecol 146:6–13, 1983.
20. Naeye RL: Nutritional/nonnutritional interactions that affect the outcome of pregnancy. Am J Clin Nutr 34:727–731, 1981.
21. Ribeiro MD, Stein Z, Susser M, Cohen P, Neugut R: Prenatal starvation and maternal blood pressure near delivery. Am J Clin Nutr 35:535–541, 1982.
22. Sibai BM, Abdella TN, Anderson GD, McCubbin JH: Plasma volume determination in pregnancies complicated by chronic hypertension and intrauterine fetal demise. Obstet Gynecol 60:174–178, 1982.

23. Goodlin RC, Dobry CA, Anderson JC, Woods RE, Quaife M: Clinical signs of normal plasma volume expansion during pregnancy. Am J Obstet Gynecol 145:1001–1009, 1983.
24. Naeye RL: Maternal blood pressure and fetal growth. Am J Obstet Gynecol 141:780–787, 1981.
25. Dhindsa DS, Metcalfe J, Hunnels DH: Response to exercise in the pregnant pygmy goat. Respir Physiol 32:299–311, 1978.
26. Naeye RL, Tafari N, Judge D, Gilmore D, Marboe C: Amniotic fluid infections in an African city. J Pediatr 90:965–970, 1977.
27. Bejar R, Curbelo V, Davis C et al.: Premature labor: II. Bacterial precursors of phospholipase. Obstet Gynecol 57:479–482, 1981.
28. Elder HA, Santamarina BAG, Smith S et al.: The natural history of asymptomatic bacteruria during pregnancy: The effect of tetracycline on the clinical course and outcome of pregnancy. Am J Obstet Gynecol 111:441–462, 1971.
29. Spiers PS, Wacholder S: Association between rates of premature delivery and intra-uterine growth retardation. Develop Med Child Neurol 24:808–816, 1982.
30. Kleinman JC, Kovar MG, Feldman JJ et al.: A comparison of 1960 and 1973–1974 early neonatal mortality in selected states. Am J Epidemiol 108:454–469, 1978.
31. Williams RL, Chen PM: Identifying sources of the recent decline in perinatal mortality rates in California. N Engl J Med 306:207–214, 1982.

Some aspects of perinatal growth: Can perinatal health be measured in kilograms?

E.R. BOERSMA, TH.M. HOORNTJE, N.H. HUTTER, P.J. OFFRINGA, J.P.H. JONXIS and R.A. SOER

Introduction

Growth in utero is a function of seed and soil. It is dependent for instance on the height of the mother, the growth potential of the foetus itself and upon the availability of a healthy intrauterine environment to fulfil this potential. The result of the interaction between these factors is a wide variation of mean birthweights between different populations, ethnic groups, geographical situations and socio-economic conditions. Extrauterine survival is expected to be related to the birthweight of the infant.

Despite numerous studies [1–9] the effect of mild to moderate maternal undernutrition on the intrauterine and subsequent growth and development *in man* remains uncertain. However, in animal experiments, severe food restriction and an artificially induced vitamin deficiency were able to produce malnourished and sometimes congenital abnormalities of the offspring [10–13].

The question arises, what should be taken as an adequate diet during pregnancy? Is it justified that total physiological requirements during pregnancy could be calculated from the sum of ordinary non-pregnant requirements and those specific to pregnancy? What is the effect of supplementary feeding during pregnancy on fetal growth and well being? Is it true that increasing mean birthweight for a population, leaving the other circumstances the same, will automatically result in a reduction of the infant mortality and morbidity? In this paper we would like to review the effect of various aspects of (mal)nutrition on maternal weight gain during pregnancy and on fetal and neonatal growth. Special emphasis is given to birthweight in relation to risk factors at birth. Where possible, information is given from data obtained in the Caribbean region, Tanzania and from other sources in the 'tropics'. As a reference, data are given from Western countries.

Nutrition versus maternal weight gain during pregnancy

Mean total weight gain during pregnancy has been studied in various countries throughout the last century. There is a wide range in maternal weight change, from a loss of some kg to a gain of 23 kg or more. 'No single figure can be regarded as 'normal' with the implication that different figures should be regarded as 'abnormal' (quoted from Thomson and Hytten [14]).

Up to the Second World War most studies came from the U.S. Average weight gain in those days was approximately 9 kg, roughly 3.5 kg lower than more recent figures. Data from underprivileged societies have shown weight gains of only 6.0 kg for Indonesia [15] and Tanzania [16], 6.5 kg for India [17], 7 kg for Ethiopia [18], 12.7 kg for Jamaica [19] and 11.5 kg for Dominica [20]. Adding together the weight of the product of conception (included placenta and amniotic fluid) and the estimated gains in the maternal reproductive systems (uterus, breasts), we can calculate a weight gain of approximately 5.4 kg for Indonesian or Tanzanian women and maximally 6.0 kg for Western countries (Table 1). Apparently the extra weight gained by the Western mother (± 6.5 kg) is due to either a surplus of extra/intra cellular water, an accumulation of fat, an increase of bloodvolume, or a combination of these factors and not to the weight of the offspring. Methods to measure the changes in body water and extracellular water during pregnancy are hampered by the problem that the maternal body can not be measured in isolation. Therefore maternal weight changes after delivery could give us some information about the volume of water retained during pregnancy. From a longitudinal study on maternal weight changes from well nourished mothers after delivery for Jamaica with a pregnancy weight gain on average of 12.7 kg [19] – similar to most industrialized countries – we could show a weight loss of 4.16 kg from the 2nd to the 28th day after delivery. This *rapid* weight loss after delivery

Table 1. Analysis of estimated weight gain during pregnancy for Caucasian and Tanzanian women.

Data	Caucasian* (kg)	Tanzanian (kg)
Fetal factors		
fetus	3.4	3.0
placenta	0.65	0.5
amniotic fluid	0.8	0.8
Maternal factors		
uterus	0.97	0.9
breasts	0.4	0.4
blood volume	1.25 ⎫	⎫
extracellular fluid	1.7 ⎬ 6.28	⎬ 0.4
fat	3.33 ⎭	⎭
Total	12.5	6.0

* Reference: Hytten and Leitch, 1971.

may indicate rather a loss of excessive water, which was retained during pregnancy, than a weight loss due to a loss of maternal fat or lean body tissue. It would be interesting to know maternal weight changes after delivery in those countries with a 'reduced' pregnancy weight gain like in Indonesia or Tanzania. But eventually, more conclusive evidence can be expected from more accurate techniques to assess changes in body composition.

In conclusion we might state that the difference in weight gained during pregnancy between the industrialized countries and most under privileged countries is to a great extent attributable to the storage of maternal water in the intra and extra vascular compartments and the storage of maternal fat and not to the formation of foetal tissue. The effect of maternal water retention on the body fluids of the foetus will be discussed later.

Maternal nutrition versus foetal growth

Evidence that inadequate diet during pregnancy has adverse effects on child-bearing is largely epidemiological and based on the fact that poorer and presumably less well fed sections of the populations have greater perinatal morbidity and mortality and smaller babies than the more affluent and presumably better fed classes. The complexity of this assumption can be illustrated by the following calculations. According to Widdowson [21], one of the most economical processes from the energy point of view is the making of a baby. The total average energy requirements for maintenance and for new body tissue synthesis by the foetus is not far from a 20,000 kcal (84 MJ). Half of these energy requirements are needed to complete the development of the foetus during the last 2 months of intrauterine life, which accounts for approximately 200 kcal (840 kJ) per day for that period. Only approximately 60 kcal (252 kJ) per day is spent during the 6th and the 7th month of pregnancy and less than 20 kcal (84 kJ) per day during the first 6 months of foetal life, as illustrated in Table 2. In Western countries [22], but

Table 2. Energy requirements for maintenance and for new body tissue by the foetus.

Fetal age (days)	Body wt (g)	Requirements (Kcal*/day)		
		Maintenance	New tissue	Total
90	100	3.5	1.0	4.5
120	200	7.0	2.0	9.0
150	400	14.0	4.4	18.4
180	1000	35.0	10.0	45.0
210	1600	56.0	57.6	113.6
240	2400	84.0	86.4	170.4
270	3100	108.5	111.6	220.1

* 1 kcal = 4.2 kJ   Calculated from Widdowson [22].

probably not to that extent in countries with reduced fat stores, an additional 40,000 kcal (168 MJ) are probably needed for laying down mainly maternal fat (the energy equivalent of 3.5 kg of fat is 34,000 kcal (143 MJ)). The majority of this fat is accumulated *before the 30th week* of gestation. At the stage of low foetal energy need, this fat store accounts for approximately 160 kcal (672 kJ) per day. Looked at it in another way, in Western countries, the estimated additional cost *throughout* pregnancy for making a baby, including the extra energy requirements for laying down maternal stores, can be calculated to account for a maximum of approximately 200–250 kcal (840–1050 kJ) daily on average. This is about one quarter of the ordinary expenditure on activity as estimated for the non-pregnant woman [23].

For non-industrialized countries, assuming a negligable storage of maternal fat, the extra daily energy requirements during pregnancy will not be more than approximately 200 kcal (840 kJ) in the last two months of pregnancy, but much less in the first two trimesters. Although not proven, the energy need of pregnancy could be met without additional supplies from the diet, just by reducing activity [24] or by a more economical process of metabolism. Some reduction of activity seems to be a physiological characteristic during pregnancy [14]. Metabolic adjustments are widespread and complex and involve a radical resetting of hypothalamic control centres with considerable effect on the proteinbinding of thyroxine and on other aspects of pregnancy metabolism [14], for instance by an increased bio-availability of different nutrients (Ca^{++}, Zn, Fe^{++}).

The effect of supplementary feeding to pregnant women with restricted nutritional intake has been studied under various circumstances [25–29]. In a well organized intervention study, often quoted, Lechtig et al. [30] showed that a total additional suppletion of 10,000 kcal (42 MJ) during the last two trimesters of pregnancy (which is equivalent to 60 kcal (252 kJ) per day) gave an average increase of 30 g in birthweight of the offspring. This would imply that for a 100 g increase in mean birthweight some 34,000 kcal (143 MJ) are needed. 100 grams new foetal tissue will contain approximately 12 g protein, 12 g fat and 75 g of water with a total caloric value of approximately 160 kcal (672 kJ). Another 30 kcal (126 kJ) are needed for the protein synthesis of this 100 g new foetal tissue [31]. Making a total of 190 kcal (798 kJ) only. This would indicate that the majority of this supplemented 34,000 kcal (143 MJ) will enter a maternal store (probably fat) or is (partially) wasted in order to achieve a 100 g increase in birthweight. Apparently, providing additional calories is a very inefficient process.

On the other hand at low levels of maternal nutrient intake the foetus can be considered to be a very efficient 'parasite' as demonstrated during the famine of the hunger winter 1944–1945 of World War Two, when basically healthy, well-nourished women were subjected to severe dietary deprivation [1]. In this study of daily food, supplies were cut down below 1000 kcal (4200 kJ) per day. A reduction in birthweight by only 200–300 g was recorded. In conclusion we may state that mean birthweight of a population with 'marginal' nutritional intake can

probably be increased by a higher nutritional intake during pregnancy (in terms of energy intake). However, the efficiency of this process is low and will most often lead to a higher maternal weight gain. Whether this increased maternal weight gain could be considered as an advantage (fat stores as a source of energy), or in case of extracellular water retention as a disadvantage (water), remains uncertain.

Birthweight versus risk factor

Increasing mean birthweight will reduce the incidence of low birthweight (<2500 g) and could reduce the risk factors and thus mortality in the perinatal period. If this assumption is correct, maternal dietary supplements during pregnancy could have a beneficial effect on the mortality in those populations of 'marginal' maternal nutrition. However this could not be proven by all studies quoted above. Two other aspects should be taken into account:
a) Reducing the incidence of low birthweight (<2500 g) by an elevation of the mean birthweight could reduce infant mortality/morbidity associated with a low birthweight, but will automatically induce a higher proportion of high birthweight babies (>4000 g) and thus increase the incidence of birth trauma with permanent brain damage to the infant. Should we take it seriously that many mothers in the unpriviliged societies prefer to have a small baby instead of a big baby?
b) Knowledge of the *gestational age* and subdivision of low birthweight infants in preterm and small for dates or a combination of these two groups is nowadays a more determinant factor in our management than the knowledge of the weight alone.

Pattern of perinatal growth in the 'tropics'

Growth rates, or velocity growth calculated in grams weight gain per kg body weight per day, are probably the best ways of expressing growth patterns in the early stages of development. Since the growth of foetuses in utero cannot be measured directly, standards for intrauterine growth can only be based on infants born alive at various gestational ages. Although it should be recognised that premature birth itself is an abnormal feature and will give an indeterminable bias in the data presented. Therefore the pattern of foetal growth as presented for Dar es Salaam, Tanzania [32] from life born infants can only be an approximation of the normal pattern of intrauterine growth. Alhough the intake of energy and proteins during pregnancy has been found to be lower [33] than the recommendations of W.H.O./F.A.O. [34], the speed of growth for weight, height and head circumference under these circumstances was greater during the last stage of pregnancy when compared to similar measurements in Montreal (Canada) [35].

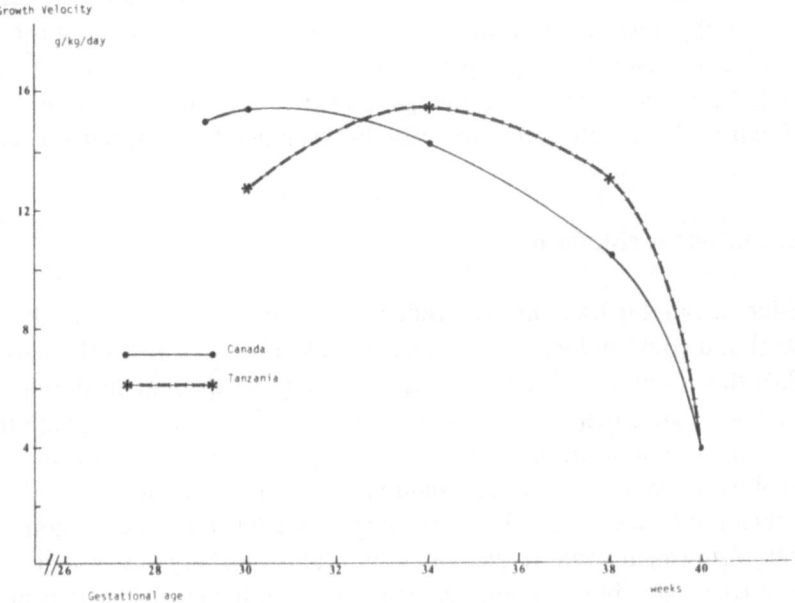

Figure 1. Prenatal velocity growth for Tanzania in comparison with Montreal. [32, 35] (grams per kilogram bodyweight per day)

This is illustrated by the weekly gain in weight, crown-heel lenght and head circumference for both sexes in Table 3 and by the velocity growth expressed in grams weight gain per kilogram bodyweight per day (Figure 1).

In both studies gestational age was assessed by the physical characteristics of the neonate. A different pattern of intrauterine growth, with a reduced speed of growth in the last stage of pregnancy was demonstrated in Ethiopia [18]. However, in this study gestational age was calculated from the last menstrual period. Information regarding the date of the last menstrual period was in the Tanzanian setting as in many other studies a less reliable tool to assess the gestational age and therefore rejected.

Postnatal growth

Postnatal studies on growth for both sexes from longitudinal or semi-longitudinal surveys from different countries with a reduced mean birthweight, but all receiving breastfeeding, as compared to an industrialized country, like the United Kingdom are reviewed by Waterlow et al. [36]. We calculated from these data the growth velocity in grams weight gain per kilogram bodyweight per day during the first 6 months of life, as presented in Table 4 and graphically illustrated in Figure 2. Included are data from the Harvard Study (USA). Although these studies

show many shortcomings and many possible sources of error, the general tendency seems clear: velocity growth is higher especially during the first month(s) of life whereas a reduced speed of growth is recorded in the following months. There is room for discussion about what these findings mean. Why this rapid weight gain of approximately 1 kg during the first month of life in countries like Tanzania, the Gambia, Nigeria, Singapore and similarly for Guatemala [37] as compared to 670 grams in the United Kingdom. A difference of more than 300 grams! At present it cannot be stated with certainty whether the increased rate of growth during the first month of life in the underprivileged countries can be explained by an increased energy intake or a reduced energy expenditure, e.g. at night when the infant usually shares the bed with the mother (reduced heat loss, nightfeedings) or a combination of both. We would like to emphasize that the most striking difference in the growth pattern of normal term infants for both sexes is focused on the first days of life as illustrated in Figure 3.

Table 3. Comparison of average intra uterine gain in weight, crown-heel length and head circumference for Dar es Salaam and Montreal for different gestational age groups.

Gestational age-groups	Average gain in weight per week of gestation (gram)		Average gain in crown-heel length (cm)		Average gain in head circumference per week (cm)	
	Montreal	Dar es Salaam	Montreal	Dar es Salaam	Montreal	Dar es Salaam
30–31 weeks	175	95	1.3	0.5	1.0	0.5
32–33 weeks	195	110	1.3	0.9	0.9	0.8
34–35 weeks	240	265	1.2	1.5	0.8	1.1
36–37 weeks	270	335	1.2	1.9	0.65	0.9
38–39 weeks	175	140	0.7	0.6	0.4	0.5

Table 4. Growth velocity in the first 6 months of life (grams weight gain per kg body weight per day).

Country	Months					
	0–1	1–2	2–3	3–4	4–5	5–6
Gambia	8.6	7.3	5.9	2.4	1.5	2.2
Singapore	9.1	7.1	4.6	3.2	2.1	1.5
Tanzania	10.5	5.8	5.5	2.7	1.4	1.6
Nigeria	10.1	6.2	4.3	3.2	1.9	1.5
mean	9.6	6.6	5.1	2.9	1.7	1.7
United Kingdom	6.1	6.8	5.3	4.2	3.4	2.6
USA (Harvard)	7.8	5.0	4.4	3.3	3.0	2.3

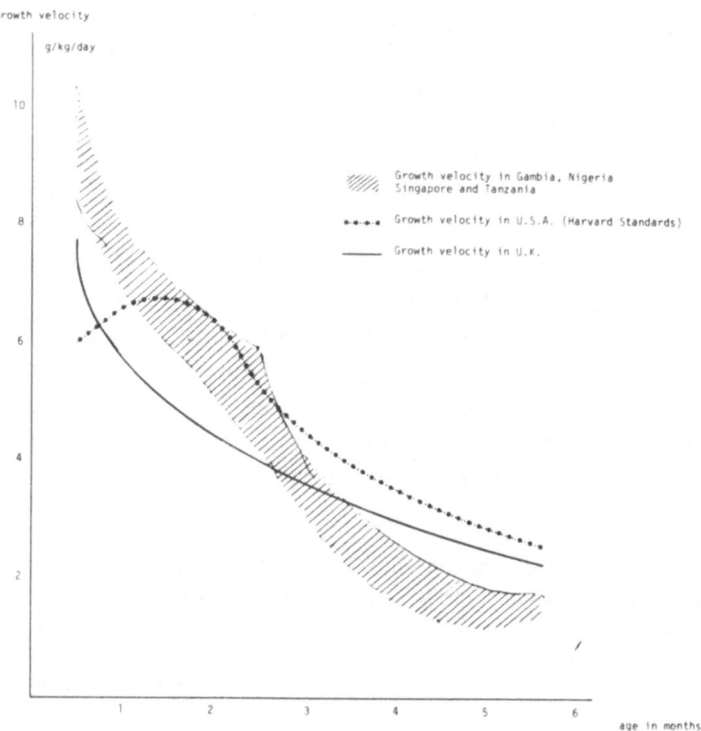

Figure 2. Post-natal velocity growth for Gambia, Singapore, Tanzania and Nigeria as compared to the United-Kingdom and the U.S.A. (Harvard). [36]

In Guatemala [37], similar to Tanzania with a mean birthweight of 2785 and 3027 gram respectively, weightloss from these infants is approximately 2–4% of the birthweght. In Dominica with a birthweight of 3252 gram, weightloss is approximately 6% of the birthweight, whereas in the industrialized countries, where the mean birthweight is approximately 3500 gram, on average 8–10%. In Tanzania and Guatemala it takes 4 to 5 days only to regain birthweight, but in Dominica it takes 7 days. In view of the fact that weight changes during the first days of life are related to total body water content [38], one factor to explain the differences in postnatal growth rate between the newborn in the industrialized and the developing countries could be that the foetus in the developing countries, like the mother, retained less body water per kg bodyweight during gestation. This will result in a reduced excretion of the excess of water in the first days postnatally.

Another factor to be considered after the first days of life, when adequate breastmilk production has been established, is the specific fatty-acid composition of the fat in breastmilk from mothers in countries with a high carbohydrate and low fat intake [39]. Dietary fat in young infants not only serves as the most

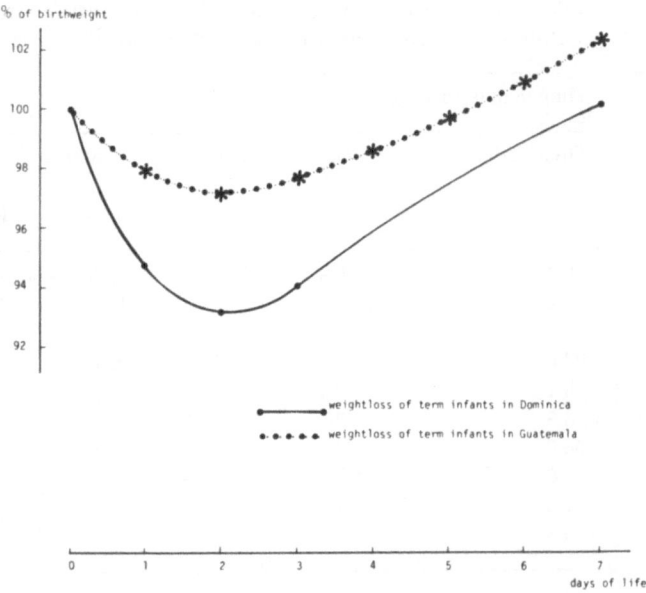

Figure 3. Neonatal weight changes as a percentage of birthweight from normal term infants in Guatemala and Dominica. [37, 20]

important source of energy but also contains nutrients essential for normal growth and development. In a study, which was conducted in cooperation with Professor Jonxis and Dr. Muskiet from the University Hospital in Groningen, the saturated fatty-acids in human milk fat from both 'rich' and 'poor' Tanzanian women contain a higher percentage of the medium-chain capric, lauric and myristic acids as compared to breastmilk fat from the Netherlands and Great Britain (Table 5). These medium chain fatty-acids are synthesized from glucose in the breast epithelial cells under circumstances of a high carbohydrate and low fat intake [40] of the mother. This specific fatty-acid composition of the fat in Tanzanian breastmilk will ensure even better intestinal absorption by the newborn infant when compared with the fatty-acid composition of human milk fat in the industrialized countries and the fat from most formula feeds. We hope to extend this research to other countries with a different feeding pattern. As far as postnatal growth is concerned, the problem remains whether we should consider the reduced speed of growth after the 3rd or 4th month as evidence of inadequate food intake and/or as, caused by, among other factors, the high incidence of recurrent infections.

We may conclude by stating that, like in many other fields of medicine, 'tropical' perinatology is different from 'Western' perinatology in many aspects. Differences are found in the physiology of the pregnant woman, the pattern of complications during pregnancy and during labour, the pattern of complications of the newborn infant during the first days of life, the physiology of the newborn,

Table 5. A comparison of the mean values for fatty acid composition of triglyceride extracted from breast milk collected from British, Dutch and Tanzanian women (9/100 g total fatty acids).

| | Human milk (mature) | | | |
| | Great Britain | The Netherlands | Tanzania | |
			'Poor'	'Rich'
C10:0 Capric	0.3	0.4	1.6	4.4
C12:0 Lauric	4.5	4.8	13.7	18.8
C14:0 Myristic	7.7	7.9	17.1	11.4
C16:0 Palmitic	27.6	26.3	23.0	11.6
C18:0 Stearic	8.1	7.1	2.3.	2.8
C16:1 Hexadecenoic	3.3	2.9	2.9	3.0
C18:1 Oleic	36.0	33.4	26.9	22.0
C18:2 Linoleic	7.0	12.4	12.4	16.4
C18:3 Linolenic	1.0	1.0	?	1.1
C20:4 Arachidonic	0.8	0.7	?	1.0

the growth pattern of the infant, the nutritional intake and many other aspects. It would be satisfying if we could convert our information about the association of poverty, age, primiparity, short stature, hypertension, smoking and probably undernutrition into knowledge of how the specific components contribute to a low birthweight infant, either preterm or small for dates. Apparently, within wide limits, the pregnant mother and the foetus are remarkably unaffected by dietary 'inadequacies'. Sofar it seems unjustified to measure perinatal health in terms of weight alone. More knowledge is required about the basic principles of 'tropical' perinatal physiology.

References

1. Smith CA: Effects of maternal undernutrition upon the newborn infant in Holland. J Pediatr 30:229–243, 1947.
2. Antonov AN: Children born during the siege of Leningrad in 1942. J Pediatr 30:250–259, 1947.
3. Sindram IS: De invloed van ondervoeding op de groei van de vrucht. Ned Tijdschr Verlosk Gynaec 53:30–47, 1953.
4. Darby WJ, McGanity WJ, Martin MP et al.: The Vanderbilt cooperative study of maternal and infant nutrition. IV: Dietary, laboratory and physical findings in 2,129 delivered pregnancies. J Nutr 51:565–597, 1953.
5. McGanity WJ, Cannon RO, Bridgforth EB et al.: The Vanderbilt cooperative study of maternal and infant nutrition. VI: Relationship of obstetric performance to nutrition. Am J Obstet Gynecol 67:501–521, 1954.
6. Thomson AM: Diet in pregnancy. 1: Dietary survey technique and the nutritive value of diets taken by primigravidae. Br J Nutr 12: 446–461, 1958.
7. Thomson AM: Diet in pregnancy. 3: Diet in relation to the course and outcome of pregnancy. Br J Nutr 13:509–525, 1959a.

8. Thomson AM: Diet in pregnancy. 2: Assessment of the nutritive value of diets, especially in relation to differences between social classes. Br J Nutr 13:190–204, 1959b.
9. Van de Rijst MPJ: Onderzoek naar de voeding van zwangere vrouwen en de gezondheidstoestand van moeders en kinderen te Amsterdam in de jaren 1950 en 1951. Voeding 23:695–751, 1962.
10. Osofsky HJ: Antenatal malnutrition: Its relationship to subsequent infant and child development. Am J Obstet Gynecol 105:1150–1159, 1969.
11. Winick M: Malnutrition and brain development. J Pediatr 74:667–679, 1969.
12. Brasel JA, Winick M: Maternal nutrition and prenatal growth. Experimental studies of effects of maternal undernutrition on fetal and placental growth. Arch Dis Child 47:479–485, 1972.
13. Rosso P: Placental growth, development and function in relation to maternal nutrition. Fed Proc 39:250–254, 1980.
14. Hytten FE, Chamberlain G (eds): Clinical physiology in obstetrics. Oxford, Blackwell Scientific Publications, 1980.
15. Humphreys RC: An analysis of the maternal and foetal weight factors in normal pregnancy. J Obstet Gynec Brit Emp 61:764, 1954.
16. Boersma ER: Perinatal circumstances in Dar es Salaam, Tanzania: studies on some physiological aspects in the tropics. Rotterdam, Bronder-Offset, 1979.
17. Venkatachalam PS, Shankar K, Gopalan C: Changes in bodyweight and body composition during pregnancy. Ind J Med Res 48:511, 1960.
18. Gebre-Medhin M: Maternal nutrition and its effect on the offspring. Uppsala, 1977.
19. Hosang N: Personal communication, 1981.
20. Sorhaindo BA, Soer RA: Personal communication, 1983.
21. Widdowson EM: Nutritional needs of the foetus and young child. In: Hambraeus L, Sjölin S (eds) The mother/child dyad. Stockholm, Almqvist & Wiksell International, pp 35–39, 1979.
22. Widdowson EM: Chemical composition and nutritional needs of the fetus at different stages of gestation. In: Aebi H, Whitehead R (eds) Maternal nutrition during pregnancy and lactation. Bern, Hans Huber, pp 39–49, 1979.
23. Beaton GH, Patwardhan VN: Physiological and practical considerations of nutrient function and requirements: Annex I. In: Nutrition and preventive medicine, WHO monograph ser no 62, 1976.
24. Tafari N, Naeye RL, Gobezie A: Effects of maternal undernutrition and heavy physical work during pregnancy on birth weight. Br J Obstet Gynaecol 87: 222–226, 1980.
25. Iyenger L: Effects of dietary supplements late in pregnancy on the expectant mother and her newborn. Ind J Med Res 55:85–89, 1967.
26. Quentin Blackwell R, Chow BF, Chira KSK, Blackwell BN, Hsu SC: Prospective maternal nutrition study in Taiwan: Rationale, study design, faesability and preliminary findings. Nutr Rep Int 7:518–532, 1973.
27. Mc Donald EC, Pollitt E, Mueller W, Hsuch AM, Sherwin R: The Bacon Chow study: maternal nutritional supplementation and birthweight of offspring. Am J Clin Nutr 34:2133–2144, 1981.
28. Rush D, Stein Z, Susser M: A randomized controlled trial of prenatal nutritional supplementation in New York City. Pediatrics 65:683–697, 1980.
29. Mora JO, De Paredes B, Wagner M et al.: Nutritional supplementation and the outcome of pregnancy. I: Birthweight. Am J Clin Nutr 32:455–462, 1979.
30. Lechtig A, Delgado H, Martorell R, Klein RE: Effect of maternal nutrition on the mother/child dyad. In: Hambraeus L, Sjölin S (eds) The mother/child dyad. Stockholm, Almqvist & Wiksell International, pp 74–93, 1979.
31. Hommes FA, Drost YM, Geraets WXM, Reyenga MAA: The energy requirements for growth: An application of Atkinson's metabolic price system. Pediatr Res 9:51–55, 1975.
32. Boersma ER, Mbise RL: Intrauterine growth of live-born Tanzanian infants. Trop Geogr Med 31:7–19, 1979.
33. Maletnlema TN, Bavu JL: Diet in pregnancy-Kisarawe study. Dar es Salaam. Nutr news 1973.
34. FAO/WHO: Energy and protein requirements. Tech rep ser nr 522, Geneva, 1973.

35. Usher R, McLean F: Intrauterine growth of live-born caucasian infants at sea level: Standards obtained from measurements in 7 dimensions of infants born between 25 and 44 weeks of gestation. J Pediatr 74:901–910, 1969.

36. Waterlow JC, Ashworth A, Griffiths M: Faltering in infant growth in less-developed countries. Lancet 1176–1178, 1980.

37. Mata JL: The children of Santa Maria Cauqué: a prospective field study of health and growth. Cambridge, MA, MIT Press, 1978.

38. Heird WC, Grebin B, Winters RW: The stabilization of disorders of water, electrolyte and acid base metabolism in newborn infants. In: Abramson H (ed) Resuscitation of the newborn infant. St. Louis, CV Mosby, 1973, p 240.

39. Boersma ER: Changes in the fatty acid composition of body fat before and after birth in Tanzania: an international comparative study. Br Med J 1:850–853, 1979.

40. Smith S, Thompson B: An evaluation of the contribution of endogenous mammary gland fatty acid synthesis to the overall composition of human milk fat. Pediatr Res 17:201A, 1983.

Maturity of the Nigerian newborn infant

S.A. OLOWE

Introduction

There are two features which will strike any paediatrician familiar with the Caucasian infant when he starts to work with the Nigerian neonate. These are: (1) very high perinatal and neonatal mortality rates and (2) a relatively advance maturity of infants weighing 2500 g or less at birth, i.e. low birth weight (LBW) infants.

Thus Morley found that whereas the overall neonatal mortality rate in Imesi-Ile was 157.6% of that in Birmingham, the mortality rate for the LBW infants in that Nigerian village was only 65.1% of that of their counterpart in the English city [1]. Similarly in a study of perinatal mortality in the University College Hospital, Ibadan, Platt was impressed with 'the lower mortality amongst the infants of booked Nigerian mothers in the lower weight group as compared with the British perinatal mortality series' [2]. In explaining their findings, these authors postulate that most Nigerian LBW infants are small for date and therefore appear more mature than white infants of the same weight group.

In trying to verify this hypothesis, one immediately encounters two problems. First, although there are many reports of the birth weight of Nigerian infants, in general, gestational age has been ignored in their analysis. The tendency has been to combine all birth weights and find the mean. The reported low average birth weights could therefore be the result of a large number of small full-term infants or of many preterm infants of appropriate weight at birth. The second problem relates to the definition of maturity. Maturity is a functional term, implying an ability of the infant to adapt to the demands of extrauterine life without artificial support. Therefore, we need a yardstick which can be used to compare objectively the maturity of the Nigerian with that of the white infant.

The objectives of this study were therefore:
1. to construct an intrauterine growth chart for a population of normal Nigerian infants, so that the chart can then be used to verify the proportion of Nigerian LBW infants that are truely small-for-date;

2. to study the development of amniotic fluid lecithin/sphingomyelin (L/S) ratio in normal pregnant Nigerian mothers as a measure of the pulmonary maturity of the Nigerian infant at various gestational ages. This is because pulmonary immaturity, manifesting as the respiratory distress syndrome (RDS), is the greatest cause of neonatal morbidity and mortality amongst the Caucasian infants [3].

Patients and methods

Four-hundred-and-thirty-six single liveborn infants delivered in the Lagos University Teaching Hospital (LUTH) between February 1975 and January 1980 were studied. All the mothers were Nigerians living in Lagos. They were from the middle socio-economic class as determined from their occupations and income. Those selected for this study had impeccable dates and began to attend our antenatal clinics during the first trimester of pregnancy. In each patient, the uterine size corresponded with the given date. Smoking is not yet common among Nigerian women and none of these mothers smoked cigarettes. They received prophylactic antimalarials throughout pregnancy. Mothers who later developed any complication were excluded from this study.

In 119 of the mothers who gave their consent to the procedure, amniotic fluid was obtained by transabdominal amniocentesis between 23 and 42 weeks of gestation. The amniotic fluid samples were analyzed for L/S ratio by the method of Borer et al. [4].

At birth the infants were examined and only those without congenital malformations were included in the study. Their gestations were calculated in completed weeks using the dates of the mothers' last normal menstrual periods. The birth weights were measured by the delivery room staff, using calibrated scales. All other measurements were made by the author within 6 to 48 hours after delivery. From these measurements, the means and standard deviations (SD) were calculated. Smoothed curves were then drawn and values for the mean ±2 SD were derived.

Results

Figure 1 shows the mean L/S ratio ±SEM obtained at each week of gestation. There was a gradual rise of the L/S ratio with increasing maturity. On the average, a mature ratio of 2.0 was obtained at 34 weeks gestation. In fact some infants had achieved this value from about the gestational age of 29 weeks.

Figure 2 shows the smoothed curve of the mean ±2 SD of the birth weights from 25 through 42 weeks' gestation. Smoothed curve values of the mean ±2 SD for crown-heel length, crown-rump length, head circumference and chest circum-

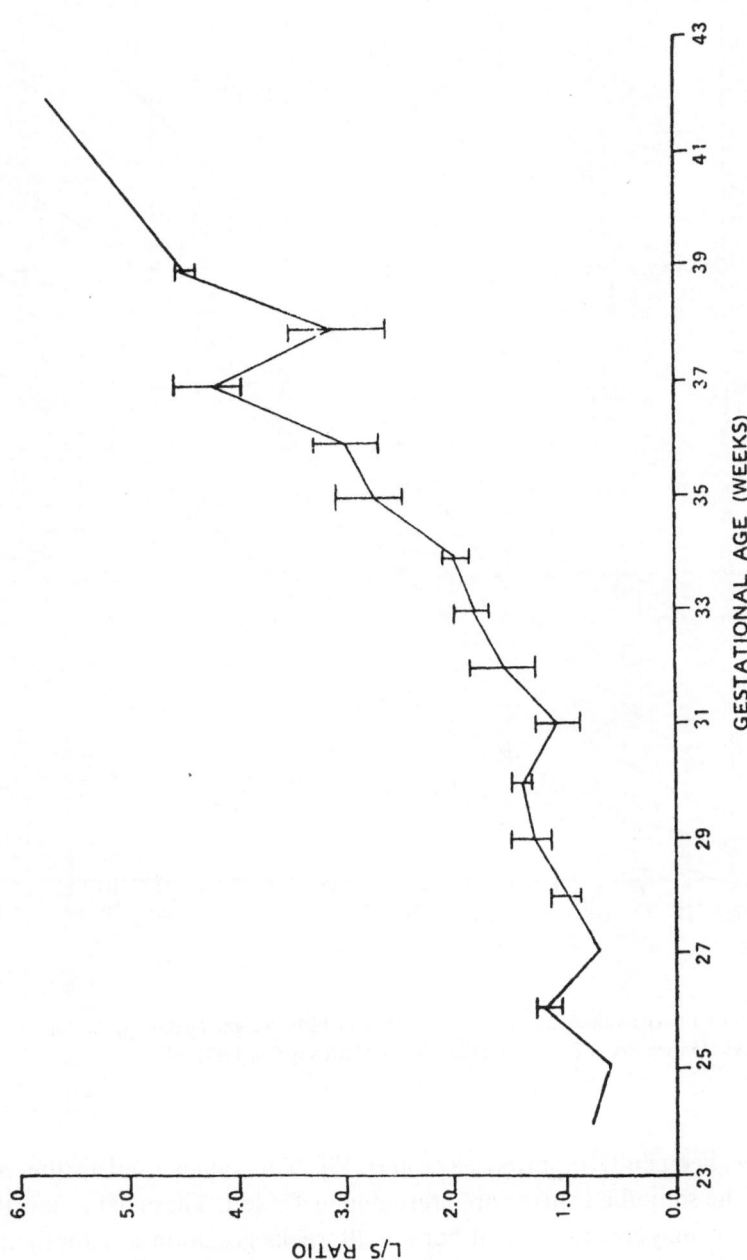

Figure 1. Mean L/S ratio (±SEM) related to gestational age (Olowe SA, Akinkugbe A: Pediatrics 62:38, 1978; American Academy of Pediatrics, 1978) [15].

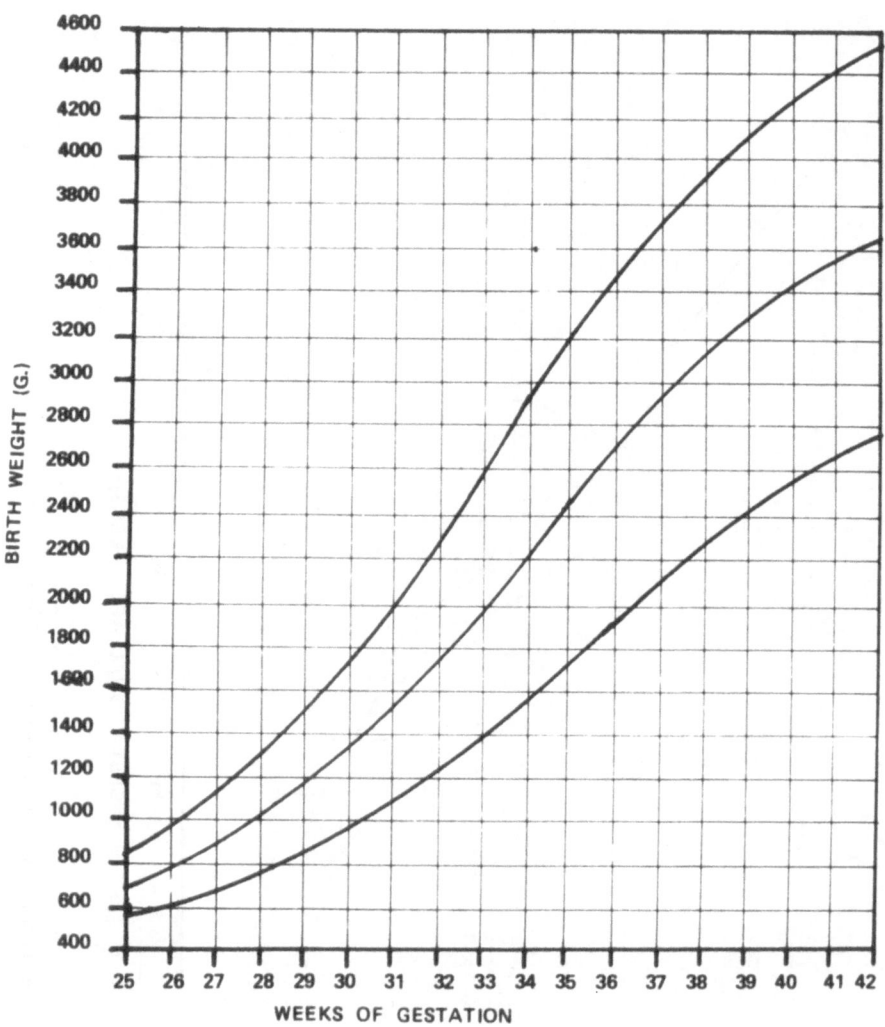

Figure 2. Smoothed curve values for the mean ±2 SD of birth weight against gestational age in completed weeks (Olowe SA: J Pediatr 99:489, 1981; CV Mosby Co, 1981) [5].

ference have been fully reported elsewhere [5]. The values used in the construction of the smoothed curves are presented in Table 1. These data show that the average normal Nigerian infant born at 40 weeks gestation has a weight of 3420 g, crown-heel length of 50.5 cm, head circumference of 35.5 cm and a crown-rump length of 33.6 cm.

Table 1. Smoothed curve measurements against gestational age.

Gestation (weeks)	Weight (g)			Crown-heel length (cm)			Head circ. (cm)			Chest circ. (cm)			Crown-rump length (cm)		
	−2 SD	Mean	+2 SD	−2 SD	Mean	+2 SD	−2 SD	Mean	+2 SD	−2 SD	Mean	+2 SD	−2 SD	Mean	+2 SD
25	600	680	760	29.5	32.5	35.5	19.0	21.0	24.0	15.7	18.5	21.3	19.0	21.2	23.4
26	640	780	900	31.0	34.0	37	20.0	23.0	24.0	16.7	19.5	22.3	20.1	22.4	24.7
27	680	880	1080	32.4	35.5	38.6	21.8	24.8	27.8	17.9	20.8	23.7	21.2	23.6	26.0
28	720	1000	1280	34.2	37.3	40.4	23.3	26.2	29.1	19.3	22.2	25.1	22.2	24.7	27.2
29	820	1160	1500	35.6	38.8	42.0	24.6	27.5	30.4	20.6	23.5	26.4	23.3	26.0	28.5
30	920	1340	1760	37.0	40.2	43.4	25.9	28.8	31.7	21.6	24.6	27.6	24.4	27.0	29.6
31	1040	1520	2000	38.2	41.5	44.8	26.9	29.8	32.7	22.7	25.7	28.7	25.4	28.0	30.6
32	1180	1740	2300	39.4	42.8	46.2	27.8	30.7	33.6	23.8	26.8	29.8	26.5	29.0	31.7
33	1340	1980	2620	40.6	44.0	47.4	28.7	31.5	34.3	24.9	28.0	31.1	27.0	29.7	32.4
34	1520	2220	2920	41.5	45.0	48.5	29.4	32.2	35.0	25.9	29.0	32.1	27.7	30.5	33.3
35	1680	2440	3200	42.5	46.0	49.5	30.2	33.0	35.8	26.9	30.0	33.1	28.4	31.2	34.0
36	1860	2640	3420	43.4	47.0	50.6	30.9	33.6	36.3	27.8	31.0	34.2	29.0	31.7	34.6
37	2080	2860	3640	44.4	48.0	51.6	31.5	34.2	36.9	28.6	31.8	35.0	29.6	32.5	35.4
38	2260	3060	3860	45.3	49.0	52.7	32.0	34.7	37.4	29.3	32.5	35.7	30.0	33.0	36.0
39	2460	3260	4060	46.1	49.8	53.5	32.3	35.1	37.7	29.7	33.0	36.3	30.3	33.3	36.3
40	2620	3420	4220	46.7	50.5	54.3	32.9	35.5	38.1	30.2	33.5	36.8	30.6	33.6	36.6
41	2780	3580	4380	47.2	51.2	55.2	33.2	35.8	38.4	30.4	33.7	37.0	30.8	33.8	36.9
42	2880	3680	4480	47.6	51.8	56.0	33.4	36.0	38.6	30.5	33.9	37.3	31.0	34.0	37.1

Discussion

Obstetric practice in Nigeria is often complicated by maternal malnutrition, infection, high twinning rate, and toxaemia [6]. All these conditions predispose to the delivery of LBW infants. The incidence of LBW infants in Nigeria is high, and has been estimated to lie between 13% in a general hospital [7] to 24.9% in a teaching hospital [8].

With such a high incidence of LBW infants, it is not surprising that the perinatal mortality rate is also very high. It is known that, in general, the lower the birth weight, the greater the mortality [9]. However, a major problem in estimating the magnitude of perinatal mortality in Nigeria is the lack of national data. But the hospital based records show that the perinatal mortality per 1000 deliveries might be as high as 52.3 in a general hospital [10] or 60.7 in a university teaching hospital [6]. These rates are very much higher than are now found among the Caucasians. In their highly industrialized and developed countries, perinatal mortality rates have fallen to levels of ten to 20 per 1000 livebriths and are still falling.

But when neonatal mortality rates are compared by weight groups, reports show that the survival of the Nigerian LBW infant is better than that of his white counterpart. To explain this paradox, it has been postulated that the Nigerian LBW infants are more mature than white infants of identical birthweights because the Nigerian infants are often small-for-date at birth [1, 2, 7].

The first problem with this hypothesis is the lack of valid intrauterine growth chart – a tool which is indispensable in the diagnosis of intrauterine growth retardation. The fact that a LBW infant thrives well after birth does not invariably mean that he is small-for-date. To make this diagnosis, one has to compare his birth weight with that of a population of normal infants born at the same gestational age in that community. Since important determinants of birth weight such as race, altitude, socio-economic status and intercurrent disease vary from one community to another, it will not be appropriate to adopt arbitrarily the standards published for some other population. We believe that our study has now satisfied the need for gestation-specific birth weight reference points for Nigeria. Our intra-uterine growth charts show that in the absence of maternal disease or environmental or socio-economic constraints, the intrauterine growth of the Nigerian infant is as good as that of the Caucasian infant (Figure 3). With these charts it should now be possible to identify the small-for-date Nigerian infant and to survey the true incidence of the abnormality in Nigeria.

The second problem with the hypothesis that the better survival of the Nigerian LBW infant is due to his reduced size at birth is the virtue which that hypothesis confers on intrauterine growth retardation. This is contrary to universal experience that when gestation is kept constant, neonatal mortality increases as birth weight decreases [11]. Also according to Butler and Bonham, LBW infants born at terms have a mortality ratio which is eight times higher than for babies weighing over 2500 g [12]. If poor intrauterine growth improves the survival

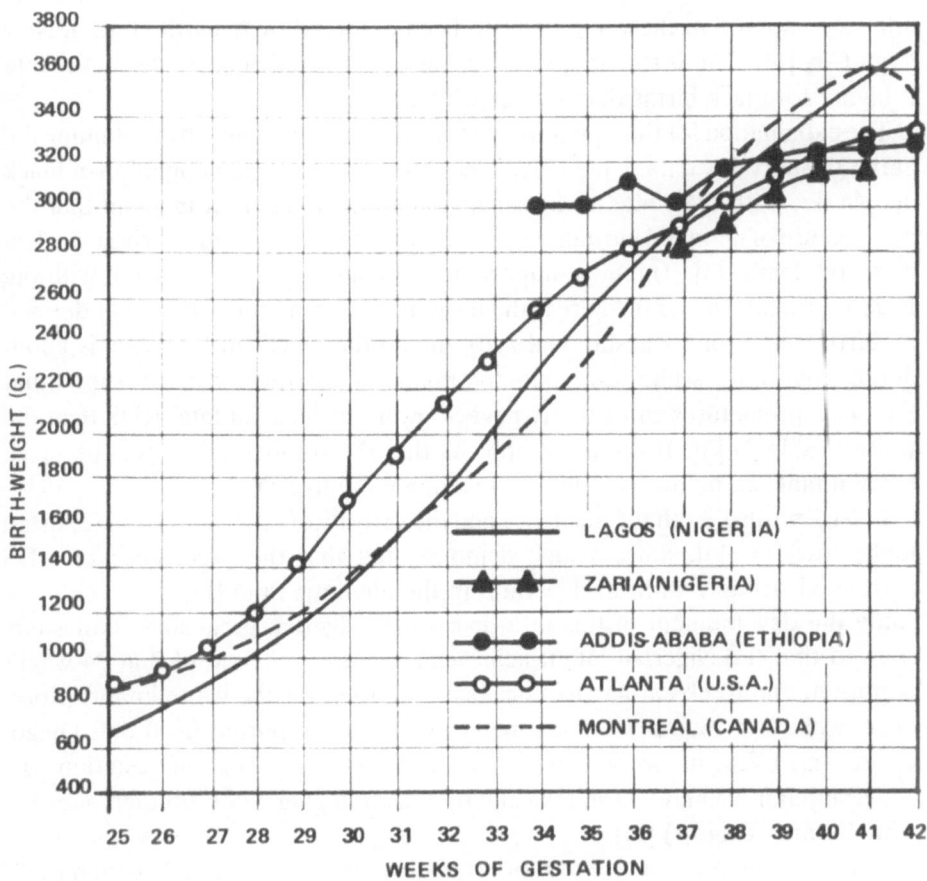

Figure 3. Comparison of the mean birth weights of black infants born in Lagos, Zaria, Addis-Ababa and Atlanta with the mean birth weights of white infants born in Montreal (Olowe SA: J Pediatr 99:489, 1981; CV Mosby Co, 1981) [5].

chance of the LBW infant, one should expect such infants born to mothers in the low socio-economic class to have a lower mortality rate than infants born to mothers in the high socio-economic class. But the reverse is the case. The figures published by North and MacDonald for Magee Women's Hospital, Pittsburgh, USA (1971–1974) show that among infants receiving the same medical care, neonatal mortality is lower for infants born to mothers in the upper socio-economic class than it is for infants of mothers of low socio-economic status (Table 2) [13]. So neither maternal poverty nor poor intrauterine growth confers any advantage on the LBW infant.

But when the neonatal mortality rates among white and black births were compared, North and MacDonald showed that in almost all LBW groups, black infants were more likely to survive the neonatal period than white infants of the same low birth weights (Table 2) [13]. A decreased mortality in black LBW infants compared to the white has also been observed by Erhardt et al. in New York City [14]. This is true in spite of the fact that overall neonatal mortality rate is higher for black births than for the white.

The explanation for this apparent contradiction may be found by examining the perinatal mortality data in the USA, a country where a large population of black people live with the white in the same environment. There it is found that the major cause of neonatal mortality is the RDS which accounts for nearly 20% of all neonatal deaths [3]. The most important aetiological factor associated with the RDS is prematurity. But whereas the incidence of prematurity (whether defined by birth weight or by gestational age) among the blacks in the USA is about double that of the white, examination of national mortality statistics shows that the black prematures consistently have a lower incidence of fatal RDS than the white (Table 3) [3]. It therefore appears that the survival factor for the black LBW infant can be found in his relative immunity to RDS.

In Nigeria also, both the incidence and the severity of RDS have been reported to be low [15, 16]. Since Gluck demonstrated that the occurrence of RDS correlated strongly with the L/S ratio in the amniotic fluid [17], we decided to study the development of this ratio in normal Nigerian pregnancy. Our study showed that the Nigerian infant achieves a mature L/S ratio of 2 at 34 weeks gestation, one week earlier than has been reported for the white infant. Moreover, when our figures were compared with those reported from San Diego, California, USA, it was observed that, at almost every week of gestation, the Nigerian infant achieves a statistically significant higher L/S ratio than does the white infant (Table 4) [15].

Thus, we find no evidence to support the hypothesis that more Nigerian LBW

Table 2. Neonatal mortality by race, birth weight and socio-economic status (ESE), Magee Women's Hospital (1971–1974)

Birth weight (g)	Neonatal mortality*			
	White		Black	
	High SES	Low SES	High SES	Low SES
500–1000	818	1000	900	861
1001–1500	446	333	230	238
1501–2000	98.4	120	50	44.9
2001–2500	24.5	28.0	0	11.3
2500	1.7	1.5	2.3	2.8
Total	8.5	13.5	15.5	19.0

* Neonatal mortality rates per 1000 live births (from the data of North AF, McDonald HM, copyright (c) CV Mosby Co, 1977) [13].

Table 3. Mortality rates by race (deaths per 1000 live births).

Neonatal deaths	1968	1969	1970
All causes/1000 TLB			
White	14.73	14.17	13.77
Other	21.53	21.42	21.43
HMD + RDS/1000 TLB			
White	2.299	2.401	2.537
Black	2.835	2.992	3.162
HMD + RDS/1000 PBW			
White	34.85	34.30	37.25
Black	18.58	21.15	22.99
HMD + RDS/1000 PBGA			
White	NA	28.83	32.52
Black	NA	16.06	17.85

Legend: TLB = total live births; PBW = premature births by weight (<2500 g birthweight); PBGA = premature births by gestational age (<37 weeks); NA = not available (Farrel PM, Wood RE: Pediatrics 58:167, 1976, American Academy of Pediatrics, 1976) [3].

Table 4. Comparison of L/S ratio in Lagos, Nigeria, and San Diego.

Gestational age (wk)	L/S ratio ± SD		p value
	Gluck & Kulovich	Present study	
23	0.44 ± 0.01	0.69	–
24	0.40 ± 0.20	0.70 ± 0.11	0.01
25	0.52	0.70 ± 0.21	–
26	0.55 ± 0.18	0.97 ± 0.34	0.05
27	0.70 ± 0.18	0.85 ± 0.18	0.20 (NS)
28	0.82 ± 0.11	0.88 ± 0.15	0.20 (NS)
29	0.62 ± 0.20	1.22 ± 0.55	0.025
30	0.82 ± 0.20	1.40 ± 0.35	0.0005
31	1.0 ± 0.48	1.09 ± 0.35	0.3 (NS)
32	1.0 ± 0.51	1.41 ± 0.76	0.10 (NS)
33	1.1 ± 0.38	1.77 ± 0.52	0.0005
34	1.5 ± 0.4	1.93 ± 0.23	0.005
35	2.1 ± 0.2	2.79 ± 0.95	0.0005
36	2.3 ± 0.3	2.83 ± 0.83	0.05
37	2.9 ± 0.6	4.20 ± 1.11	0.0005
38	3.5 ± 0.7	3.76 ± 1.47	0.3 (NS)
39	3.8 ± 1.2	4.46 ± 0.18	0.025
42	5.2 ± 1.4	5.73	–

(Olowe SA, Akinkugbe A: Pediatrics 62:38, 1978, American Academy of Pediatrics, 1978) [15].

infants survive the neonatal period because of intrauterine growth retardation. Rather, it would appear that the survival factor can be found in his more mature lung at birth, a characteristic which is probably shared by black LBW infants in the USA. We therefore believe that efforts directed at reducing the incidence of LBW and small for date infants in Nigeria would further increase the survival rate of these infants and decrease the present high perinatal and neonatal mortality rates in the country.

References

1. Morley D: Paediatric priorities in the developing world. London, Butterworth & Co. (Publishers) Ltd, 1973.
2. Platt HS: Perinatal mortality and maturity of the Nigerian newborn. MD thesis, University of London, 1970.
3. Farrell PM, Wood RE. Epidemiology of hyaline membrane disease in the United States: analysis of national mortality statistics. Pediatrics 58:167–176, 1976.
4. Borer RC Jr, Gluck L, Freeman RK et al.: Prenatal prediction of the respiratory distress syndrome (RDS). Pediatr Res 5:655, 1971.
5. Olowe SA: Standards of intrauterine growth for an African population at sea level. J Pediatr 99:489–495, 1981.
6. Nylander PPS: Perinatal mortality in Ibadan. Afr J Med Sci 2:173–178, 1971.
7. Lesi FEA: The incidence of prematurity in Lagos, Nigeria. West Afr Med J 16:132–134, 1967.
8. Adelusi B, Ladipo OA: Preterm and other babies with low birthweights in Ibadan. Trop Geogr Med 28:316–322, 1976.
9. Usher R: Clinical implications of perinatal mortality statistics. Clin Obstet Gynecol 14:885–925, 1971.
10. Sogbanmu MO: Perinatal mortality and maternal mortality in General Hospital, Ondo, Nigeria. Use of high risk pregnancy predictive scoring index. Nig Med J 9:123–127, 1979.
11. Lubchenco LO, Searls DT, Brazie JV: Neonatal mortality rate. Relationship to birth weight and gestational age. J Pediatr 81:814–822, 1972.
12. Butler NR and Bonham DG: Perinatal mortality. The first report of the 1958 British Perinatal Mortality Survey. Edinburgh, Livingstone Ltd, 1963.
13. North AF, MacDonald HM: Why are neonatal mortality rates lower in small black infants than in white infants in similar birth weight? J Pediatr 90:809–810, 1977.
14. Erhardt CL, Joshi GB, Nelson FG et al.: Influence of weight and gestation on perinatal and neonatal mortality by ethnic group. Am J Pub Health 54:1841–1855, 1964.
15. Olowe SA, Akinkugbe A: Amniotic fluid lecithin/sphingomyelin ratio. Comparison between an African an a North American community. Pediatrics 62:38–41, 1978.
16. Azubuike JC, Izuora GI: Incidence of idiopathic respiratory distress syndrome (IRDS) among neonates in Enugu. Nig J Paediatr 4:24–26, 1977.
17. Gluck L, Kulovich MV: Lecithin/sphingomyelin ratios in amniotic fluid in normal and abnormal pregnancy. Am J Obset Gynecol 115:539–546, 1973.

Neonatal intensive care in the developing countries: conservative or aggressive approach

S.R. DAGA and A.S. DAGA

Introduction

Modern neonatal intensive care symbolises sophistication, and high cost automatically follows. The projected requirements in terms of money, manpower and material involved put this treatment virtually out of reach for the developing countries. However, delivery of basic care, which is available to everyone in form of breastfeeding, thermoregulation by simple devices and prompt treatment of infections, can make a sea of a difference to the number of survivors.

1. Cost considerations

The exorbitant amounts of money spent on neonatal intensive care are really frightening. Here are some of the figures.

United States

1. Annual costs of neonatal intensive care units (NICU) in the U.S. were more than $1.5 billion [1].
2. The model budget for neonatal regional care centres for 8000–12,000 deliveries per year was $2.637 million [2].
3. Average cost per NICU admission was $10,000 [1].
4. Average cost per day was $500 [1].
5. For babies weighing less than 1000 g,
   (a) total costs per survivor were $40,287 [3];
   (b) daily costs of care were $825 [3];
   (c) costs adjusted per normal survivor were $88,058 [3].

Canada

Costs of care till discharge from NICU per baby with 1000–1499 g birth weight totaled $ (Can) 142,000 [4].

France

Cost per life saved without handicaps amounted to Fr. 4600 [5].

India

The annual model budget for NICU with 25–30 beds in India is recommended to be $ 200,000 with $ 150,000 as a non-recurrent and $ 50,000 as a recurrent expenditure [6].

Here are some reactions to the expenditure on neonatal care in affluent countries:

(a) 'Neonatal intensive care was found to be the highest priced treatment' [7].

(b) 'We must choose how to spend our limited dollars'.

(c) 'Parlous plight of the country's economy is common knowledge'.

Amidst such figures and opinions, our experience is likely to give a welcome respite. The model budget for a NICU in our own country, which is very much a developing country, has been found by us to be a luxurious one. We got this impression while studying the cost effectiveness of our unit.

2. Planning and evaluation of NICU

Planning of the NICU

Our unit has been in operation for over two decades, and average admissions are approximately 350 per year. A little less than half of these admissions are the inborn admissions from approximately 2500 deliveries per year. The remaining admissions are the outborn babies, transported from a radius of about 40 km of which approximately 50% are within 6 hours, 40% between 6 to 12 hours and 10% after 12 hours of birth. Most of them on admissions are hypothermic, appreciable number are hypoglycaemic and not an insignificant number acidotic due to delayed and bad transport.

About 5 years ago we started working to a plan. Lack of formal training in neonatology for the doctors and nurses, an unfavourable ratio of nurses to babies and inadequate facilities to diagnose and manage the problems of very preterm babies, however, did not detract from giving very basic care in terms of the following:

(a) ensuring mother's milk for most of the babies, (b) keeping the environment warm with simple devices and (c) prompt detection and treatment of diarrhoea.

(a) Ensuring mother's milk for most of the babies. We only acted as catalysts in bringing the mothers and babies closer and mothers were keen to feed the babies. Previoulsy the babies used to get breast feeds only between 8 AM and 8 PM to ensure adequate rest for the mother, soon a place was provided to the mothers where they could relax and feed the babies when the feed was due. More than 95% of these babies started getting their own mothers' milk.

(b) Keeping the environment warm. The unit is not air-conditioned and of course there are no radiant warmers. The nursery is divided into $3\,m \times 4\,m$ cubicles. Each cubicle has ordinary room heaters costing $\$15$ each and the temperature in cubicle with babies less than 24 hours old is maintained around $33°\,C$ and in others around $31°\,C$. In winter there are two room heaters at night and one during day. During other seasons one heater provided constantly at night and intermittantly during the day was found to be adequate. The absence of baby incubators for the past 2 years has not been felt, except while managing babies less than 1000 g.

(c) Prompt detection and treatment of diarrhoea. It took 3 years to feel death from diarrhoea to be a thing of the past. In the immediately preceding year, 10% of the admissions died of diarrhoea. All cases of diarrhoea were treated as infective ones. Primary sensitivity was sought in the index case. Thus the choice of a drug was available within 24 hours. This helped in choosing the right drug for subsequent cases.

In dehydrated babies oral rehydration by human milk has been successfully achieved for the past 4 years. Intravenous fluids were given only to babies in shock and for a minimum period. All the babies with diarrhoea received oral sodium bicarbonate in quantities depending on the severity of the case.

Cost studies

Cost studies were done in 1978 and again in 1980, i.e. before and after the human milk era, and the results were as follows:
1. Capital expenditures:
    Building: $\$7500$;
    Durable goods (furniture, utensils, instruments and equipments): $\$15,300$;
    Non-durable goods (linen, glassware): $\$3400$.
    Total: $\$26,200$.
2. Recurrent expenditures:
    Staff salary: $\$11,500$;

Milk and medicines: $2,500.

Total: $14,000.

In 1980 milk and medicine expenditures decreased to $1650; the rest remained unchanged.

Table 1. The distribution of health care expenditures.

Year	Average cost per bed per day on milk and medicines	Average bed occupancy (Total beds 20)
1978	0.6	11
1980	0.35	12

Causes of death in weight category <1000 g (1982).

Cause	Deaths (no.)	Cause specific mort. rate (%)
I.C.H.	9	47.36
Bronchopneumonia	2	10.52
Prematurity	3	15.78
H.M.D.	2	10.52
Sepsis	1	5.26
Gross I.U.G.R.	1	5.26
Apnoea	1	5.26
	19	

Leading cause of death was I.C.H.

89% deaths occurred within 24 h.

Showing yearly admissions (no.) and mortality (%).

Year	Admissions (no.)	Mortality (%)	Annual % decline
1978	374	55.8	
1979	306	53.2	2.6
1980	312	42.5	10.7
1981	336	33.0	9.5
1982	435	27.4	5.6

Effectiveness studies

Table 2. Showing yearly admissions (no.) and mortality (%).

Year	Admissions (no.)	Mortality (%)
1978	374	55.8
1979	306	53.2
1980	312	42.5
1981	336	33.0
1982	435	27.4

Thus mortality has shown a progressive decline.

Table 3. Showing yearly admissions (no.) and mortality (%) among inborn and outborn babies.

Year	Inborn adm. (no.)	Inborn mort. (%)	Outborn adm. (no.)	Outborn mort. (%)
1978	120	43.3	254	61.8
1979	152	44.7	154	61.6
1980	144	33.3	168	51.7
1981	177	24.2	159	42.7
1982	219	20.0	213	37.0

Thus the mortality has dropped in both inborn and outborn categories.

Table 4. Showing yearwise deaths (no.) early (<72 h) vs. late (>72 h).

Year	Admissions (no.)	Early deaths		Late deaths	
		(no.)	(%)	(no.)	(%)
1978	374	143	38.2	68	18.1
1979	306	78	25.4	75	24.5
1980	312	86	27.5	47	15.0
1981	336	74	22.0	37	11.0
1982	435	85	19.5	39	8.9

Thus there has been progressive decline in early as well as late deaths.

238

Table 5. Showing yearwise admissions (no.) and mortality (%) in weight category 1000–1250 g.

Year	Total adm.	Inborn adm.	Outborn adm.
1978			
Admissions (no.)	59	16	43
Mortality (%)	86.4	68.75	93.0
1979			
Admissions (no.)	48	18	30
Mortality (%)	75.0	61.1	83.3
1980			
Admissions (no.)	44	16	28
Mortality (%)	79.5	68.7	85.7
1981			
Admissions (no.)	54	19	35
Mortality (%)	66.6	78.9	60.0
1982			
Admissions (no.)	55	22	33
Mortality (%)	45.0	27.0	57.0

Causes of death in weight category 1000–1250 g (1982).

Cause	Deaths (no.)	Cause specific death rate (%)
Bronchopneumonia	8	32
I.C.H.	8	32
H.M.D.	3	12
Prematurity	3	12
Twin-twin transfusion	2	8
Sepsis	1	4

Leading causes of death were bronchopneumonia and I.C.H.
68% deaths within 48 h.
76% outborn.

Table 6. Showing early admissions (no.) and mortality (%) in weight category 1260–1500 g.

Year	Total adm.	Inborn adm.	Outborn adm.
1978			
Admissions (no.)	108	26	82
Mortality (%)	69.4	65.3	70.7
1979			
Admissions (no.)	77	28	49
Mortality (%)	55.8	42.8	63.2
1980			
Admissions (no.)	74	27	47
Mortality (%)	51.3	37.0	59.5
1981			
Admissions (no.)	65	25	40
Mortality (%)	35.3	36.0	35.0
1982			
Admissions (no.)	101	35	66
Mortality (%)	27.0	17.0	32.0

Causes of death, weight category 1260–1500 g (1982).

Cause	Deaths (no.)	Cause specific death rate (%)
Bronchopneumonia	7	25.9
Prematurity	5	18.5
I.V.H.	4	14.8
Sepsis ± N.E.C.	7	25.9
H.M.D.	1	3.7
Others.	3	11.1
	27	

Leading causes of death were bronchopneumonia, sepsis, I.V.H.
66% died within 48 h.
77% were outborn.

Table 7. Showing yearwise admissions (no.) and mortality (%) in weight category 1510–2000 g.

Year	Total adm.	Inborn adm.	Outborn adm.
1978			
Admissions (no.)	159	61	98
Mortality (%)	32.7	22.9	38.7
1979			
Admissions (no.)	141	88	53
Mortality (%)	39.7	38.6	41.5
1980			
Admissions (no.)	140	67	73
Mortality (%)	28.5	22.3	29.7
1981			
Admissions (no.)	121	68	53
Mortality (%)	17.3	8.8	28.3
1982			
Admissions (no.)	163	83	80
Mortality (%)	21.0	18.0	25.0

Causes of death weight category 1510–2000 g (1982).

Cause	Deaths (no.)	Cause specific death rate (%)
Bronchopneumonia	10	28.5
Prematurity	8	24.2
I.C.H.	7	22.8
H.M.D.	3	8.5
Sepsis	2	5.7
Other	5	14.25
	35	

Leading causes of death were bronchopneumonia, prematurity and I.C.H.
62% died within 48 h.
57% were outborn.

Table 8. Showing yearwise admissions (no.) and mortality (%) in weight category >2000 g.

Year	Total adm.	Inborn adm.	Outborn adm.
1978			
Admissions (no.)	20	5	15
Mortality (%)	35.0	20.0	40.0
1979			
Admissions (no.)	11	6	5
Mortality (%)	27.2	33.3	20.0
1980			
Admissions (no.)	41	28	13
Mortality (%)	21.9	21.4	23.0
1981			
Admissions (no.)	69	56	13
Mortality (%)	14.4	12.5	23.0
1982			
Admissions (no.)	88	70	18
Mortality (%)	12.5	10.0	22.0

Causes of death weight category >2000 g (1982).

Cause	Deaths (no.)	Cause, specific death rate
Asphyxia	4	36.36
Sepsis	3	27.27
I.C.H.	2	18.18
Birth trauma	1	9.09
Anencephaly	1	9.09

Asphyxia, sepsis, I.C.H. were leading causes of death.
54% died within 24 h.
63% inborn.

Relationship of mortality rate and birth weight.

Birth weight (g)	Mortality rate		
	General	Within 48 h	Outborn
<1000	67.85	89	–
1000–1250	45.45	68	78
1260–1500	26.70	66	77
1510–2000	27.0	62	57
>2000	12.5	54	37

Progressive decline as weight increases.
Maximum within first 48 h.
More in outborns (except 2000 g).

Table 8. Continued.

Leading causes of death in different weight categories.

Birth weight (g)	Leading causes
<1000	I.C.H., prematurity, bronchopneumonia, H.M.D.
1000–1250	Bronchopneumonia, I.C.H., prematurity, H.M.D.
1260–1500	Bronchopneumonia, sepsis, I.C.H., prematurity
1510–2000	Bronchopneumonia, prematurity, I.C.H.
>2000	Asphyxia, sepsis, I.C.H.

Thus tables 5, 6, 7 and 8 show that there has been a general progressive decline in all mortality in all the weight categories among inborn as well as outborn babies. However mortality among babies <1000 g remained unchanged at 85–90%.

Table 9. Showing yearly still births per thousand live births.

Year	Live births (no.)	Still births (no.)	Still birth rate
1978	2010	81	40.5
1979	2249	62	27.9
1980	2242	52	23.1
1981	2273	40	18.2
1982	2504	28	11.2

Thus there has been progressive decline in the still birth rate.

Table 10. Showing yearly early neonatal deaths (<7 days) per thousand live births.

Year	Live births (no.)	Neonatal deaths (no.)	E.N.D.R. early neonatal death rate
1978	2010	37	18.5
1979	2249	53	23.5
1980	2242	39	17.3
1981	2273	32	14.6
1982	2504	28	11.2

Thus early neonatal death rate has progressively declined.

Table 11. Showing deaths due to infections for the year 1978 and 1980.

Infection	1978			1980		
	Episodes (no.)	Deaths (no.)	Case fatality rate (%)	Episodes (no.)	Deaths (no.)	Case fatality rate (%)
Diarrhoea	95	41	43	32	8	25
Septicaemia	9	6	66.6	1	1	100
Umbilical sepsis	4	1	25.0	1	1	100
Pyoderma	6	–	–	2	–	–

Thus diarrhoeal episodes and diarrhoeal deaths declined by 1980.

Table 12. Showing periodicity of diarrhoeal episodes.

Month	1978	1980
January	9	5
February	15	–
March	7	–
April	6	–
May	13	–
June	5	15
July	11	8
August	9	6
September	6	4
October	4	–
November	5	–
December	5	–

Thus diarrhoeal episodes started making appearance in epidemics rather than being endemic.

Table 13. Showing follow up of babies discharged between January–April 1982.

Admissions	148
Discharges	113
Deaths during hospital stay	35
Transferred after brief observation	8
Regular follow up for one year	57
Responded to reminders & found well	21
Found doing well on home visiting	12
Families untraceable	12
Deaths after discharge	3

Table 14. Showing hospital stay (days) in different weight categories.

Year	1000–1250 g	1260–1500 g	1510–2000 g	>2000 g
1980	33.2	23.8	12.9	7.6
1981	24.5	19.7	12.8	4.2
1982	16.5	15.7	12.1	3.3
1983 (April to Aug.)	16.1	9.8	6.7	5.1

Thus hospital stays in all categories have declined progressively.

Another notable saving has been in the nursing hours. Earlier 45–50% of the duty hours were spent on either preparing or administering the feeds to the babies, now only 10% of the time spent on feeding the babies. Soon we went a step ahead. Babies taking mothers' milk by spoon and gaining weight were managed in postnatal ward. This resulted in drop in bed occupancy rate from 11 in 1980 to 7 in 1983, and nurse to baby ratio from 1.5:1 to 1:1.

Summary

Thus basic care in the form of breast feeding, thermoregulation and prompt treatment of infection resulted in saving of lives, saving of money, saving of nursing hours and reduction in hospital stay. Since breast feeding was continued upto 1 year, the post-neonatal mortality was even less than the general population, although these were the high risk infants.

In the year 1979 and 1980 much effort was made to convince the authorities to provide extra nursing staff, air-conditioning of the unit, better laboratory facilities, blood gas analysers, ventilators etc. However, the requests could not be granted due to financial constraints. Thus we became conservative without any option. However, we have now realised that it was a bliss in disguise. We have learnt that a lot could be achieved with the existing facilities. The reassessment of cost effectiveness in 1980 reaffirmed our belief and we have become conservative by choice and the belief is strengthening with time.

Secondly, it would be too optimistic to believe that the transport of the babies is going to improve dramatically in a near future, nor is it going to be cost beneficial. In the face of suboptimal quality of transport, upgrading the NICU in quality is going to meet with limited success. In short with reasonable goal in mind, conservative care has a lot to offer where NICU mortality is very high.

Summary and recommendations

1. Breast feeding, thermoregulation and prevention of infections can reduce NICU mortality substantially.
2. These can be achieved at a very low cost.
3. It is strongly felt that conservative care in this form can bring down the mortality to 15 per cent.
4. Further drop cannot be achieved without good transport facilities, ventilator therapy and matching obstetric services.
5. Breast feeding saves nursing hours.
6. Maternity ward can be effectively used as an intermidiate care nursery.

References

1. Phibbs CS, Williams RL, Phibbs RH: Newborn risk factors and costs of neonatal intensive care. Pediatrics 68:313–321, 1981.
2. Committee on Perinatal Health: Toward improving the outcome of pregnancy, White plains, N.Y. 1976. National Foundation, March of Dimes.
3. Pomerance JJ, Ukrainski CT, Ukra T, Henderson DH, Nash AH, Meredith JL: Cost of living for infant weighing 1000 g or less at birth. Pediatrics 61:908, 1978.
4. Boyle MH, Torrance GW, Sinclan JC, Horwood SP: Economic evaluation of neonatal intensive care of very low birth-weight infants. N Engl J Med 308:1330–1337, 1983.
5. Chapalain MT: Perinatality: French cost-benefit studies and decisions on handicap and prevention. In: Ciba Foundation Symposium 59 (New series) Amsterdam Excerpta Medica, 1979, pp 755–761.
6. Recommendations on neonatal care in India, 1981, p 88.
7. Schroeder SA, Showstack JA, Roberts E: Frequency and clinical description of high-cost patients in 17 acute care hospitals. N Engl J Med 300:1306–1309, 1979.
8. Davies PA: Perinatal mortality. Arch Dis child 55:833–837, 1980.

Determinants of fetal growth and early postnatal growth in a rural area of Indonesia

A. ALISJAHBANA and A. USMAN

Introduction

Prenatal and postnatal growth are influenced by biological factors of the mother as well as her socio-economic conditions. Reports from most countries show more affluent families have a higher mean birthweight and a lower percentage of low birth weight (LBW) infants [1]. Various studies on the relationship of social environment and birthweight also stress the importance of the social environment although it is difficult to classify any specific social factors that might contribute to the percentage of LBW [1, 2].

Information on fetal growth is mostly indirect, using retrospective data from birth records. Data using gestational age are usually applied in developed countries. Contrary to this, in developing countries, particularly in rural areas where knowledge is poor and illiteracy is high, gestational age from maternal menstrual history is difficult to obtain [3, 4].

Other constraints in obtaining data from birth records in rural areas, are poor reporting and recording because of the high percentage of home deliveries and deliveries carried out by traditional birth attendants [4].

At present, there are no official standards for Indonesian fetal growth and previous studies on birth weight distribution have also not been related to gestational age. Reports available are mostly from Teaching Hospitals where more abnormal deliveries are made and referral cases are delivered.

Fetal growth in humans is affected by a host of factors, including maternal age, parity, birth interval, gestational age and sex of the infants. These factors are considered basic to all pregnancies. Other factors, which may be considered to be abnormal and may appear only in some pregnancies, can be categorized into three groups: fetal factors, complication of pregnancy and environmental factors [2, 5]. Compared to infants born in Teaching Hospitals, fetal factors and medical complications of pregnancy, showed a relatively lower incidence in rural areas [4]. Consequently, biological and environmental factors are more important. Included in environmental factors are the socio-economic circumstances, and

women from poor socio-economic circumstances in particular may exhibit some of the behaviour shown below [2]:
1. delivery before 20 and after 35 years of age;
2. lack of antenatal care;
3. high parity;
4. low maternal weight gain during pregnancy.

Other factors of some importance are:
1. illiteracy or a low level of education;
2. low income;
3. poor living standards.

The aim of the present study is to examine the effects of maternal, biological, nutritional and environmental factors on fetal growth in a rural area, rather than on the statistics of normally grown fetuses.

The subjects were infants born during the perinatal mortality and morbidity survey carried out in 3 locations in Bandung, West Java between 1978 and 1980. This survey was sponsored by the WHO-SEARO. One of these locations was the district of Ujung-Berung, a rural area 15–20 km outside Bandung. The altitude of the survey area was approximately 600 m above sea-level. The total population studied was approximately 40,787 of which 16.5% were females of reproductive age (15–44 years). Occupational distribution showed a high percentage of farmers and unskilled labourers. Unemployment is high at a rate of 20.5% for males over 15 years of age. The total fertility rate for married women in one survey area was 5.9; experiences of child death was universal and nearly two-thirds of the women over 30 years of age had experiences of child loss [7]. The educational level of married women in the project area showed more than 79.8% as having received some years of primary schooling; the illiteracy rate was 12.7%. The crude birth rate was 38‰ population, the crude death rate 13.2‰. Perinatal mortality rate 45‰ deliveries and the infant mortality rate was estimated to be 120‰ live births. Maternal mortality rate on the other hand, was 1.7‰ live births.

The causes of perinatal deaths were mainly asphyxia and tetanus. The total incidence of LBW was 14.7%, while the total mean birth weight was 2975 grams.

Maternity and methods

Information on age, parity, birth interval as well as antenatal educational status was collected by research midwives living in the survey area. Maternal anthropometric measurements including weight, height, mid-upper-arm circumference (MUAC) were taken. Because of some difficulties, continual measurement of weight gain during pregnancy was not done, but the weight at 32 weeks of gestation was taken. Birth weight, birth length and head circumference were obtained mainly during the first 24 hours of life, and in approximately 20% of cases this information was collected within three days of delivery. An infant weight balance, checked daily for zero adjustment, and a modified infantometer with the infant flat on his back and legs extended were used to measure crown to heel lengths. Head circumference was measured with a fibre-glass tape at the largest fronto-occipito circumference.

The gestational age was available in only 1796 single live born infants (78.8%). Therefore data on fetal growth on this group of infants were only analysed for the 10th, 50th and 90th percentiles. A follow-up throughout the neonatal period was carried out on only 1750 infants still alive at 28 days. On this group of infants, weight increase during the neonatal period was calculated.

In the survey area nearly all infants were breastfed and those who were not were mostly infants who were small or sick and who died in the neonatal period. These infants were excluded from the analysis.

Results

The total mean birth weight in this series of 2278 single live born infants was found to be 3009 grams, while the percentage of low birth weight was 13.1%. Infants with known gestational age showed a mean birth weight of 2968 grams at term (37–42 weeks), and mean gestational age of 39.8 ($\pm$1.3) weeks.

Anthropometric measurements at birth

Fetal growth of single live born infants in the survey area was measured in weight, length and head circumference and estimated between 32 and 43 weeks of gestation. Infants with less than 32 weeks gestation were excluded because of their low number and infants with congenital malformation were also excluded. Weight–length ratio was calculated according to the Rohrer's ponderal index [2, 8]. The index measures how heavy the baby is for its length and age; the larger numbers portray a heavy-for length and the smaller numbers describe an infant who is thin for its length. The 10th, 50th and 90th percentiles were calculated for each anthropometric measurement and the results were compared with the results of a survey carried out on infants from better socio-economic conditions. The data on the last group of infants were the result of a survey carried out in 1976 on live born single infants from middle and upper socio-economic classes born in a Maternity hospital in the urban area of Bandung. Included were infants of mothers with known last menstrual period and without any signs of complications during pregnancy. The urban survey was carried out in order to obtain a standard intrauterine growth index for Indonesian infants in Bandung [6].

Fetal growth curves of infants born in the rural area were compared with growth data from the urban area and revealed results shown in Figure 1.

The 10th, 50th and 90th percentiles for each week of gestation of infants from

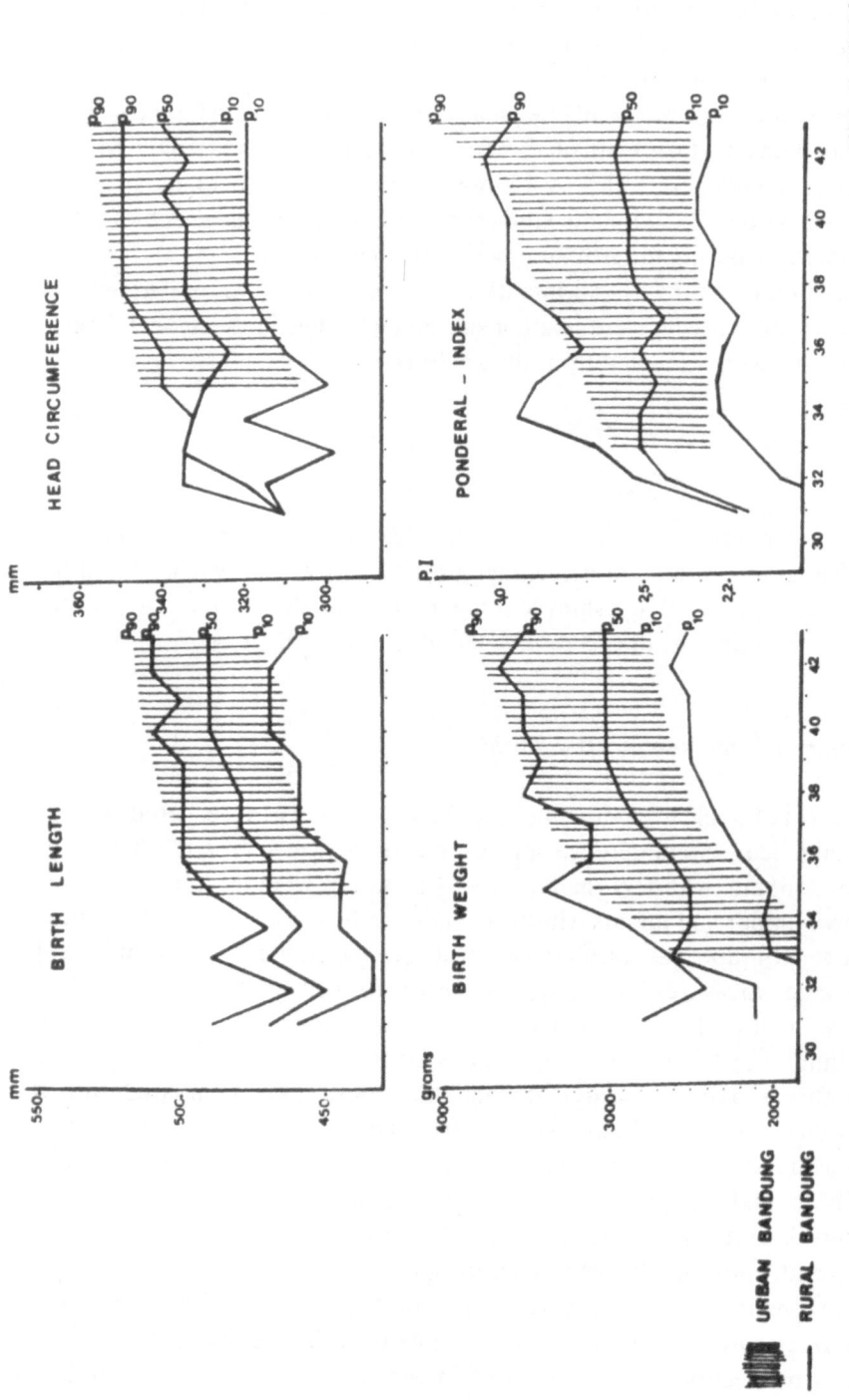

Figure 1. Percentiles of intrauterine growth in weight, length, head circumference and weight–length ratio of infants from rural and urban areas of Bandung.

the rural area were plotted against the intrauterine curves of infants from the urban population with better socio-economic conditions. It can be seen that there was little difference in the growth curves although the rural infants showed slightly lower curves. It is interesting to find a flattening of the growth curves after 36 weeks of gestation in all measurements but the difference is not significant, in rural infants. Irregularities in the earlier gestational weeks may be due to the difficulties in evaluating the gestational age which was based on interviews. Another factor is the few cases of short gestation.

To give some international comparison, the mean birth weights of rural infants was compared to Colorado data which was not expected to be very different from the Indonesian population [6,9]. The result showed nearly similar mean birth weight in the shorter periods of gestation and a flattening of the growth curve near term of rural Bandung infants.

Relationship of maternal factors and birth weight

Mean birth weight and percentage of low birth weight is often used to evaluate the influences of independent variables on fetal growth. Figures 3 and 4 illustrate this relationship among maternal biological factors on birth weight and percentage of LBW.

Figure 3 shows the relationship between maternal parity, and mean birth weight. The curves are similar to those in Figure 4 for maternal age. The mean birth weight increases with increasing parity and the percentage of low birth weight falls as parity rises, except in high parity where an increase in the percentage of low birth weight is shown.

The relationship between maternal nutritional status and birth weight can be seen in the Figures 5, 6 and 7. For this purpose maternal height, mid-upper-arm circumference (MUAC) and weight at 32 weeks of gestation was used for evaluation.

Maternal height, MUAC and weight showed a relationship which is similar among each variable. Compared to maternal height, MUAC and weight at 32 weeks showed a better relationship.

Maternal weight at 32 weeks of gestation shows a relationship strongly associated with low birth weight and with women with the highest weight gain having the highest mean birth weight.

The mean weight of pregnant women at 32 weeks of gestation was 49.9 kg while the mean weight of non-pregnant Indonesian women in the reproductive period ranged from 40–47 kg [10, 11]. Low weight in non-pregnant and non-lactating women was found particularly in rural areas. These data give the impression that weight gain during pregnancy was not very high in this area. More specific research is needed to investigate the relationship of weight gain and mean birth weight, as this survey was unable to demonstrate the relationship between pre-

252

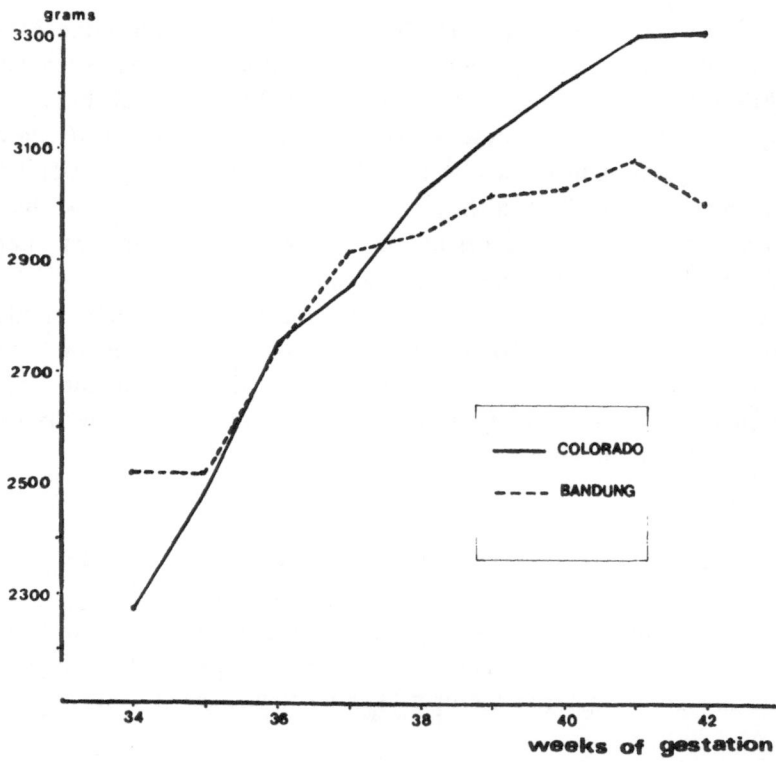

Figure 2. Comparison between mean birth weight of rural infants and Colorado's data.

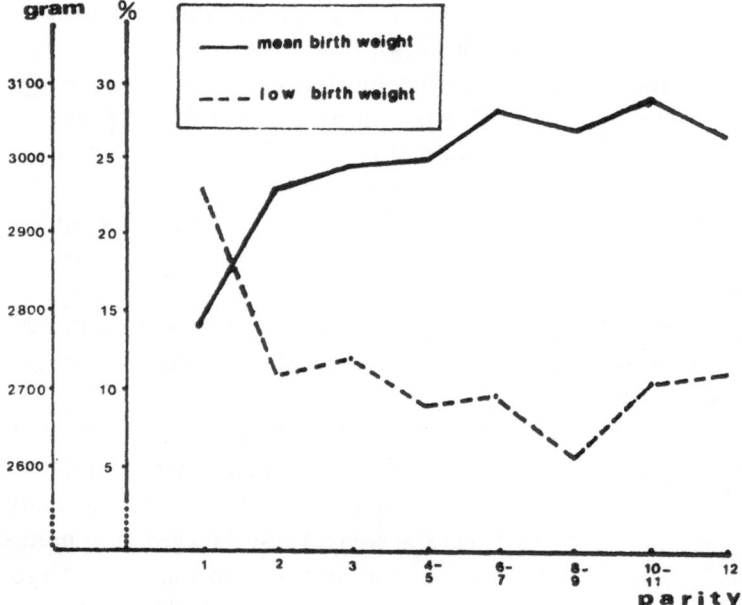

Figure 3. Relationship between maternal parity, mean birth weight and low birth weight.

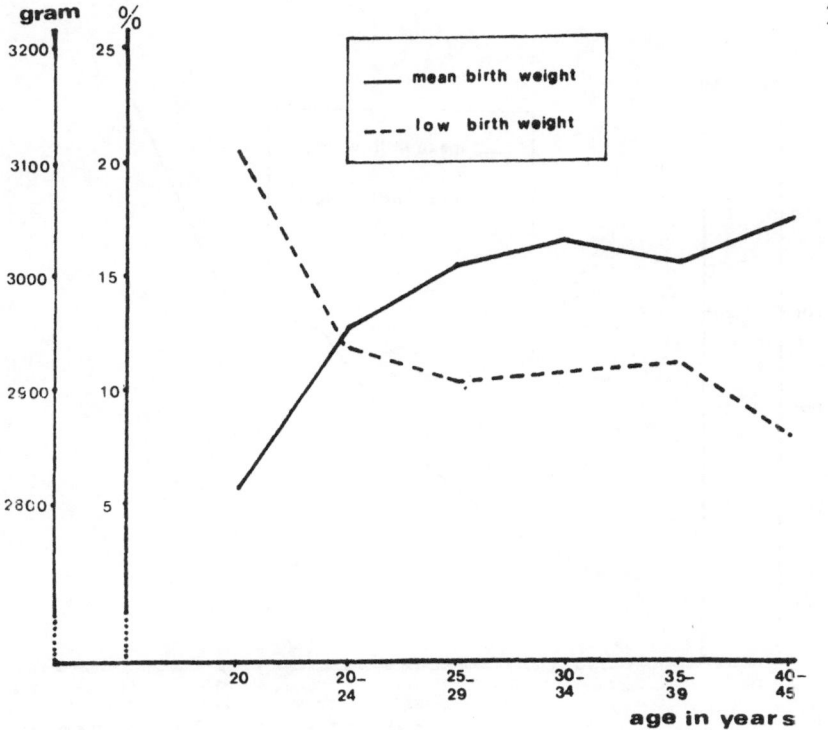

Figure 4. Relationship between maternal age, mean birth weight and low birth weight.

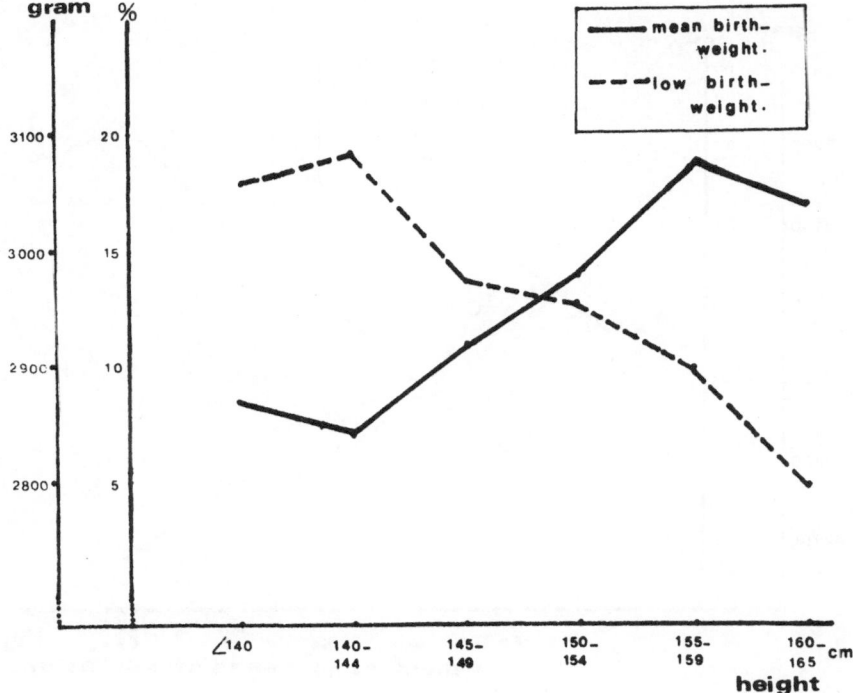

Figure 5. Maternal height, mean birth weight and low birth weight.

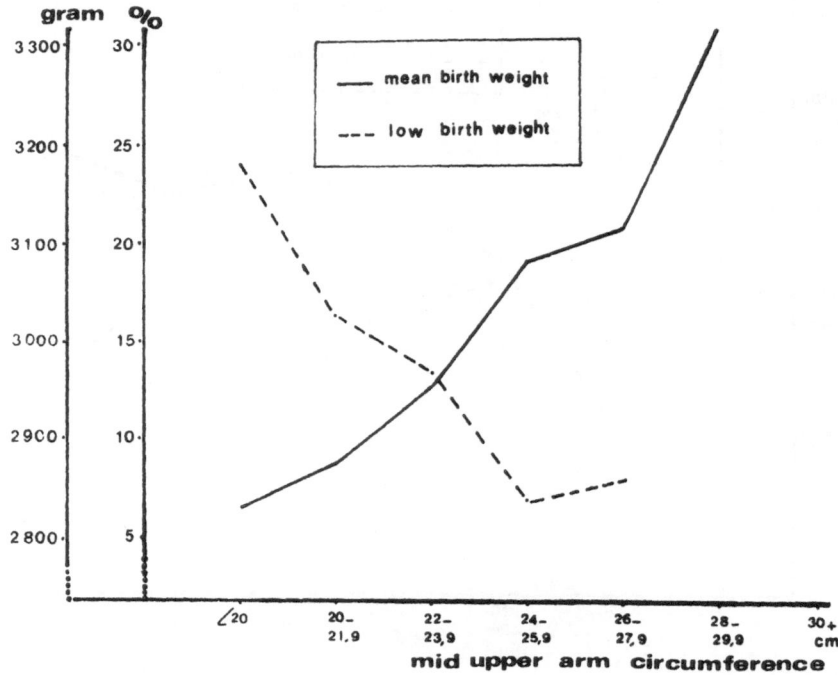

Figure 6. Maternal MUAC, mean birth weight and low birth weight.

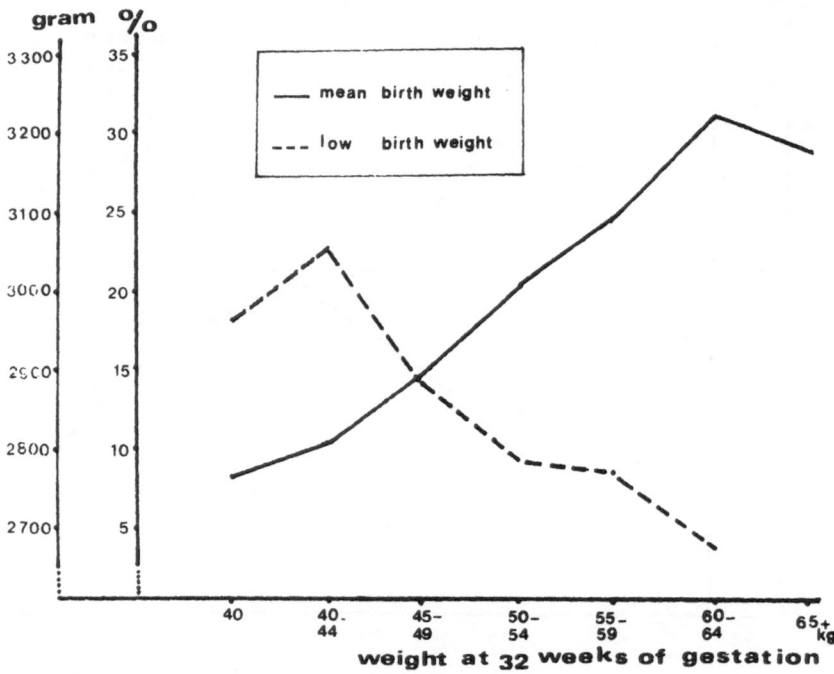

Figure 7. Maternal weight at 32 weeks gestation, mean birth weight and low birth weight.

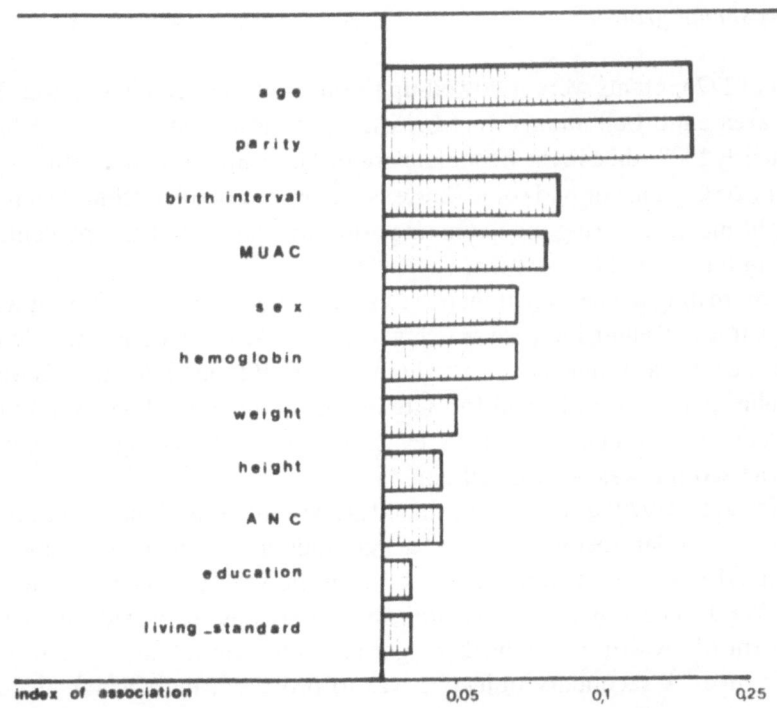

Figure 8. Factors associated with low birth weight.

pregnancy weight and mean birth weight.

It is well known that low birth weight is a universal problem and in all populations it is the single most important determinant of the chances of the newborn to survive and to experience healthy growth and development

Therefore it is of particular importance to understand the relationship of low birth weight to each specific variable.

Multiple regression analysis was carried out to isolate the relationship of 11 individual factors to low birth weight and rank the individual factors in order of their importance as determinants of low birth weight.

As can be seen, maternal age, parity, birth interval, sex of the infants and Hemoglobin concentration are the strongest determinants followed by weight and height. Factors such as antenatal care, education and socio-economic conditions are at the bottom of the list. Multiple regression analysis indicated in Figure 8 cannot explain the observed associations with LBW. The coefficient correlation is found to be $R^2 = 0.09$ or $R = 0.299$, which means that all these factors are statistically not significant as determinants of low birth weight at level of significance $p = 0.05$.

Early postnatal growth

A total of 1775 infants were followed-up throughout the neonatal period. In the survey area almost all infants were breastfed; of those who refused any kind of food, nearly 100% died in the neonatal period. These infants had a birth weight of less than 2000 grams or had some illnesses and were excluded from the analysis.

Weight increase during the neonatal period was calculated as a percentage of the mean birth weight.

It is interesting to see weight increase as a dependent variable of birth weight. In this survey, weight increase was highest if mean birth weight was low and showed a decrease as mean birth weight increased. It is possible that this was due to a higher percentage of small-for-date infants in the lower birth weight group and needs further investigation as evaluation of gestional age by means of Dubowitz scoring was not carried out.

Martell et al. (1979) developed postnatal growth curves for infants of Caucasian mothers of similar socio-economic backgrounds in Montevideo. Tables were constructed based on a new criterion: mean growth velocity per weight unit (MGU/WU). The object of designing this curve was to provide data for an assessment of growth of low birth weight and full term infants in their normal weight range. A secondary objective was to provide a method for evaluating growth velocity. The author stated that these growth curves can be used to evaluate weight gain in developing countries [12].

If postnatal growth of infants in the rural area survey was plotted on Martell's curve the results in Figure 10 would follow.

It can be seen that weight gain of the rural infants in the first month of life is within the adequate range. For larger infants weighing more than 4000 grams, the weight gain showed a sharp decrease reaching an insufficient weight gain at percentile 25.

The total mean weight gain for infants in the survey area, during the neonatal period was 843 grams, which is not statistically different with the mean weight gain of 816 grams in Martell's series for infants with an initial weight between 1400–4000 grams ($p > 0.05$). Fomon stated that 'failure to thrive' should be defined as a rate of gain in length and/or weight less the value corresponding to twice standard deviation of the mean during an interval of at least 56 days for infants less than five months of age [12]. Contrary to this statement, Martell et al. define insufficient weight gain as weight gain less than percentile 25, which is near one standard deviation of the mean. Ruth Lawrence suggests that in managing the breastfed infant a careful medical evaluation should be provided for infants who do not regain weight by 3 weeks of age or gain at a rate below the 10th percentile beyond one month of age [13].

Mean weight gain for the rural area was found to be 843 grams while one standard deviation is 245 grams. Using Mantell's criteria this study used weight gain less than 600 grams as criteria for insufficient weight gain, and the infant was

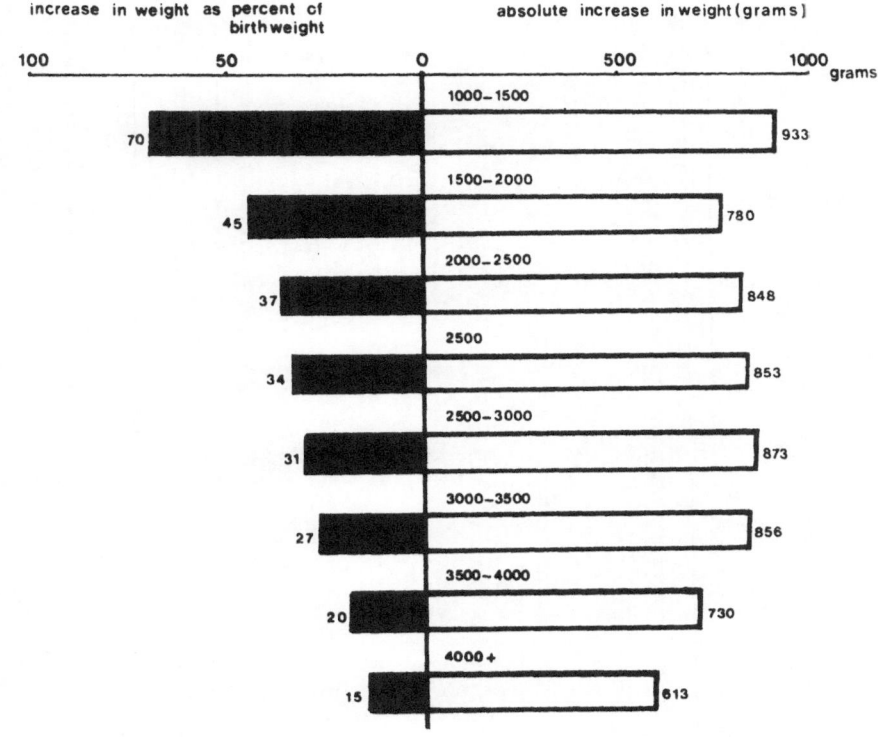

Figure 9. Weight increase over the first 28 days of life.

considered at risk. Maternal factors and infants associated with insufficient weight gain is shown on Table 1. The total number of infants with insufficient weight gain were 112 infants or 6.3%.

As can be seen, there is no significant difference in the mean anthropometric measurements of the mother. Mothers in this area, who had infants with insufficient weight gain showed a lower hemoglobin concentration, and the difference is statistically significant. Infants from lower living standards were significantly higher in the insufficient weight gaining group. The main factor influencing infant weight gain is birth weight. The group with insufficient weight gain had a significant higher percentage of low birth weight infants.

Discussion

All studies of fetal growth have errors in determination because of the difficulties in measuring anthropometric parameters exactly. This is especially true in rural areas of developing countries like Indonesia, particularly because pregnant women are not sure of their last menstrual period. This error may be com-

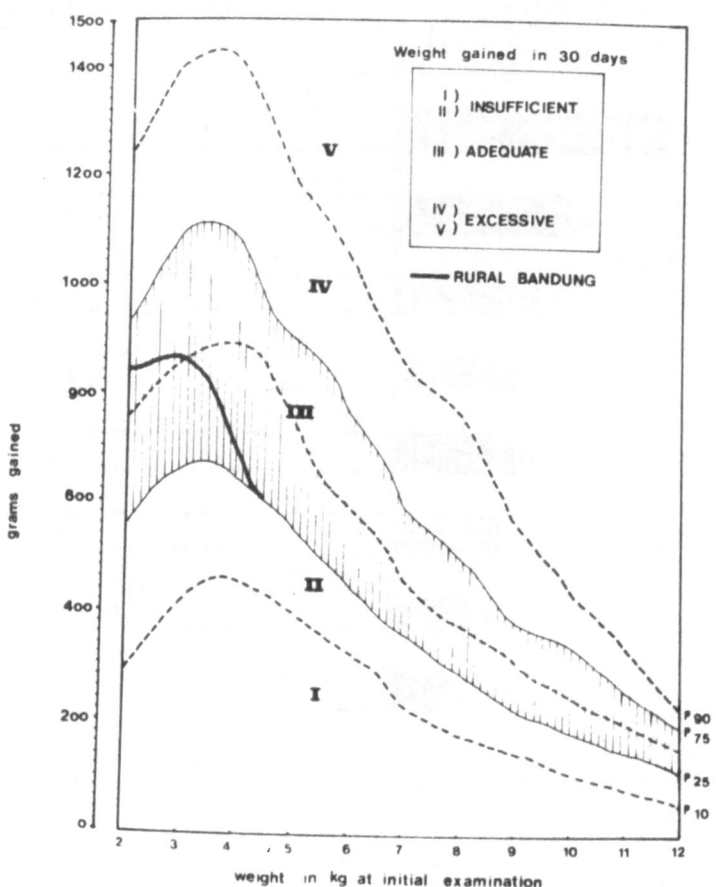

Figure 10. Weight gain of rural infants in the first month of life plotted on Martell's growth curve.

Table 1. Factors associated with insufficient weight gain.

Variables	Weight gain		Significant at p = 0.05
	<600 g	≥600 g	
Maternal factors			
Mean age	26.2 (±6.1)	26.1 (±6.3)	NS
Mean parity	3.25 (±2.6)	3.87 (±2.7)	NS
Mean height (cm)	149.4 (±4.6)	149.3 (±4.5)	NS
MUAC (cm)	22.1 (±2.3)	22.5 (±1.6)	NS
Hemoglobin (g/dl)	10.8 (±1.7)	11.2 (±1.7)	S
Poverty (%)	26.8	24.7	S
Infant factor			
Low birth weight (%)	25.9	11.2	S

Legend: NS = Not significant; S = Significant.

pounded by vaginal bleeding in early pregnancy or because of occurrence of pregnancy during lactation [3, 8].

Evaluation of fetal growth in these areas is facing other problems because so far no standard measurement of fetal growth for Indonesia is available due to poor reporting and recording of births and birth weights. Available data come mostly from (teaching) hospitals. Nevertheless, this survey attempted to analyse infants with known gestational age and compare it with unpublished data of infants born in hospital/maternity clinics under better socio-economic conditions. The survey was carried out in Bandung during 1976. The results show that fetal growth for weight, length and head circumference in the earlier weeks of gestation were similar or slightly lower than the urban population. Rural infants growth curves cease slightly near term. A more obvious difference was found if fetal growth pattern of rural infants was compared to the Colorado data. Mean birth weight after 32 weeks of gestation was nearly the same until the infants reached 36 weeks of gestation, showing a ceasation of growth near term. This result shows some similarity with Singer et al. and Brueton as quoted by Taha S.A et al.; they found intrauterine growth in African babies ceases in late pregnancy and that growth rate is less from 32 weeks to term compared to Caucasian levels at the same gestational age [3]. The result may suggest that more infants not involved in the study were born small for gestational age or had experienced intrauterine growth retardation near term. These findings may also explain why weight gain in the first 28 days, particularly for low birth weight infants in this study was higher compared to Martell's study [12] and showed in fact a 'catch up growth' frequently found to be small for gestational age infants early in postnatal life [15].

Many factors, such as maternal biological, environmental and nutritional status, are known to affect fetal growth jointly or independently [14]. Multiple regression analysis carried out to rank the order of relationship, showed higher association between maternal age and parity as well as nutritional status. Contrary to expectation living standards, antenatal care and maternal education appeared to play only a minor role.

Characteristics of mothers between the groups with sufficient and insufficient weight gain infants were not very different regarding their biological and nutritional condition except the Hb concentration of the mother. Poverty is significantly associated with insufficient weight gain, as is the case with low birth weight.

The public health implications of the observed association between maternal biological and antropometric measurements and low birth weight may provide a basis to build indicators predicting the risk of mothers being delivered of low birth weight infants. Beside these factors, anemia and poverty increase the risk of insufficient weight gain in the early postnatal period. These indicators are crucial for improving the efficiency of MCH programs.

Acknowledgements

We wish to thank Ir Totowarsa for his statistical assistance and collaboration.

References

1. Petros-Barvasian A, Behar M: Birthweight and reproductive pattern. SAREC Report no. R2:59–60, 1978.
2. Miller CH, Merritt AT: Fetal growth in humans. Yearbook Medical Publishers INC, London, 1979.
3. Taha SA: Normal foetal growth in the Sudan. J Trop Pediat Env Chld Hlth 24 (5):226–229, 1978.
4. Alisjahbana A, Suroto-Hamzah E, Tanumidjaya S, Wiradisuria S, Abisudjak B: Final report V. Perinatal mortality & morbidity and low birth weight. The Pregnancy outcome in Ujung-Berung, W.Java, 1983.
5. Alberman E: Sociobiological factors and birthweight in Great Britain. The epidemiology of prematurity. Urban & Schwarzenberg, Baltimore, pp 145–156, 1977.
6. Alisjahbana A, Suroto-Hamzah, Suganda T: Fetal growth in Bandung (unpublished data) (1977).
7. Alisjahbana A et al.: Final report II. Perinatal mortality and morbidity and low birth weight: Background information and retrospective survey in Ujung-Berung. 1981.
8. Lubshenco: The high risk infant. WB Saunders, Philadelphia, 1976.
9. Intrauterine growth as estimated from liveborn birth weight data at 24 to 42 weeks of gestation.
10. Karjati S, Kusin JA, de With C: Maternal nutrition and birth weight distribution in a rural area of Madura. Paper presented at the Workshop on the Interrelationship of Maternal & Infant Nutrition in Surabaya 26–27 April, 1983.
11. Widya Karya Nasional Pangan dan gizi, Lombaga Ilmu Pengetahuan Indonesia, Maret 1979.
12. Fomon SJ et al.: Food consumption and growth of normal infants fed milk based formula. Acta Paediatr Scan Suppl 202:1, 1971.
13. Lawrence RA: Breast feeding a guide for the medical profession. CV Mosby, London, 1980.
14. Hardy JB, Mellits ED: Relationship of low birth weight to maternal characteristics of age, parity, education and body size. The Epidemiology of Prematurity Urban & Schwarzenberg, Baltimore, pp 105–117, 1977.
15. Davies DP, Platts P, Pritchard JM, Wilkinson PW: Nutritional status of light-for-date infants at birth and its influence on early postnatal growth. Arch Dis Childh 54:703–706, 1979.
16. Martell M, Gaviria J, Belitzhy R: A new method for evaluating postnatal growth in the first two years of life. Bull Pan Am Health Org 12 (4):370–379, 1979.

The pregnancy monitoring chart: an approach to reduce the prevalence of low birth weight by village cadres

S. MARTODIPURO

Introduction

To improve the health status of the community, the Ministry of Health of Indonesia has set up the National Health System. It contains the policy and strategy on how to manage and develop health delivery in the country. A set of indicators and targets has been determined to assess its achievements [1].

One of the stated targets is to reduce the prevalence of low birth weight (LBW) from the present figure (14–20%) (Sarwono, 1977) by half [2]. In order to achieve this target, an instrument – a pregnancy monitoring chart – has been developed (Martodipuro, 1982) [3]. Indeed, appropriate technology is required to implement the chart in the field, and the chart contains the most important components to monitor the mother, in order to undergo a safe delivery of a healthy baby.

The chart is simple to use and designed to be understood by the layman, like members of women welfare organizations or village cadres. Of course, a certain amount of training is necessary as well as continuous supervision by health workers and the midwives.

The use of this chart will be optimized if supplementary feeding programs are given for those who show failure to follow the curves in the pregnancy monitoring chart. Otherwise it is nothing more than a tool for health education to increase the awareness of pregnant mothers. If it is used properly, it serves as an instrument for selection of the high risk cases of pregnant mothers as well.

Background information

It is generally accepted that there is a strong relation between nutrition of pregnant mothers and the outcome. Food shortage during war and famine have had an influence on the reproductive behavior of the community. Amenorrhoe became common, birth rate decreased and the birth weight during these periods decreased 50–500 grams.

Fetal growth is influenced more by undernutrition in late pregnancy than it is in the first months. It is also influenced by the life style and habits of the mother. Moreover, hard work during pregnancy consumes more calories and is disadvantageous for the fetus. In particular, working in an upright position will reduce placental flow. In late pregnancy it is advisable for pregnant mothers to get sufficient rest in order to promote placental flow (Thomson, 1983) [4].

Other non-nutritional factors causing low birth weight are smoking and possibly the small stature of the mother and low body weight. Short intervals of pregnancy and repeated pregnancies are also mentioned as causes of low birth weight. The relation of factors can be summarized in the following scheme.

Situation analysis

Hospital figures of low birth weight varied from 12–20%, whereas reports from the field showed a wider range of 6.6–22%, varying from place to place [2, 5, 6]. The high figures of low birth weight in the hospital cases are due to the referred cases of complications of pregnancy and to the wide range from the field due to the difference of sample taken in the study.

The high prevalence of low birth weight may be related to the high figure of perinatal deaths, which range between 43.9 per 1000 live births in the field and 150 per 1000 in the referral hospitals [7], to the high infant mortality rate (IMR), which is 91 per 1000 live births [8], or to the high neonatal death, which is $1/_3$ to $1/_2$ of the infant mortality [6].

Although not directly related to low birth weight, another important factor is the maternal mortality rate (MMR). The figure of MMR is 20–40 per 10,000 deliveries in hospitals of middle and high socio-economic class clients to 120–200 maternal deaths in referral hospitals. The high figures of maternal deaths should actually be recalculated, the mothers who did not deliver in the hospitals should also be added to the denominator, since they are in the region of the referral hospitals.

Another possible factor causing low birth weight is undernutrition with or without anaemia of the pregnant mothers. According to a household survey conducted in 1980 (Pundarika et al.), it was found that 70% of pregnant mothers suffer from anaemia [8]. Kardjati (1977) in a nutrition study reported a high prevalence of undernutrition of pregnant mothers (69%) [9].

The pregnancy monitoring chart

The pregnancy monitoring chart was based on the asumption that during the 1st, 2nd and 3rd trimesters, the weight gain of a pregnant mother is respectively $1^1/_2$ kg, $3^1/_2$ kg and 5 kg for singletons [10]. A total weight gain of 12.5 kg is considered normal. The weight gain is assumed to be similar for mothers with different initial body weight before pregnancy so that parallel curves are printed in the graph [3].

This chart can be used for mothers with recorded date of last menstruation and without the data of the beginning of gestation. It will be very useful if the initial body weight prior to pregnancy was known, or at least several records of body weight. By monitoring the weight gain of the pregnant mother and plotting it in the graph, it can be seen whether it follows the curve or not.

If the weight gain is according to the curve, a mature pregnancy is expected to deliver a baby of 3 kg or more. If the weight gain deviates too much from the curve, action must be taken. If the dots form a horizontal line, the pregnant mother should be examined for possible underlying diseases or may need supplementary feeding. The ideal situation would be to support the mother if she was economically weak, during the last semester in particular.

If the dots form a very steep line, the possibility of a twin pregnancy or hydramnion should be considered. The weight gain may reach 15 kg in total or more; so preparations could be made for and by the family. The most important consideration is to explain and motivate the pregnant mother and the family to ensure a healthy and strong baby. If the mother expects to give the baby a good start, she must try to improve her food intake. She has also to take a rest during the day, preferably to lay down in order to improve the placental flow, which is beneficial for the growth of the fetus.

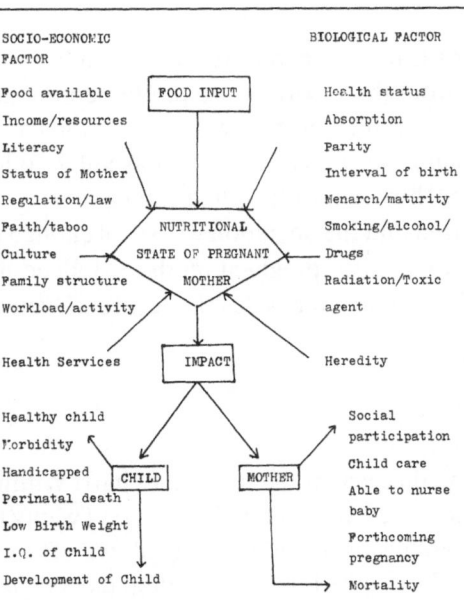

Table 1. The influence and impact of nutritional state during pregnancy.

Additional food given should combine proteins, fat, carbohydrates and vitamins. As a matter of fact, any food is useful so long as it gives additional calories. It is advisable to give iron and folic acid tablets too, since 70% of the pregnant mothers suffer from anaemia [8].

Other items to be monitored are the hemoglobin content of the blood, blood pressure, edema, albumin in urine and, of course, the pregnancy itself. Tetanus toxoid immunization should also be completed. The chart also provides questions to select high risk pregnancies. These questions can be filled in by layman, but of course the answers need to be checked by the midwife. The outcome of the pregnancy should be recorded whether it ends in abortion, stillbirth, livebirth or any other possibility.

To estimate the date of delivery, an obstetric calender is provided, simplified with units of weeks, by drawing a straight line downwards. Since people like to use the lunar calender, an adjusting mechanism is set up by drawing the verticle line further downwards.

Test of the chart

The chart was tested in two ways:

1. Testing whether the monitoring chart is workable

Two hundred records from a maternity clinic were taken as a sample. The body weights obtained from the records were plotted on the graph of the chart. The assumptions were: (a) if the dots follow the curve, the baby born will have a birth weight of more than 2500 grams; (b) if the dots fail to follow the curve, the baby born will have a birth weight of less than 2500 grams.

The results showed that the deviation was small enough to tolerate and that the chart can be used to monitor pregnant mothers. Indeed physical and laboratory tests should also be conducted besides the record of weight gain of the mothers.

2. Field testing the chart

Another maternity clinic was asked to use the chart. Within a period of 6 months, 133 records were collected and sent to the author. Twenty records were discarded due to incomplete filling and could not be analyzed. The outcome was, 2 twins, 7 low birth weights, 39 weighed between 2501 and 3000 grams, 56 weighed 3001–3500 grams and 9 weighed 3501 grams or more.

Notes of the 7 low birth weights:

1. Case 1, 32 years, $G_{XI}P_{60045}$, male baby, 2500 g/48 cm.

Dots according to the curve, delivery 4 weeks ahead.

2. Case 2, 32 years, G_IP_0, female baby, 2400 g/48 cm.
   Body weight in last months decreased, 17 days ahead.
3. Case 3, 20 years, $G_{II}P_{10001}$, female baby, 2370 g/45 cm.
   Dots are not according to the curve.
4. Case 4, 25 years, $G_{III}P_{20102}$, male baby, 2500 g/49 cm.
   Weight gain 15 kg, edema +, hydramnion?
5. Case 5, 19 years, G_IP_0, female baby, 2450 g/46 cm.
   Caesarian section, body weight 39,5 kg, no weight gain.
6. Case 6, 24 years, G_IP_0, male baby, 2500 g/48 cm.
   Dots according to curve, height 143 cm, weight 42 kg.
7. Case 7, 20 years, $G_{II}P_{00010}$, male baby, 2350 g/47 cm.
   No record of last menstruation, premature?

In all 7 cases, reasonable causes were found to explain the low birth weight in these cases.

Use of the chart by village cadres

Female cadres are selected for this purpose. They are voluntary workers from the community and are unpaid by the government. For a community of 2000 people, usually with 400 households, about 15 cadres are needed. They are trained by giving a set of self-learning modules to identify pregnant mothers and how to select the high risk cases.

Once a month, the midwife of the health center visits the village. The village cadre should refer the pregnant mothers to the midwife. The weighing of the pregnant mothers are conducted by the cadres and recorded in the chart. The midwives are provided with some simple laboratory tools, i.e. Talquist test for hemoglobin, combistix for albumin and glucose test in the urine. Of course also a funduscope and tensimeter. The traditional birth attendant is also included in this activity.

With this approach almost all pregnant mothers could be reached and prenatal care given. Only those who are in the first months of pregnancy are missed. The suggested four times prenatal care in the field could also be achieved. The high risk cases identified by the cadres will be reexamined by the midwife and appropriate preparations for the delivery could be arranged.

To increase the knowledge and awareness of the pregnant mothers a simulation game about mother and child health is given. The use of it should be assisted by the cadres. It is a snake and ladder game. The winner is not the one who reached the finish at the top first, as a matter of fact the main idea was the explanation of, and reasoning why, fines, and rewards are given for the pictures. Nutrition and health education is included in the game.

Evaluation

The pregnancy monitoring chart contains many items to be evaluated. Indeed, it is an ongoing project, so it is only a small part of the scheme of evaluation. Within six months of the study, one hundred and fifty cases of pregnancy have been identified, sixty mothers have delivered their babies. In order to see improvements in the outcome of the pregnancies, the data are grouped in trimesters, so that they can be compared later on. Group 0 are the cases of delivery in April–June 1983; group 1, the cases in the period of July–September 1983.

The items to be evaluated are the recording of history taking, what has been examined, the mother's body weight and birth data of the baby. If it is complete a score of 10 is given.

History taking consists of height, age, weight before pregnancy, parity, number of children alive, number of operations, eclampsia, cardiac or renal disease, repeated abortions, bleeding, premature birth, last menstruation recorded and others. Examination and treatment include blood pressure, urinanalysis, edema, hemoglobin, tetanus toxoid vaccination two times. Birth data of baby include sex of the baby, birth weight, kind of attendant and falling off umbilical stump. Also weekly weighing of the baby is conducted until 6 weeks of life. Data from group 0 are compared with group 1 in Table 2.

Discussion

Until now certain indicators have been used to assess the activities and process of MCH programs. These may be grouped into the assessment of inputs, which include the facility of health center and subcenter, staffing, operation costs and community participation, a process which consists of training, supervision and monitoring. The outputs are measured with the coverage of services, i.e. care of underfives, prenatal, natal and postnatal care, high risk selections and referral cases.

It would be ideal if, following an intervention, we could see the impact directly. Unfortunately, this is not the case; it takes time to see the outcome of the activity.

Table 2. Score of completeness of recording by village cadres, group 0 versus group 1.

	Group 0 n = 47	Group 1 n = 26
History taking	4.81	6.90
Examination	6	8.56
Body weight of mother	1.95	4.29
Birth data of baby	7.88	7.90

By involving the village cadres, they can actively participate in following up mothers from the beginning of pregnancy, delivery and the baby until the age of one month, one year, or even until childhood. The cadres will thereby contribute to the collection of data on stillbirth, livebirth, perinatal death, neonatal death, infant death, child death, maternal death, etc.

Indeed, in order to have complete data, continuous and tight supervision of the village cadres by health workers is needed. A mechanism for reporting should be set up and standardized. This means that the activities of the village cadres should also be supported by appropriate management of the health workers.

The figures presented in this paper only show how the result of the study will be reported later on. A statistical test has not yet been done; so no conclusions can be drawn. However, the idea of using village cadres to monitor pregnant mothers in the area has been put forward. There are, however, further issues to be raised: Are they able to do the work correctly? Is the curve in the pregnancy monitoring chart proper? Are there additional variables to be included in the chart? Or should it be simplified?

In this monitoring activity, nutrition of the mother is assumed to be one important determinant of low birth weight, and the body weight gain is used as the indicator which is visible and measurable. Other possible causes like small stature and low body weight of the mother are uncontrolable, and smoking is uncommon among Indonesian women.

Laboratory examination in the field presents a problem. If the midwife should do it by herself, the use of simple methods should be considered, i.e. Talquist test for hemoglobin and combistix for urinanalysis. Otherwise the involvement of a laboratory assistant is required; these personnel are available in the health center but may not be in subcenters.

From this preliminary evaluation the impression is that the use of village cadres, patience and repeated training and tight supervision are unavoidable. So, a retraining scheme is scheduled; it will include the skill of recording and also weighing the mothers and babies.

References

1. Departemen Kesehatan RI: Pemantapan dan Pengembangan Sistem Kesehatan Nasional. Jakarta, 1981.
2. Sarwono E: Perawatan Bayi Berat Badan Lahir Rendah. Beberapa Masalah Perinatologi di Indonesia.
3. Martodipuro S: Introduksi Kartu Monitor Ibu Hamil. MOGI 8(3):155–162, 1982.
4. Thomson AM: Maternal nutrition in pregnancy and lactation. EJPS Workshop, Surabaya, April 1983.
5. Alisjahbana A: Pola Penyakit dan Sebab Kematian Bayi di Bandung dan Sekitarnya. Workshop on the Interrelationship of Maternal and Infant Nutrition Surabya, April 1983.
6. Sri Kardjati, Kusin JA, de With C: Maternal nutrition and birth weight distribution in a rural area

of Madura. Workshop on the Interrelationship of Maternal and Infant Nutrition Surabaya, April 1983.

7. Soeprono: Aspek Kebidanan Dalam Meningkatkan Kesejahteraan Ibu dan Anak. Mimbar 1983. Peningkatan Kesejahteraan Ibu dan Anak, Jakarta, Augustus 1983.

8. Pundarika R et al.: Household survey 1980, Badan Penelitian dan Pengembangan Kesehatan, Departemen Kesehatan Republik Indonesia, Jakarta, 1981.

9. Sri Kardjati, Kusin JA, de With C: East Java nutritional studies. Report I. School of Medicine University of Airlangga, Surabaya, 1977.

10. Castello MA: Getting ready for parenthood. A manual for expectant mothers and fathers. Collier Books, New York, 1962 (1st edn).

The mother-infant dyad in Madura, Indonesia: nutritional aspects

J.A. KUSIN and S. KARDJATI

Introduction

Malnutrition is still widely prevalent in developing countries. The clinical stages of malnutrition are generally encountered in toddlers of 1–3 years of age [1]. However, growth retardation starts at around the fourth month [2] whereas the peak of child mortality appears to be at infancy, especially in the peri- and neonatal periods [3, 4]. As the chances of survival for the infant are greatly determined by birth weight, particularly in developing countries, it is quite likely that low birth weight, or impaired fetal growth, is an important cause of infant death [5]. This observation has resulted in a resurgence of interest in maternal nutrition during pregnancy in relation to fetal growth and outcome of pregnancy. For similar reasons much attention is now being paid to lactation performance and the factors influencing volume and composition.

The nutritional aspects of the mother-infant dyad has been reviewed on several occasions [6–15]. From these reviews it can be concluded that the limited information available from developing countries is conflicting. Obviously, the consequences of malnutrition among women in the reproductive period depend upon the type, duration and severity of nutritional deprivation as well as the many other factors influencing the women's biological performance.

To assess the inter-relation between mother and infant with respect to nutrition, growth and development, the East Java Nutrition Project was started in 1975.

Selective results from the surveys and preliminary data from the longitudinal study will be presented. Detailed information of the surveys have been reported in East Java Nutrition Studies, Report I–III, obtainable from the authors.

Nutritional surveys

To assess the prevalence and geographical distribution of malnutrition among

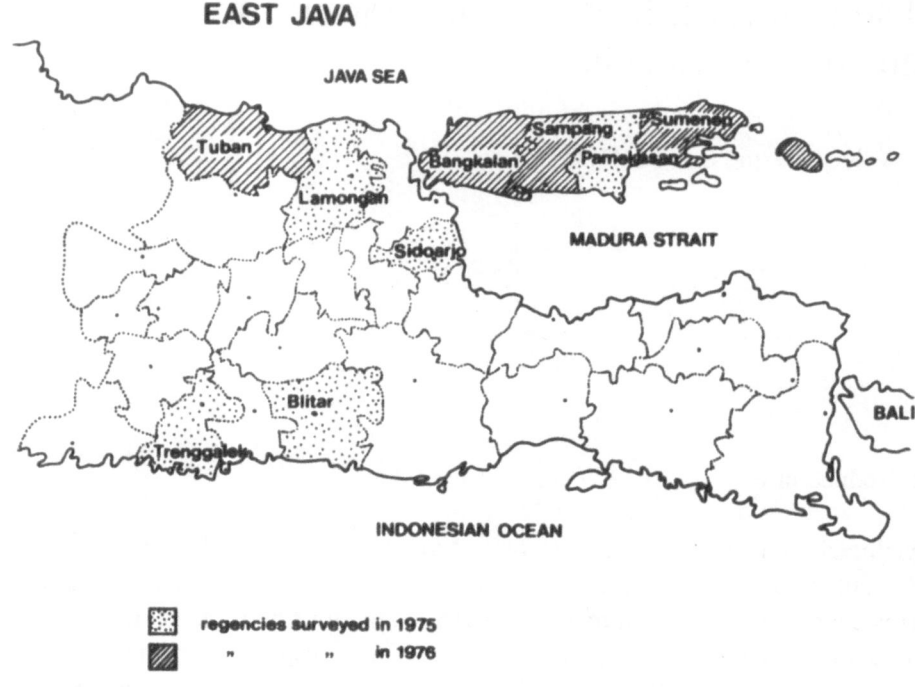

EAST JAVA

JAVA SEA

Tuban

Lamongan

Bangkalan Sampang Sumenep

Pamekasan

Sidoarjo

MADURA STRAIT

Blitar

BALI

Trenggalek

INDONESIAN OCEAN

▨ regencies surveyed in 1975
▨ " " in 1976

Map East-Java.

mothers and preschool children in East Java, two surveys were conducted in 1975–1976 in nine regencies of which four were located on the island of Madura (Map). Since the problem was most serious in Madura [16, 17] in the year following the surveys foods consumed by mothers and preschool children were measured in Madura and in the regency with the lowest prevalence of malnutrition and mortality for comparison [18].

Data on child mortality and feeding practices were obtained by interviews. Weight and length were measured according to standard techniques [19]. Foods cooked for and eaten by mothers and preschool children during one whole day were measured by weighment. Conversion into energy and nutrients was done using the Indonesian Food Composition Table.

In this presentation only relevant results from Madura will be discussed.

Characteristics of mothers

Madurese women are short and slim (Table 1) and their average height is 148 cm. The mean weight of non-pregnant, non-lactating mothers was 41.2 kg and of lactating mothers 42.1 kg. Although the number of pregnant women examined was small, from these cross-sectional data it appears that weight gain during pregnancy was low, i.e. about 6 kg. It is reflected in the larger percentage of pregnant women in the last trimester having a weight-for-height less than 80% of a local reference.

The staple diet in this area consists of rice mixed with maize and fish and to a lesser extent vegetables and pulses. In the central area cassava is the staple food. The amount of food eaten by mothers was not influenced by physiological state and during pregnancy and lactation, when food requirements are higher, these women did not eat more. Obviously daily intake in energy was very low while protein intake was marginal.

Child mortality

No death registration was available in the villages; to gain an impression of the pattern of child mortality, mothers were asked how many children were born, how many died and the child's age at death.

From the total of child deaths, 19% occurred in the perinatal period, 18% at 8–28 days and 37% at 1–11 months of age. In comparison, the death rate after infancy was low (Table 2). When child mortality was grouped by parity, an upward trend cound be seen, suggesting maternal depletion.

Table 1. Characteristics of mothers in Madura (survey data).

| | Non-pregnant, non-lactating | Lactating | Pregnant, trimester | | |
			1	2	3
Number examined	988	494	25	39	58
Height, cm (mean ± SD)	148 ± 5.0	148 ± 4.9		148 ± 5.6	
Weight, kg (mean ± SD)	41.2 ± 5.8	42.1 ± 4.8	41.5 ± 5.6	42.7 ± 3.6	47.9 ± 5.3
Weight-for-height ≤80% local reference[a]	8%	3%	6%	6%	11%
Number examined	407	381		90	
Energy intake, kcal/day	1450	1600		1500	
Protein intake, g/day	41	44		40	

[a] Indonesian reference for non-pregnant women in 90% international reference.
For pregnant women, the local reference is calculated.

Breastfeeding practices

In rural areas prolonged breastfeeding is still customary (Table 3). At the time of the interview almost all infants were being breastfed and those who were not given mother's milk in the first few months were considered special cases. Either the mother was sick or the mother's milk was witheld because the previous child had died while it was still on the breast. According to local belief mother's milk is than assumed to be unsuitable for the child.

Energy and protein intake of infants

The most striking observation was that infants are fed solid foods from the first

Table 2. Child mortality according to age at death and parity (survey data).

Child mortality	Percentage
Age at death	
perinatal	19
8–28 days	18
1–11 months	37
12–23 months	11
2 years	5
3– 5 years	3
5–15 years	6
By parity	
1– 3	13
4– 6	24
7–10	35
≥11	43

Total number of child deaths: 1585.
Total number of children born: 6213.
Child mortality = percentage of children born.

Table 3. Breastfeeding pattern in Madura (percentages): survey data.

Age groups (months)	n	Excl. B.f.	Mixed feeding	No. B.f.
0–6	99	11	83	6
7–12	165	8	84	8
13–18	139	5	75	20
19–24	105	1	50	49
25–48	462	–	15	85

Mixed feeding = breastmilk + complementary foods.

month onwards. Complementary foods consist of banana and rice in the first two months, and rice in the next six months. Some fish and vegetables are introduced towards the end of the first year. They provided on average 100 kcal and 1.4 g protein per day in the first months, quite a large amount of rice and banana! Intake doubled in the following two months (about 200 kcal and 3.3 g protein), but a very small increase was observed in the eight months thereafter (Table 4).

Infant growth

To give an impression of the pattern of growth, mean weight and length of Madurese infants have been expressed as a percentage of the Harvard Standard in Figure 1. Weight was comparable with the reference in the first two months, but progressively deviated thereafter until it was about 80% by the age of one year. Length wavered in the age group 1–4 months, but stabilized at about 94% of the reference at 5–12 months.

From the survey data a hypothetical model of the mother-infant dyad can be deduced. Apparently in this agrarian community, fertility is uncontrolled and food intake during pregnancy is marginal. It is quite likely that low birth weight is prevalent, which would partly explain the high mortality in the first month of life. High mortality will maintain a high number of pregnancies at short birth intervals in traditional agrarian communities, leading to progressive deterioration of the nutritional status of pregnant women. The relation between child mortality and parity seems to support this assumption.

Table 4. Daily intake of energy and protein from complementary foods of infants in Madura (survey data).

Age-groups in months	n	Statistics	Energy		Protein (g)
			kcal	kJ	
<1	14	Mean	99	414	1.4
		S.D.	61	225	1.0
1–2	17	Mean	212	887	3.3
		S.D.	113	472	1.7
3–5	49	Mean	247	1033	4.1
		S.D.	125	523	2.8
6–8	49	Mean	287	1200	5.5
		S.D.	124	519	4.2
9–11	55	Mean	324	1355	6.5
		S.D.	125	523	4.5

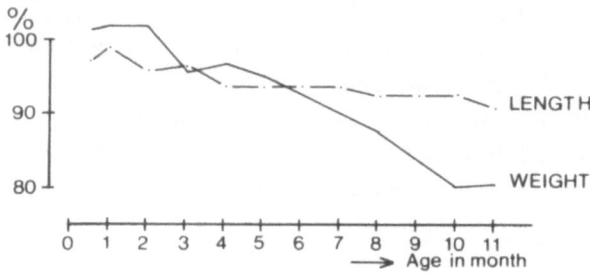

Figure 1. Mean weight and length of infants in Madura expressed as percentage of Harvard Standard (survey data).

Since little fat reserves are built up during pregnancy and food intake during lactation does not compensate for the low energy stores, mothers may be right in assuming that they need to complement their low milk yields with solids in order to satisfy the infant's dietary requirements. However, the early supplementation in an unhygienic environment carries the danger of weanling diarrhoea. The resulting diarrhoea–malnutrition vicious circle is likely to be the cause of infant mortality after the first month.

In the hypothetical model, impaired fetal growth and poor lactation performance due to malnutrition of the mother during pregnancy and lactation are assumed to be the key variables influencing infant survival and growth.

The East Java pregnancy study

To test these hypotheses an experimental study is being conducted in three villages in the regency Sampang, Madura from 1982–1985. It is assumed that improvement of energy intake during pregnancy by providing a supplement of about 500 kcal per day during the last trimester will reduce the incidence of low birth weight and hence peri- and neonatal mortality. It is also expected that women will start the lactation period with larger fat reserves. The resulting increase in breast milk yield will promote infant growth, postpone the introduction of complementary foods and reduce infant mortality.

Before the experimental study was started baseline data were collected with regard to habitual dietary intakes during pregnancy and birth weight distribution in the period August 1981–November 1982. Since the experimental part has just started, only results of the baseline period are presented. Preliminary data of feeding practices, growth and mortality will also be given.

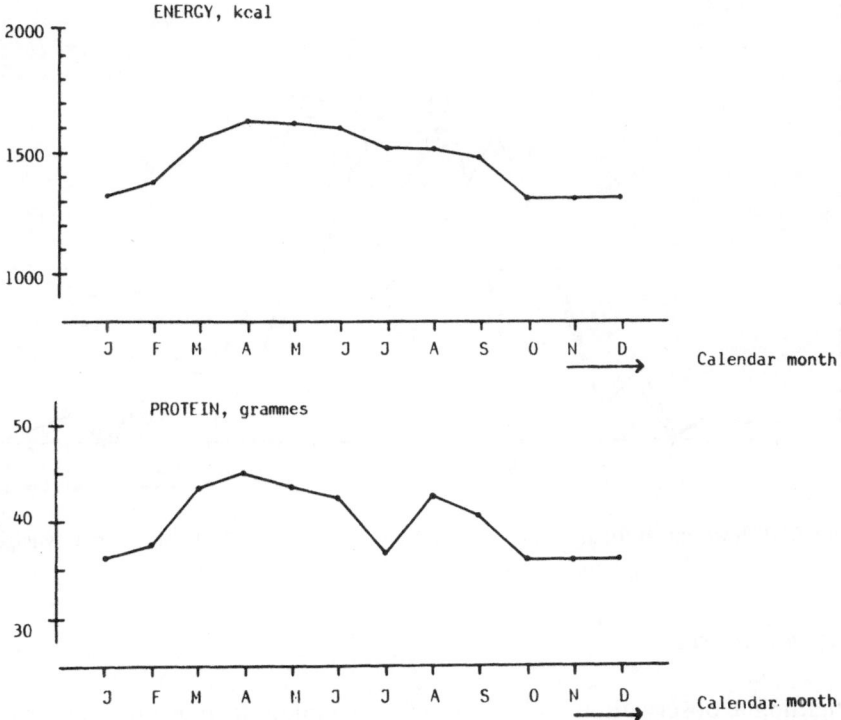

Figure 2. Seasonal pattern in daily energy and protein intake of pregnant women in three villages of Madura.

Energy and protein intake of pregnant women

Food consumed by 243 women was measured by weight assessment on three consecutive days in pregnancy months 5 and 6; 7, 8 and 9. The mean daily intake in energy (about 1500 kcal) and protein (about 40 g) were similar throughout pregnancy. The pattern by calendar month is shown in Figure 2. There seems to be a peak in the months March–June and a trough in the period October–January.

Birth weight distribution

In the baseline period 432 single live births were reported, of which 382 birth weights were measured within 24 hours after delivery. Mean birth weight for males and females was 2.83 kg and 2.84 kg respectively, with a standard deviation of 360 g. The distribution is shown in Figure 3. The percentage of low birth weight (less than 2500 g) was 12% for the three villages combined. For the villages Gulbung, Apaan and Aengsareh the incidence was 14%, 14% and 8% for males and 18%, 7% and 7% for females.

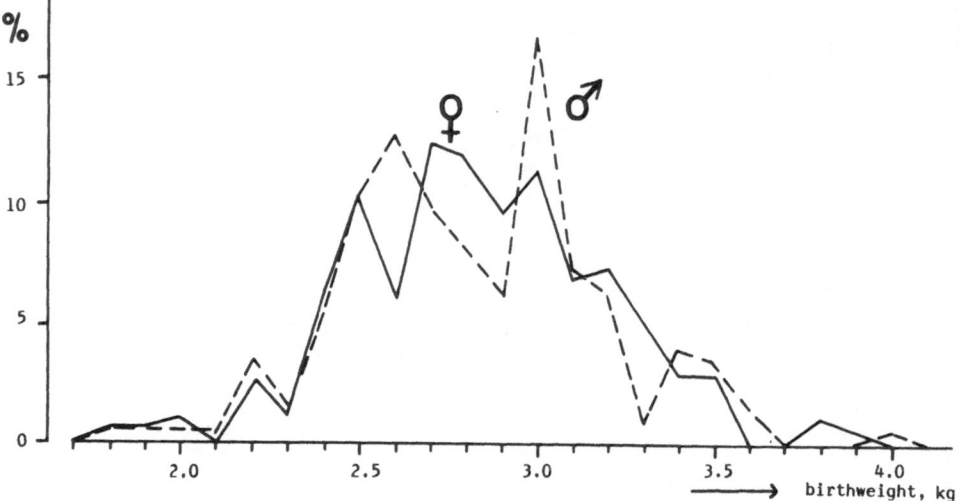

Figure 3. Birthweight distribution for male and female singleton live-borns in three villages in Madura.

Feeding practices

Longitudinal observations and interviews about infant feeding practices resulted in similar data as recorded during the surveys (Figure 4). Force-feeding was, however, not followed by diarrhoea as assumed in the hypothetical model. Only two of the 70 neonates had diarrhoea of 1–2 day duration in the fourth week postpartum.

Infant growth

The growth curves of infants, measured 1–7 times in the period October 1982–March 1983 are shown in Figure 5. Madurese infants were slightly shorter (0.4 cm) but much lighter (400 g) at birth than North American infants. They grew at the same rate as their US counterparts during the first two months but growth wavered progressively from then onwards and seemed to come to a standstill between 6 and 9 months.

Child mortality

In the 21 months from 1 September 1981 to 1 June 1983, a total of 97 children died. The highest percentage were still births and deaths in the first week (34%); neonatal mortality accounted for 44% of the total number of deaths; another 44% died in the following five months but none after 24 months of age (Table 5).

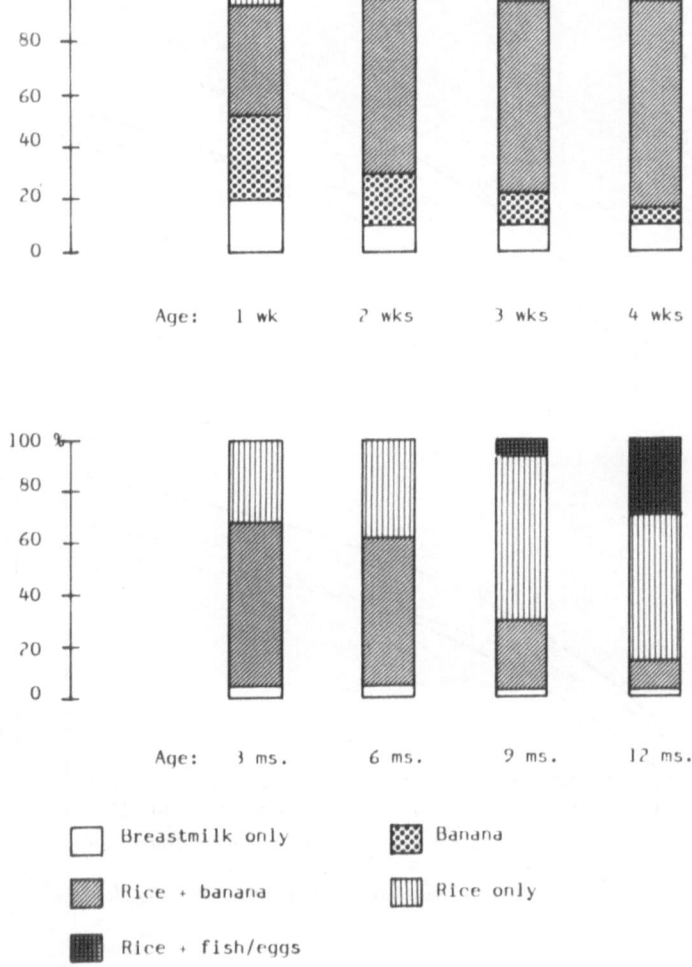

Figure 4. Type of complementary foods (percentages).

Table 5. Child mortality by age at death in three villages in Madura (longitudinal data).

Age	n	Percentage
perinatal	33	34.0
7–28 days	11	10.3
1– 3 months	21	21.6
4– 6 months	22	22.7
7–12 months	9	9.3
13–23 months	2	2.1
over 2 years	0	0.0

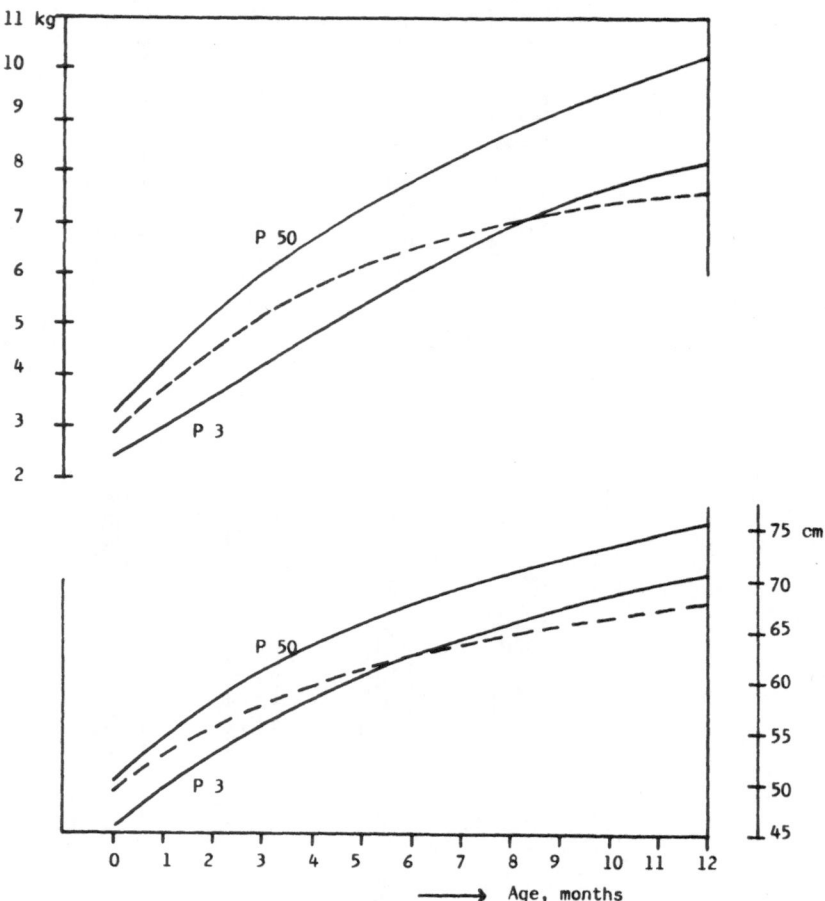

Figure 5. Weight and length of infants in Sampang compared with NCHS Reference.

Causes of death were not verified by the doctor in all cases. Roughly one can say that infants with a birth weight of less than 2200 g, whether premature or small for age, will die. Breastfeeding fails due to low sucking frequency and poor sucking vigour. Tetanus neonatorum was a cause of death in only two infants, although almost all deliveries are done by traditional birth attendants who, in spite of health education, continue to put a mixture of ash, salt and bettel leaves on the stump of the umbilical cord. The anti-tetanus vaccination of pregnant women, which started with the project, proved to be successful.

In the first half of infancy untreated upper respiratory infections, fevers of unknown origin and diarrhoea appear to be the main causes of death in this sequence of importance.

It is important to note that mortality after the age of six months was comparatively low, though growth retardation was quite serious!

Comments

Many factors influence infant growth and survival. The survey data suggest that maternal undernutrition during pregnancy and lactation may be an important cause of infant mortality whereas the insufficient quantity and quality of complementary foods are factors related to growth retardation.

The results of the longitudinal observational study conducted in three villages in Madura confirm the basic assumption of the East Java Pregnancy Study. Energy intake during pregnancy is very low for a large part of the year and the prevalence of low birth weight is about twice that of industrialized countries.

With respect to infant feeding practices and growth, the real problem is not breastfeeding but the type and amount of complementary foods. The timing of its introduction does not appear to be a reason for concern and force-feeding is not related to diarrhoea. Unless other ill effects are proven (reduction of breast milk yield for instance) counter-action is not necessary. It is still not clear why mothers introduce complementary foods so early. It may be that they wrongly interpret the infant's cry as a 'hunger' cry due to insufficient breast milk. This is understandable since exclusively breastfed infants cry more often to be fed than those given a semi-solid meal. When asked, mothers give the following responses as a reason for force-feeding: 'the baby is hungry. I don't have enough milk'; 'the baby sleeps for hours after a meal'.

In spite of early supplementation of breast milk, retardation of growth, or 'slow' growth, is more the rule than the exception. Mothers do not worry about it, mainly because the baby does not look abnormal; both weight and length are affected, and the baby remains proportionally well-fed. So far growth monitoring does not trigger action by the mother although nutrition education is given! The amount of foods given, appears to be governed by the infant's size rather than by it's age. Moreover, there are constraints with respect to increasing the amounts of a locally made weaning food for infants. Mothers do not have time to feed the infant more than twice a day. Other ways should be found to address this problem and one avenue could be a modification of the most appropriate local snacks made and sold in the villages.

If in the short term one is mainly concerned about child survival, the emphasis in our area has to be on methods which will prevent low birth weight and to the provision of simple treatment via an *active guidance* to mothers by village workers. Medical treatment is given free of charge by the project, but our experience is that having health services available does not necessarily lead to the use of these services by the community. Minor illnesses are too common and mothers only seek treatment after the illnesses have become serious.

References

1. DeMayer EM: Protein energy malnutrition. In: Beaton GH, Bengoa JM (eds) Nutrition in preventive medicine. WHO, Geneva, pp. 23–54, 1976.
2. Waterlow JC, Ashworth A, Griffith M: Faltering in infant growth in less developed countries. Lancet ii:1176, 1980.
3. Puffer RR, Serrano CV: Patterns of mortality in childhood. PAHO Scientific Publication No. 262, Washington DC, 1975.
4. Puffer RR, Serrano CV: Birthweight, maternal age and birth order: three important determinants in infant mortality. PAHO Scientific Publication No. 294, Washington DC, 1975.
5. Sterky G, Mellander L (eds): Birthweight distribution – an indicator of social development. SAREC Report No. R2, Uppsala, 1978.
6. National Academy of Sciences: Maternal nutrition and the course of pregnancy. Washington DC, 1970.
7. Symposium on malnutrition and infection during pregnancy: determinants of growth and development. Am J Dis Child 129:419–463; 549–580, 1975.
8. Colloquium on prenatal and perinatal nutrition. Arch Latino-Amer. Nutr. XXVII (Suppl. 1), June 1977.
9. Mosley WH (ed): Nutrition and human reproduction. Plenum Press, New York, 1978.
10. Jelliffe DB, Jelliffe EFP: Human milk in the modern world. Oxford University Press, 1979.
11. Hambraeus L, Sjolin S: The mother/child dyad, nutritional aspects. Symposia of the Swedish Nutrition Foundation XIV. Almqvist & Wiksell Intern, Stockholm, 1979.
12. International workshop on effect of maternal nutrition. Panajachel, Guaetemala. Arch Latino-Amer Nutr XXIX (Suppl. 1), 1979.
13. Aebi H, Whitehead RG (eds): Maternal nutrition during pregnancy and lactation. Nestlé Foundation Publ. Series no 1, Hans Huber, Bern, 1980.
14. Workshop on Nutrition of the Child: Maternal nutritional status and fetal outcome. Am J Clin Nutr 34(4) Suppl., 1981.
15. Dobbing J (ed): Maternal nutrition in pregnancy – eating for two. Academic Press, London, 1981.
16. Kardjati Sri, Kusin JA, de With C, Sudibia IGK: Feeding practices, nutritional status and mortality in preschool children in rural East Java, Indonesia. Trop Geogr Med 31:359, 1979a.
17. Kusin JA, Kardjati Sri, de With C, Sudibia IGK: Nutrition and nutritional status of rural women in East Java. Trop Geogr Med 31:571, 1979.
18. Kardjati Sri, Kusin JA, de With C: Food consumption and nutritional status of pre-school children and mothers in Sidoarjo and Madura. East Java Nutrition Studies, Report III, December 1979b; Airlangga University, Surabaya/Tropical Institute, Amsterdam.
19. Jelliffe DB: The assessment of the nutritional status of the community. WHO Monograph Series no 53, Geneva, 1966.

Erythrocyte glucose-6-phosphate dehydrogenase (G6PD) deficiency and neonatal hyperbilirubinaemia

CHAP-YUNG YEUNG

Introduction

Erythrocyte Glucose-6-Phosphate Dehydrogenase (G6PD) deficiency is common among several ethnic groups such as the Sephardic Jews, the Mediteranean people, the Negroes and the orientals including the Chinese [1]. The incidence in southern Chinese populations is estimated to be between 3.7 and 5.5% [2, 3]. In the neonatal period, severe hyperbilirubinaemia has frequently been associated with the condition. A number of precipitating factors have been identified but in the majority of cases acute haemolysis is often spontaneous and unprovoked [4].

This communication reports the various features of neonatal hyperbilirubinaemia associated with G6PD deficiency in Chinese infants.

Materials and methods

Chinese infants who were referred to the paediatric services of Queen Mary Hospital, Hong Kong for hyperbilirubinaemia (above 10 mg/dl), over a 2-year period (1981/82) are included in this study. The fluorescent spot test, which has been proven to be a reliable screening test [5], is used for detecting erythrocyte G6PD deficiency state.

Results

11.4% (80/704) of infants who developed bilirubinaemia above 10 mg/dl were associated with erythrocyte G6PD deficiency (Table 1). The enzyme deficiency was associated with a significantly higher incidence of severe hyperbilirubinaemia compared to the other causes. Two of the four infants who developed kernicterus were also from the G6PD deficient group. Enzyme deficient infants who developed neonatal jaundice had a more prolonged course and acute haemolysis often occurred beyond the first week of birth. 24 infants were found to have low haemoglobin levels (less than 15 gm/dl in the first 2 days and 12 gm/dl thereafter) but without evidence of external blood loss. This criteria was used as presumptive evidence of haemolysis. Their features were significantly different from the other 46 who did not show evidence of haemolysis. Infection, herb exposure and inhalation of naphthalein vapour were associated with significantly higher incidence of severe hyperbilirubinaemia necessitating exchange transfusions among G6PD deficient infants. The type of infections are discussed.

Discussion

G6PD is the entry enzyme to the Hexose Monophosphate (HMP) shunt. This is the only pathway in the RBC for the generation of NADPH which is an important reducing agent protecting the red cells from oxygen damage. Deficiency in this enzyme therefore renders the erythrocyte to increased haemolysis when exposed to oxygen and various drugs. A large number of drugs have been identified to cause severe haemolysis [6]. Up to now, there is no effective way of preventing this process.

This study has identified a number of important factors which could precipitate acute haemolysis in G6PD deficient infants. Infection appears to be the single most important factor, followed by exposure to naphthalein vapour and Chinese herbs. As predicted in a previous study in 1973 [7], the improved social economic status and health care programs in Hong Kong have been associated with a marked reduction of the severity of neonatal jaundice in the past few years. Among G6PD deficient infants, the incidence of severe haemolysis with resultant brain damage has also markedly reduced. With further improvement of neonatal care including early identification and prompt treatment of infection, as well as

Table 1. Neonatal hyperbilirubinaemia (1981–82) (QMH).

Associated condition	Incidence		Exchange transfusion	
	No.	%	No.	%
ABO incomp.	116	16.5	19	16.4
G6PD def.	70	9.9	16	22.9
ABO + G6PD	10	1.4	4	40
Cephalhaematoma	18	2.5	2	11
Infection	36	5.1	12	33.3
LBW	157	22.3	13	8.3
Non-specific	297	42.2	17	5.7
Total	704	–	83	11.8

improved public health education to avoid the various precipitating factors, the severity of neonatal hyperbilirubinaemia in G6PD deficient subjects will probably be further minimised.

The present study has confirmed an earlier finding [7] that infection is an important cause of neonatal jaundice. This study has also demonstrated a statistically significant association between infection and severe hyperbilirubinaemia in both G6PD deficient and normal subjects. Such association between infection and G6PD haemolysis have been noted in adults who developed typhoid fever [8] and virus hepatitis [9]. These workers have suggested that with prompt control of the infection, the triggering mechanism for haemolysis by the typhoid fever could be prevented [8]. If a similar phenomenon is true for neonatal sepsis, early diagnosis and prompt treatment of neonatal infections may also avert the haemolytic effect of these infections.

The traditional belief and folklore practices of Chinese have significantly affected the G6PD deficient infants. As shown in this study, a number of infants have been given herbal medicine before the haemolytic jaundice occurred. Although the direct relationship between herbs and haemolysis is not entirely known, a recent study in our laboratory indicated that two of the four commonly used herbs in the neonatal period are shown to induce significant Heinz body formation in vitro. This may infer a genuine predisposition to acute haemolysis in vivo. As 40% of the southern Chinese mothers believe in giving their babies herbs 'to get rid of the placental toxin' [10], improved health education is urgently needed to avoid the unnecessary morbidity and often mortality resulting from misuse of these herbs.

Most parents continued to use naphthalein mothball as an insect-repellant to preserve old clothings and blankets. Many patients shown in this study who developed haemolysis and one of the two who developed kernicterus, were victims of such practice. Again this can be prevented through improved public health education.

Table 2. Neonatal hyperbilirubinaemia (1981–82) (QMH).

Associated conditions	Serum bilirubin (mg/dl)			
	10–20	20.1–25	25.1–30	>30
ABO incomp.	97	14 (1)	5	–
G6PD def.	54	6	4	6[a] (2)
ABO + G6PD	6	1	2	2
Cephalhaematoma	16	2	–	–
Infection	24	6	5	1
Non-specific	428[b] (1)	25	1	–

[a] 4 with S.B. >40 mg/dl; 2 had encephalopathy.
[b] 4 VLBW had E.T. at S.B. less than 16 mg/dl.
( ) = Bilirubin encephalopathy.

Among infants who developed low haemoglobin levels suggestive of haemolysis very little abnormality could be detected from the peripheral blood smear besides a fairly high number showing evidence of thrombocytosis. There were no unusual features in the morphology of the red cells apart from the occasional demonstration of Heinz bodies.

Several workers have raised questions recently as to the need of exchange transfusions in term infants who developed hyperbilirubinaemia [11, 12]. Some have suggested that the cut-off point for exchange transfusion may not be as low as 20 mg/dl as it has been traditionally practised. The present study and an earlier experience [7] provide some evidence to support the traditional practice and raise warning against deviation from such. It can be noted from this present report that of the three term infants who developed kernicterus, one had bilirubin level of only 23 mg/dl although the other two had levels exceeding 40 mg/dl. In a previous report [7] on 152 kernicteric infants, the serum bilirubin levels ranged between 22.3 and 50 mg/dl with an average of 35.4 mg/dl. 50% of the kernicteric infants in this large series had their serum bilirubin levels fall between 22.3 and 35.4 mg/dl range. A common feature in these two studies was the presence of a number of identifiable factors such as the infection, herb exposure and so on, associated with the hyperbilirubinaemia. It may be true that infection or other factors have played an additional role in the development of the kernicterus. But as long as these factors are still operational in the tropical and developing countries, to adopt exchange transfusion guidelines which may not be applicable to one's own community would be very risky and unwise. The present study together with my previous report provide an example to illustrate these points.

In the two-year period of the present study, 80 infants required admission to the hospital for significant hyperbilirubinaemia; of these, 20 necessitated exchange transfusions. With an estimated catchment from 800,000 population to

Table 3. Kernicterus in Chinese infants with B.W. >2.5 kg.

Infants	Number		Kernicterus		Death
Associated condition	1969/71	1981/82	1969/71[b]	1981/82	1969/71
ABO incomp.	414	94	–	–	–
SB[a]	157	17	51	1	3
G6PD def.	241	70	–	–	–
SB[a]	130	19	58	2	13
Cephalhaematoma	40	16	–	–	–
SB[a]	12	2	3	–	1
Non-specific	1051	297	–	–	–
SB[a]	275	17	40	–	12

[a] SB = Serum bilirubin level above 20 mg/dl.

[b] Average S.B. = 35.4 mg/dl (22.3–50 mg/dl).

our paediatric service, and an estimated incidence of enzymatic deficiency between 3.7 and 5.5%, this number represents 13–19% of the G6PD deficient infants who required hospital paediatric care, and a significant proportion (20/80) of them required intensive neonatal care. During the same study period, 28 children beyond the neonatal period required admission to the hospital with various illnesses associated with G6PD deficiency state. Most of them were showing features of acute haemolysis and anaemia requiring top up transfusions besides treatment for their other associated illnesses. Many of these had known precipitating factors notably exposure to herbs and aspirin containing drugs. Massive health education campaign in Hong Kong has been launched to identify G6PD deficient infants and to issue warning notes to advise parents and physicians against certain drugs and herbs, and to educate the public to be aware of the potential risks and hazards related to the enzymatic deficiency. Since launching the campaign, it was gratifying to see that there was a significant drop of indiscriminate use of herbs and patent medicine by parents in recent months.

Conclusion

Erythrocyte G6PD deficiency is still an important health hazard in Hong Kong. It is related to a high incidence of neonatal hyperbilirubinaemia, it is still accountable for a number of kernicterus due to sudden severe haemolysis, it is prone to develop haemolysis following infectious exposure to herbs and naphthalein mothball vapour.

References

1. Beutler E: Abnormalities of the hexose monophosphate shunt. Semin Hematol 8:311, 1971.
2. Yue CK, Strickland M: Glucose-6-dehydrogenase deficiency and neonatal jaundice in Chinese male infants in Hong Kong. Lancet 1:350, 1965.
3. Chan TK, Todd D, Wong CC: Erythrocyte G6PD deficiency in Chinese. Br Med J 2:102, 1964.
4. Yeung CY, Field E: Phenobarbitone therapy in neonatal hyperbilirubinaemia. Lancet 2:135, 1969.
5. Yeung CY, Lai HC, Leung NK: Fluorescent spot test for screening G6PD deficiency in newborn babies. J Pediatr 76:931, 1970.
6. Gilman PA: Hemolysis in the newborn resulting from deficiencies of red blood cell enzymes. J Pediatr 84:645, 1974.
7. Yeung CY: Neonatal hyperbilirubinaemia in Chinese. Trop Geogr Med 25:151, 1973.
8. Chan TK, Chesterman CN, McFadzean AJS, Todd D: The survival of G6PD deficiency erythrocytes in patients with typhoid fever on chloramphenicol therapy. J Lab Clin Med 77:177, 1971.
9. Chan TK, Todd D: Haemolysis complicating viral hepatitis in patients with G6PD deficiency. Br Med J 1:131, 1975.
10. Yeung CY: unpublished data, 1981.
11. Lucey JF: Bilirubin and brain damage. Pediatrics 69:381, 1982.
12. Watchko JF, Oski FA: Bilirubin 20 mg/dl = vigintiphobia. Pediatrics 71:660, 1983.

Training and teaching – Primary health care systems

CHAIRMAN: R.G. HENDRICKSE

Training of overseas paediatricians in the U.K.: Relevance to primary child health care

J.P. STANFIELD

Many of us in paediatrics in U.K. are concerned about what we can best offer towards assisting our overseas paediatric colleagues in the training of their postgraduate doctors. What will be supplementary rather than substitutional to their own rapidly developing programmes? What is of relevance to their own problems and particularly to primary child health care? Have we anything to offer here?

I used to believe the answer was 'No'. My own training as a paediatrician and, until fairly recently, that of many others in U.K. was very much curative, secondary/tertiary, hospital, high technology based. I was brought up in former days to regard what was then called primary health care, general practice or child welfare, as primitive and less than challenging of a doctor's ability! I learned what a mistake I had made in the third world.

The reasons for this were many. Perhaps the chief one was that the health of our children in U.K. had been affected enormously by the improvement of child life and environment from influences at work long before the need for specifically health based interventions. We inherited the luxuries of a better quality of life and so we slept. Tetanus neonatorum was eradicated before maternal immunisation with toxoid was necessary. The incidence of many other infections was on the downgrade before vaccination appeared on the scene, hence our agony over pertussis vaccine and the present epidemics. Malnutrition was a shadow of what it must have been before food and milk was available for all. Virus disease, metabolic abnormalities, genetic disorders were filling our wards and enough to fill our time and thoughts completely.

I have no doubt we will be hearing from Roy Brown how he and I and many others woke up when we joined our colleagues in Africa, Asia and South America.

The time came when I returned to U.K. and I thought there surely could be little relevance in the U.K. for training postgraduates for the needs of child health in their own countries. I remember Dick Jelliffe referring to the problems of child health in U.K. as compared with those in Uganda as 'picayune'. How could there be relevance in the direction of our services, the opulence of our resources and standards of living and the nature of our training which already had led many of our best graduates at Makerere in the exact opposite direction from primary health care?

I have now worked for about as long again in U.K., in Glasgow and Newcastle and I believe we were wrong. I have become increasingly aware of strands of similarities which have common denominators in both worlds though the numerators may be very different. I have measured and outlined contours of disadvantage which we can use as a milieu of relevance in training postgraduates from the third world. I have come to understand 'training' from a very different viewpoint than the traditional filling of empty containers.

I would like to share this experience very briefly with you now. Common denominators:

Last week I was listening to a lecture given at the centenary of a childrens hospital of one of our big cities, by a surgeon who was talking on cost reduction policies in the child health service, in particular paediatric surgery. He was emphasising how paediatricians and nurses must wake up to the necessity for changes towards reducing costs, and the importance of examining new equipment, techniques, and interventions on the basis of cost-benefit. Did we need to keep children in hospital for so long? Could we operate more cheaply, or more effectively for the same cost? What about reusing disposable equipment? Wasn't oral rehydration cheaper than intravenous lines? Déjà vu! we have much to learn from each other yet.

Similarities are less easily seen in the content of our problems than in the attitudes and methods needed to detect, measure, analyse, interpret apply and evaluate their magnitude and remedy. As far as content goes our disadvantaged communities in inner city or remote rural areas still provide a poverty of health in children and of health services appropriate for them which resemble to some small degree that of the third world. Stunting, rickets, diarrhoeal disease, deprivation, child abuse, low birth weight, emotional disturbances and poor achievement are some of the problems very prevalent still.

The child health service in U.K. provides many more common denominators. Maternal and child health is split between the three major elements of the health service, local authority, hospital and general practice. General practice takes a fair amount and, as general practitioners are independent contractors, the quality and adequacy of child health services are very patchy. In some of the inner city areas they are totally inadequate. In many of these areas pilot projects are being developed by the local authority or even the University Departments of Child Health, as for instance in two or three particularly deprived areas in Glasgow and one area in Newcastle. There is a large wastage of resources, absence of cost benefit attitudes as already mentioned, overlooking of the felt needs of people particularly in obstetric practice. Hospital delivery has reduced the perinatal mortality but also interfered with brast feeding, rooming in and a number of other mother child needs, and a proper balance needs restoring. The principles and practices of our 'training' programme.

So in Newcastle we set about developing a programme for overseas postgraduates with the emphasis on primary maternal and child health care. We decided to use the milieu of the community in which we worked, warts and all. In fact we blessed the warts for they made it easier to share with others who might think such disfigurements only afflicted them. The 'training' would be aimed at post postgraduates, that is the more senior graduates who had passed through their immediate postgraduate education and qualifications. The traditional course structure is avoided.

The philosophy behind this approach is as follows:

i. The training experience should tend to support or supplement local postgraduate training rather than displace it.

ii. The best means of acquiring knowledge is in doing rather than hearing or seeing.

iii. Strands of relevance are to be found between paediatric practice and problems in Britain and in the third world. The strands show up best in the attitudes and methods of every day activities during the process of making a clinical or community diagnosis, constructing protocols, developing appropriate measurements, collecting and analysing data, ordering and presenting reports, deriving and applying conclusions.

iv. Simulated problems may be intellectually stimulating to solve, but it is more satisfying and perhaps more memorable to be involved in finding needed answers to current local problems especially if there is the added opportunity to apply and evaluate the results.

v. Study of one's own community and its health services by someone new from outside, unimpeded by any preconceptions, is often very revealing.

vi. As a corollary to this, study of someone else's community and its health services may enable clearer insights into one's own situation on return home. This is certainly the experience of many of us who have been abroad.

The programme of training is based on participation. Graduates are given a problem to solve or a task to accomplish on their own with supervision and guidance from tutors. In most instances graduates have come in groups from WHO, the Institute of Child Health in London, and the International Childrens Centre in Paris, as examples. The tasks set might include the evaluation of a training programme or a sector of the MCH services or the elucidation of factors affecting the health of mother or child depending on the graduate's particular interest or requirement. The studies are selected by the graduates or the tutors and concern questions to which answers are needed. This ensures that we stand to learn and benefit from the findings as much as the graduate. Both the methods of study and results are presented, and the conclusions examined to see how they apply in Newcastle. The graduates have an additional task to reflect on how they might apply to their own situations. By this means we hope they learn as much about process as about outcome of study. Introductory seminars set the background. Terminal examinations are replaced by presentations of their conclusions to both colleagues and tutors.

Let me describe four examples of such 'training' programmes to illustrate what we tried to do.

One postgraduate from Thailand undertook a comparison study in the use and usefulness of home based child health records in Newcastle and Bangkok. Time unfortunately did not allow her to share in the modifications of the Newcastle record which her findings had helped to suggest. At the moment another Commonwealth Fellow from South India is completing this evaluation.

One seminar, repeated annually, has had as its chief objective an introduction to the construction and application of a research design in the field of maternal and child health. About 15 postgraduates are divided into pairs and given topics sufficiently circumscribed to yield observations of value within the month of the seminar and varied enough to cover a large spectrum of maternal and child health in Newcastle. Titles of some of these projects in the last three years are:

'The role of the "chemist" in the primary health care of children;

The effect of a hospital admission of a child on the family;

A comparison of the mobility of handicapped children using calipers and wheeled chairs;

Attitudes of mothers and staff in a maternity teaching hospital towards breast feeding;

Attitudes of mothers to the management of a perinatal death in hospital some time after the event;

Traditional customs still surrounding pregnancy and delivery in Newcastle;

Management of diarrhoea and vomiting in children in Newcastle with special reference to oral rehydration'.

During the final evaluation of the value of these seminars many of the participants have emphasised the importance of the experience in discovering methods of finding answers to real practical problems and in interpretation and presentation. The shortage of time is a handicap but necessitates the recognition of defining priorities and appreciating limitations which insufficient data place on conclusions. Our own insights into some of these problems have undoubtedly benefitted as a result of these projects.

Another group of seminars, involving a similar number of senior postgraduates from South East Asia for about the same time, has been concerned with examining the role and training of the main categories of staff in the MCH services in and around Newcastle. Each group have identified patterns of services in which they have found similarly qualified staff often playing very different roles. By interviewing patients and staff they have reached some understanding of the effectiveness and adequacy of these services. Then they have tried by further interviews and observations to assess the appropriateness of the training of the different cadres of staff for the needs and demands of the services.

Conclusions are shared at the end of the seminar concerning their perceptions of our training and services in maternal and child health and the relevance of the method of study and their observations to their own problems and practice. They have found advantages applicable to their own situation in the methods used in Newcastle of involving patients in the management of their own health problems; they have been appalled at the lack of integration of our MCH services and the failure to properly utilise the training and potential of midwives!

Finally a further seminar was conducted with the International Childrens Centre in Paris on methods by which seven major child health problems in Newcastle had been identified, measured and effectively or otherwise remedied. Each pair of graduates looked at one problem area and there was some dismay when they were handed their tasks. They had anticipated a seminar with lectures and discussion groups. They did not expect to be visiting clinics and homes, interviewing staff and patients, attending court cases and sitting in on case conferences. In the plenary sessions at the end of the month most of the presentations showed an appreciation of the importance and the methods of arriving at a community diagnosis. Given time they felt sure they could apply the method to their own circumstances.

This method of 'training' has enabled full participation in a learning experience which has been found to be refreshingly new to most and has aroused interest in its potential. Participants and tutors have become more aware of the relevance of what we share rather than how we differ on matters relating to maternal and child health. We have worked as colleagues and the learning has been mutual and that is surely where we should be heading.

Thanks are due to Professor J.K.G. Webb and my colleagues in the Department of Child Health and in the Maternal and Child Health Services of Newcastle, and to many overseas postgraduate colleagues whom it has been our privilege to serve, and without whom this work would never have been done. The author was supported by a grant from the Overseas Development Administration of the British Government.

Nutrition in primary health care: functional analysis

A. PRADILLA

1. Defining and quantifying malnutrition

The term 'malnutrition' is used in reference to a number of diseases, each having a specific nutrient-related etiology (e.g. protein, iodine, calcium, etc.), and each being defined as a metabolic imbalance at the cellular level between the supply of macro- and micro-nutrients and energy and the body's demand for them to ensure maintenance, function and growth.

Malnutrition can be prevented by modifying, or removing altogether, blocks to normal nutrient and energy flow at any of several possible stages, from food availability to absorption to final metabolism; and it can be treated by increasing or decreasing cellular nutrient and energy supply. Malnutrition can be produced experimentally, with clearly defined anthropometric, clinical and biochemical symptoms and signs.

The body's first response to nutrient imbalance is adaptation. In cases of severe or prolonged stress, however, adaptation fails and the symptoms and signs just referred to begin to appear. It is at this stage that malnutrition becomes a medical problem, by itself as well as in conjunction with other closely interlinked conditions of illness.

These are a number of health and non-health factors that can interfere with nutrition and energy flow at any stage, chief among which, in conditions of deficit malnutrition, are:

(a) reduced national or regional food availability (the result of natural or man-made disasters, for example);
(b) reduced family food availability (poverty being a major cause);
(c) reduced individual food availability (most often for dependent persons, e.g. children, the aged and infirm, often a function of the time other family members can devote to their care; cultural dietary practices; in addition to complications arising from conditions (a) and (b) above);
(d) reduced food intake (based on decreased appetite of whatever origin, and conditions (a) through (c) above);

(e) reduced energy and nutrient absorption (intestinal infections or other causes);

(f) increased nutrient and energy loss (enteropathy, renal damage, development of fistulae, environmental stress, etc.);

(g) increased nutritional requirements (owing to fever, activity levels, physiological conditions, etc.);

(h) decreased or abnormal metabolism (metabolic abnormalities, genetic metabolic diseases, cellular damage, etc.);

(i) decreased capacity in the nutrient transport system during pregnancy (resulting from infections or other illnesses).

Malnutrition, as defined above and measured by anthropometric indicators, continues to be a major public health problem in both developing and industrialized countries. Its principal manifestations in the former (stunting and wasting) and in the latter (obesity) have a considerable negative impact on chances of survival and general welfare.

Crude data collected in recent years, on the basis of national surveys and nutritional status surveillance systems, have made possible the preparation of geographically disaggregated global and national nutrition analyses. For example, data have been compiled concerning low birth weight, nutritional anaemia in women, and stunting and wasting in preschool children. Table 1 presents the most recent estimates of the prevalence of these conditions by geographical region.

The age distribution of nutritional deficiency prevalence has also been explored given that the immediate epidemiological factors influencing the growth of children under six, and the associated factors of acute and chronic malnutrition, vary considerably from one year to the next. The significant variations in prevalence for different types of malnutrition, both within and between countries, support the view that the factors determining each are largely dependent on specific environmental conditions (see Figure 1).

2. Maintaining perspective on the multisectoral approach to malnutrition

While it is generally accepted that the control of malnutrition is dependent on action in virtually all sectors, the management of truly multisectoral interventions has proved difficult in practice in the majority of cases.

The concept of multisectorality, as it is traditionally employed, seems to imply that a given action should necessarily have the same effect on malnutrition prevalence for all groups everywhere. If this may be so in isolated instances, experience suggests that the need for each sector's participation, and the specific role it has to play, varies considerably according to the epidemiological factors encountered and their interaction at family, community and national levels. As an example, at one extreme, deficit malnutrition in industrialized countries is influenced essentially by psychosocial factors, genetics and individual dietary

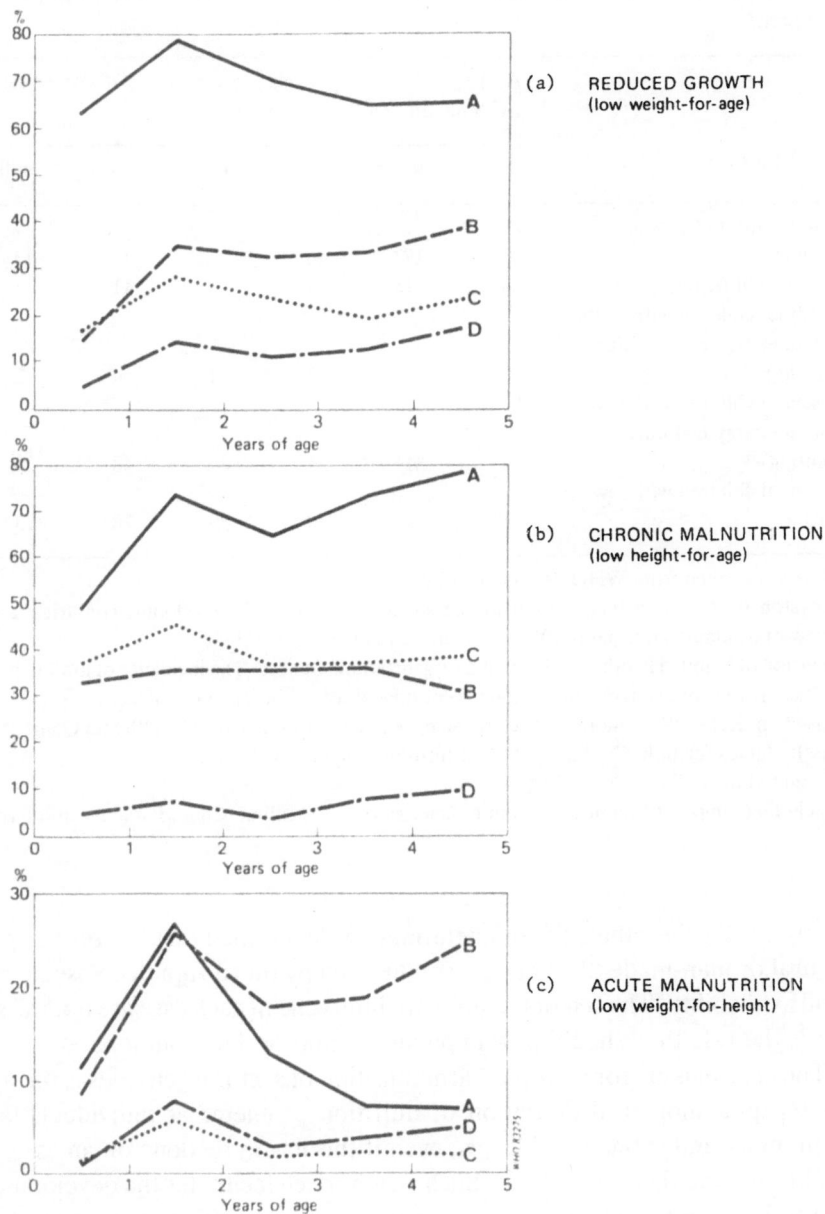

Figure 1. Age specific prevalences of low weight-for-age (reduced growth), low height-for-age (chronic malnutrition) and low weight-for-height (acute malnutrition) in four child populations of different socio-economic and cultural background. Prevalences are shown in per cent of children having values below the mean minus 2 standard deviations of a reference population. (This figure taken from WHO document A36/7).

Table 1. Estimated prevalence and number of cases of nutritional deficiency in developing countries, by region.*

	Asia (without China)		Africa		The Americas[e]	
	%	millions	%	millions	%	millions
Women with nutritional anaemia[a]	58	172	40	37	17	13
Birth weight below 2500 g[b]	27	13	15	3	11	1
Preschool children with acute protein energy malnutrition (wasting)[c]	16[d]	33[d]	7	4	4	2
Preschool children with chronic protein energy malnutrition (stunting)[c]	40[d]	81[d]	35	24	43	20
Preschool children with low weight[c]	47[d]	94[d]	30	20	28	13

* This table taken from WHO document A36/7.

[a] Royston E: The prevalence of nutritional anaemia in women in developing countries: a critical review of available information. World Health Stat Quart 35 (2), 1982.

[b] Division of Family Health, World Health Organization, Geneva. The incidence of low birth weight: a critical review of available information. World Health Stat Quart 33 (3), 1980.

[c] Based on: Keller W, Filmore C: The prevalence of malnutrition. World Health Stat Quart 35 (4) (in press). Values for India: Kerala Statistical Institute, unpublished data.

[d] Weighted for India.

[e] Excluding temperate countries of South America (i.e. Argentina, Chile, Paraguay and Uruguay).

practices. At the other, factors determining deficit malnutrition resulting from natural or man-made disasters are conditioned by the abrupt decrease in overall food availability. The sectors required to intervene in each case are not the same, nor is the role they should play in pursuit of appropriate solutions.

The critical issue for a proper harmonization of sectoral activities is the appropriate epidemiological definition of nutrition problems at individual, family, community and subnational levels, even if this has to be done on an essentially qualitative and theoretical basis. Such an approach facilitates the development of sectoral nutrition strategies aimed at overcoming or modifying the specific factors interfering with the nutrition process, and helps to order the time sequence of interventions. In addition to timing, some sectors may have a more important role to play at the national level, others at an intermediate level, and still others at the local level.

3. Health sector options in primary, secondary and tertiary malnutrition prevention

With its potential for vastly increased coverage through an integrated system of service delivery, primary health care (PHC) offers the best opportunity for the health sector to reach those persons who are most in need of preventive or curative services that have a positive impact on nutritional status.

Growth monitoring is a core nutritional activity in PHC in view of the sensitivity of this indicator as a reflection of overall child well-being and, by extension, of the quality of the environment in which the child lives. Growth monitoring is not an end in itself; rather it represents a particularly useful entry point, during periods of high individual risk, for introducing both preventive and curative health measures.

Depending on conditions encountered, the principal health sector options, singly or in combination, include treatment, referral, and individual and family counselling on the probable effects on health of a particular course of action. The aggregation of such information at community and subnational levels permits a relatively precise identification of those groups on whose behalf special action is required.

Of the possible health sector options following on growth monitoring, a number are directed towards specific age groups such as those listed in Table 2

Table 2. Examples of health sector options in reference to specific age groups.

Problem	Indicator	Associated factors	Health sector options
Intrauterine	Poor weight	Maternal illness	Early diagnosis and management; preventive actions for prevalent disease
Malnutrition	Gain during pregnancy	Excessive energy output for intake	Education if constraints not from outside health, facilitate women's activities; promotion of higher dietary intake
	Low birth weight for gestational age	Size of mother	Activities related to next generation of women
		Smoke, alcohol other drugs	Increase awareness, facilitate behaviour changes
		Age, frequency of pregnancies, number of pregnancies	Increase awareness, facilitate family planning
		Genetic, congenital	Genetic counseling

Table 2. Continued.

Problem	Indicator	Associated factors	Health sector options
		Insufficient intake of specific nutrients	Detection and management; food enrichment, dietary changes
Infant/ young child malnutrition	Inappropriate weight or height gain	Insufficient dietary availability	Increasing awareness of need for extra energy during lactation; increasing awareness of need for supplementation after 4–6 months of age; referral for food aid; facilitating through community action time for child care when maternal needs outside the house are pressing for family survival
		Insufficient intake	Increasing awareness of need for psychosocial stimulation; dietary management during disease or convalescence – to overcome lack of appetite
		Excessive losses or increased requirements	Early diagnosis and management of disease including diet; preventive measures for prevalent diseases in the area
		Excessive intake or unbalanced diets	Awareness of risk, alternative management and control – special dietary management
		Insufficient intake of specific nutrients	Early detection and management; food supplementation/enrichment
Youth and adult malnutrition	Inappropriate weight/height gain	Chronic illness	Early diagnosis, management; preventive measures
	Weight losses	Insufficient dietary availability and excessive energy output	Generally due to factors outside the capacity of health sector; health sector role to advocacy for action of others
		Psychosocial, drugs	Early diagnosis, management
	Excessive weight gain	Cultural, psychosocial	Increase awareness of risk; dietary or medical management

together with nutritional status indicators and associated factors. It is clear that the effect of health sector activities on malnutrition is not unlimited; other factors can easily neutralize the benefits normally accruing from interventions of the health sector or otherwise limit family choices. Each activity (column 4) is directed towards solving a specific problem (colomn 1).

Basic to the successful delivery of PHC intervention programmes is the presence of a corps of appropriately trained community health workers. In the light of the foregoing, the general nutrition training provided these workers, and their supervisors and trainers, requires careful consideration from two points of view; first, training programmes should emphasize the important direct and indirect role all health interventions in PHC play, where improvements in overall nutritional status are concerned. Such awareness is important for countering a common tendency to view the purpose and effect of individual activities in isolation. Second, such training should be thoroughly task-oriented and based on the practical resolution of everyday problems in a field environment.

WHO has begun to develop guidelines for nutrition training, using the modular approach, on the basis of a definition of the specific problems faced by community health workers. These guidelines are demonstrating their value for increasing health workers' awareness of the interdependence of the various interventions for which they are responsible, and, consequently, for improving their effectiveness in delivering nutrition services to those in need. Their problem-solving orientation assigns a dual purpose to increasing health workers' effectiveness within the context of national health system development: continuing training for PHC workers, as well as guidance to communities and community health workers on practical problems arising in connexion with all aspects of PHC, are viewed not only as means for increasing system coverage, but also for improving the quality of services rendered.

Primary Health Care in the hospital

Z. ISANI

Introduction

The only way developing countries can achieve the target of 'Health for all by year 2000' is through Primary Health Care.

What is Primary Health Care?

The International Conference on Primary Health Care at 'Alma Ata' defines it as essential health care based on practical, scientifically sound and socially acceptable methods and technology made universally accessible to individuals and families in the community through their full participation and at a cost that the community and the country can afford to maintain at every stage of their development in the spirit of self reliance and self determination.

Two things stand out very clearly in this definition:
1. No mention is made of hospital care;
2. The individual and the community are no longer being cared for but have become people involved in their own care.

Before we can discuss the role of 'Hospital in Primary Health Care' it is important to define the framework on which primary health care services are to be based depending on the social, medical, political, and developing circumstances existing in the particular community.

In order to define this framework on the living conditions in Pakistan, I would like to present the following statistical data (Table 1).

The following problems arise from these living conditions:
1. High infant mortality (100 per thousand);
2. High perinatal mortality (40 per thousand. Of these deaths, 30% are due to tetanus);
3. High maternal mortality (10 per thousand);
4. Malnutrition (70% of children under age 5 are malnourished, 10% in Grade III);

5. Diarrhoea: Every child under 2 years of age will have anything from 2 to 6 attacks per year; 40–50% of our total deaths are due to diarrhoea;
6. High incidence of infectious diseases such as, polio, whooping cough, tetanus, tuberculosis, diptheria, measles; and other conditions such as malaria, typhoid, hookworm infestations, etc.

Incidence of infectious diseases in Pakistan (Table 2).

Tables 3–5 present some data from the National Institute of Child Health in Karachi. These data define the components of Primary Health Care in Pakistan which are as follows:

1. Promotion of breast feeding;
2. Oral Rehydration Therapy in diarrhoea;
3. Immunization against 6 common diseases;
4. Use of growth charts, especially to detect invisible malnutrition;
5. Birth spacing (family planning);
6. Training of traditional birth attendants;
7. Improving sanitation and water supply;
8. In some areas in the North, prevention of goitre becomes an integral part of the programme.

Primary Health Care, as it is known today, is practically non-existant. In

Table 1. Statistical data about living conditions in Pakistan.

Area	796,000 km^2
Population	85 Million (70% rural)
% under 15	45
% under 5	18
Literacy rate	20%
Crude birth rate	41 per thousand
Crude death rate	13 per thousand
Growth rate	3%
Access to safe water supply	27%; rural 3%
Sanitation	No sanitation in rural area
G.N.P. per capita	U.S. $300

Table 2. Incidence of infectious diseases in Pakistan.

Name of the disease	Annual incidence in children	Estimated annual mortality in children
Measles	987,552	20,000
Polio	22,207	6,638
Tetanus	47,735	47,167
Whooping cough	262,246	4,958
Diptheria	14,211	12,181
Tuberculosis	71,809	12,181

Pakistan there are several reasons for this:

1. Demographic pattern: M.C.H. services have to look after 60–70% of the population and sufficient staff is not available.
2. Rurality: 70–80% of the population live in the rural areas.
3. Politically strong urban sector of the population.
4. Lack of resources.
5. Unbalanced distribution of resources (urban/rural). 80% of the budget goes on medical education. The medical graduate teaching is confined to the hospital with no exposure to the community and a curricula which stresses curative and diagnostic medicine.
6. Faulty planning: The planners are usually doctors who have been hospital trained but have very little knowledge of community problems. For instance, we have a research programme for cancer and cardiovascular diseases but not for nutrition. We are training 4500 doctors annually, most of whom will be providing services in the rich urban centres. Like other developing countries

Table 3. Deaths of children under the age of 1 year in 1982 (total admissions, 2536; total deaths, 298).

Disease	No.	Percentage
Diarrhoea with P.C.M.	123	41.3 } 48.7
Diarrhoea alone	22	7.4
Resp. infections	28	9.4
T.B. meningitis	15	5
Miscellaneous	110	36.9

Table 4. Neonatal deaths (excluding tetanus) (total admissions, 744; total deaths, 201).

Cause	No.	Percentage
Low birth weight + R.D.S. + I.V.H.	113	56.3
Cerebral anoxia	21	10.4
Pneumonia	21	10.4
Septicemia	16	8
Miscellaneous	30	14.9
Total	201	100

Table 5. Deaths due to neonatal tetanus (from Dec. 1982 to Aug. 1983).

Total admissions	120
Total deaths	42
Percentage	35

we also suffer from a top heavy pyramid with most manpower being at the higher professional catagories.

The ratio of doctors to primary health care workers is 4:1.

Having said all this, I now come to the actual topic of Hospital and Primary Health Care.

Although as stated, no mention of the word 'hospital' was made at the Alma Ata Conference, as things exist at the moment in Pakistan, hospitals should be an integral part of the primary health complex, for without proper supervision the primary health care centres will be in danger of falling into the trap of 'second class medicine for second class citizens'.

Hospitals are mostly located in the urban areas. At one end of the spectrum they are highly sophisticated, built on the western style; at the other end, they are poorly managed, overcrowded, filthy and ill equipped.

The present day role of the hospital depends upon the size, situation and whether or not they are teaching institutions. By and large, they only just fulfil the basic needs of a patient, such as crisis care and drugs, with some sophistication in a few cases.

Result: The problem is ongoing and the patient keeps coming back to the hospital. No effort is made to solve the basic problem and meet the social needs.

In other words, hospitals are really not playing any 'role' in Primary Health Care. However, this situation is changing and hospitals and doctors are working with health workers to achieve the target of 'Health for all by the year 2000'. Their cooperation is vital, for as Halfdan Mahter puts: 'In theory you can practice primary health care in spite of the doctors. In reality, if they decide to fight it, I think they will win'.

The role of hospitals in Primary Health Care is therefore as follows:
1. Encouraging community participation;
2. Actively providing direct support to primary health care (education, supervision, referral);
3. Orientating physicians and other health personnel;
4. Supporting research.

I would now like to illustrate why hospitals in Pakistan can play a major role in Primary Health Care and I would go as far as to say that hospitals will decide the failure or success of Primary Health Care.
1. 80% of the budget is spent by the hospitals. Part of this budget could be earmarked for Primary Health Care.
2. The senior physicians working in these institutions are in a position to get some concessions from the Government, the local politicians and the international agencies. Since primary care is a very topical subject these days, a lot of help is avaitable.
3. Since people respect hospitals as places equipped with the latest medical knowledge, methods of preventive therapy instituted here have a better

chance of being accepted outside the hospital, e.g., in the use of ORS in the treatment of diarrhoea.

4. Directors and heads of hospitals are in a better position to get the support and guidance of the local 'elders', and without their help primary health care can never succeed. Since very little effort and money has been spent on the health of the rural people, they are always suspicious that the 'do-gooders' have an ulterior motive, such as asking for votes in elections, or coming from family planning departments. However, hospital needs, are beyound suspicion and are more likely to succeed where other workers have failed.

I belong to one of these prestigious institutions and would like to give you a brief resume of the Primary Health Care services carried out in my hospital. Since the Government, health planners and doctors dealing with children are committed to 'Health for all by the year 2000', all hospitals are now to a lesser or greater extent involved in Primary Health Care.

1. Healthy baby clinic and under 5 clinic: These clinics are run by health visitors and supervised by doctors. Activities carried out are:
   (a) promotion of breast feeding;
   (b) advice on weaning;
   (c) weaning food demonstration;
   (d) use of growth charts.
2. Immunization is carried out against the six common diseases (measles, tuberculosis, diptheria, pertusis, tetanus and polio).
3. Oral rehydration therapy: Children with mild and moderate dehydration are admitted to this ward, for a couple of hours. Here the mothers are taught how to recognize dehydration and how to use oral rehydration therapy.
4. Family planning services.
5. Education and training:
   (a) doctors, undergraduates and postgraduates: Emphesis is laid on teaching postgraduates. Undergraduate training is not satisfactory as paediatrics is not a major subject in our medical curricula and hence student attendance is poor. We are fighting against this and hopefully in future paediatrics will be given its due importance.
   (b) health visitors and paramedics: All the above activities are in fact carried out by the health visitors who come to us in the course of their training.
   (c) community health workers.
   (d) we also hold symposia and conferences in the remote areas where the main theme is always primary health care.
   (e) preparing documentary films and talks for the various mass medias.
6. Contributions to research: Research is being carried out on ORS and diarrhoea.
7. Training mothers to look after preterm babies and neonatal tetanus. Our intensive baby care units are largely run by mothers resulting in a better survival rate and these methods can be used in the peripheral centres.

8. Community outreach: The hospital staff runs an M.C.H. Centre in Meh-moodabad which is an urban slum and we hope to increase such detachment areas. The other sister institution at Dow Medical College looks after 3 villages which are basically farming communities and has had good results. Criteria for referral are defined, maintaining the flow in both directions.

With the leadership provided by the hospital, the areas covered by primary health care are gradually increasing.

Utilisation of child health services in developing countries

A. BAMISAIYE

Introduction

Evidence world-wide indicates that those who need health services the most, the urban and rural poor, use them the least. Because the health care system is not in contact with the mass of the people, technical interventions, such as immunisation, or major advances such as oral rehydration therapy for diarrhoea, are limited in their effectiveness.

The basic problem for the rural and urban poor is lack of modern health services available to them. Where they do exist, however, they are far from being fully or properly utilised [1]. The problem of low utilisation rates is often obscured by the appearance of overflowing clinics and harassed, seemingly overworked staff. Only when use patterns are related to a denominator, in other words when rates of health service coverage are calculated, does the problem emerge clearly.

Data from the service run by the Institute of Child Health and Primary Care in Lagos may be used to illustrate this point. During the first year of operation of an integrated preventive and curative service, we registered for primary care service over 3000 pre-school age children, by means of a home-based referral system. The volume of work this involved meant that the clinic was full every day and staff felt themselves working to capacity. However it was important to remind ourselves at the end of the year that this number of children registered represented only 40% of the estimated 7500 pre-school age children in the target population of 30,000 people resident in the area surrounding the clinic.

Moreover, scrutiny of our records at the end of the first year illustrated that the use made of the service by the first 3000 children registered was far from the levels our service objectives envisaged. Forty per cent of these children had only ever attended the clinic once, for the registration visit and had not even started the immunisation programme. Only 15% of the children registered in the first year had completed three doses of DPT and polio vaccine [2].

Nearly ten years later we have registered 80% of our eligible pre-school population. However these children are still not using our service as we hoped.

Coverage with three doses of DPT and polio vaccine is 42% and only 22% of children are completely immunised by one year of age. Attendance figures for 1976–8 indicated that only 23% of children 0–1 year of age, the most vulnerable group, had visited the clinic monthly. During 1982–3 the ratio of well to sick visits was one well visit for every six visits for curative care [3].

For the last ten years we have been struggling to understand the dynamics of service utilisation by the community, trying to ascertain the factors which act to depress use of our service and hence achievement on our part of optimum service coverage. We have found it useful to conceive of utilisation as limited by the *availability, accessibility,* and *acceptability* of health services. We consider that the task of the health worker in developing countries is to develop strategies, relevant to the constraints identified, for promoting contact between the service and the community and for increasing the effectiveness of the services offered [4, 5].

Service availability

The overwhelming majority of the poor in developing countries have no modern health services available to them. This is partly because the economic resources devoted to health services by governments in the developing world are extremely meagre, nearly half such nations devoting less than U.S. $ 3 per capita per annum to health [6]. The situation is worsened by a reliance on high-cost, high technology curative care facilities which tend to be concentrated in urban areas. In Ghana, 40% of health expenditure is devoted to specialised hospitals which serve only 1% of the population [7]. In Nigeria, the Federal Ministry of Health estimated that in 1975 national coverage with modern medical care was only 25%, the population excluded from care being essentially that 80% resident in the rural areas [8]. For the developing world as a whole, less than 10% of those born each year ever see a health worker [9]. Thus, WHO concludes that prior to 1980 less than 10% of children in these countries were receiving any immunisation against the six most common childhood diseases [10].

The provision of a health facility in a remote rural area is only one step in making a service available for use. A service must also be staffed, equiped, supplied with essential items, drugs and vaccines and linked into a system of referral, support and supervision. Moreover these resources must be continuously available for a service to function such that people will use it. A careful study in Ghana showed that in the two health districts surveyed, *all* resources (staff, supervision, transport, referral, supplies) fell short of the absolute minimum for adequate service delivery. The study also documents how service attendance fell immediately the community realised that essential drugs and vaccines were lacking at a particular clinic [11]. In Guatamela, the non-utilisation of widely distributed rural health posts was studied. The health posts were found to be under-equiped and short of essential drugs. The author found that the *only* medical items in adequate supply were syringes, wooden tongue depressors, thermometers and cotton swabs [12].

The logistics of supplying drugs, vaccines and other essential items may overstrain the limited managerial capacity of ministries of health in developing countries, who generally do not have the resources or the experience to serve widely dispersed primary health clinics [13]. However, the consequence of failure to supply needed resources is non-utilisation of service, since in our experience an empty drug cupboard equals an empty clinic. Without regular supplies the health worker cannot compete with the traditional healer (in the country side) or the chemist (in the cities). At least their stock in trade is always available [14].

Thus, not only do an estimated two thirds of the population in developing countries not have services available for use, those that do may have a building and (not always) staff with very few activities going on because of non-availability of essential resources and poor training and supervision of personnel.

Service accessibility

Factors limiting the access of a community to a health service have been extensively documented. Geographic access is important since use of health services diminishes sharply with distance [15, 16]. Three to five kilometers appears to be the limit people are prepared to walk to a health facility, yet in rural areas health centres may be expected to serve an area of a thousand square kilometers [6]. Bad roads, inadequate transportation systems and heavy seasonal rains contribute to the disincentive effect of distance on service use [17]. If people are afraid, or in pain, great efforts may be made and considerable distances travelled to get care [18]. In rural Northern Nigeria it is not unknown for a woman in labour to be taken for 3 days by donkey before a motorable road to the hospital is reached [19]. These kinds of desperate efforts are less likely to be made for children, who die so easily. If they are, it will be for curative care for an acute illness.

Health service use may also be limited by problems of economic access. In developing countries direct costs, in the form of a fee-for-service are usually low, or non-existent, for government child health services. However, the poorest and least educated may be intimidated into paying for services which should be free [10]. Such corrupt practices may be relatively rare in fact but contribute to the 'reputation' of a service on which people base their decision whether to use it or not.

Indirect costs for service include transportation to and from the health facility and the opportunity cost of attending the service. By the latter is meant the money lost from trade, farming or employment by clinic attendance. The loss of a day's earnings may be vitally significant in terms of the extremely narrow budgetary limits within which the poor of the developing world have to operate [21–24].

This is particularly the case in situations where women head households or, as in West Africa, are expected to shoulder considerable economic responsibilities for the care of children [25]. A study of the opportunity cost to mothers interviewed in the ICH clinic in Lagos revealed that 90% of the mothers would have been engaged in trade, had they not come to the clinic that day, from which their profit would have been 2–3 naira (approx. U.S. $2–3).

Health services must also be functionally accessible to a population [5]. By this is meant that integrated care (curative, preventive and promotive) should be available on a continuing basis to a population, whenever they need it and provided by an appropriately organised health team. In practice, this principle is very often ignored. The study of health services in Ghana, previously referred to, concluded that clinics were organised in such a way as to make utilisation of services as difficult and time-consuming as possible [11]. For example, a service with which we are familiar in Lagos separates preventive and curative care with respect to time, place and staff. It has a patient flow pattern so complex that a mother attending for the first time with an ill child would have to pass through no less than thirteen service points. Moreover, despite the presence of eleven fully qualified nurses, every child attending is required to be seen by the one doctor on duty, thus ensuring a wait of six to seven hours for those mothers at the end of the queue. Such examples of lack of functional access may be repeated endlessly throughout the developing world.

The health service system must also be culturally accessible, that is the technical and managerial methods used should be in keeping with the cultural patterns of the community [5]. Where women live in purdah, or seclusion, after marriage this obviously requires that community-based workers also be female. And yet community health aides recruited in Kaduna State, in the Muslim North of Nigeria, are 90% male, as are community health workers in one region of India [26]. These are clear instances of culturally inappropriate methods of delivering services, which result in low levels of use of these home based workers.

The cultural context in which a service operates may often contain elements which act to depress service use, particularly among mothers and young children who need services the most. Where women are secluded after marriage, the permission of the husband must always be obtained for any absence from home, including attending a clinic or hospital. Permission may be refused for preventive and promotive care, since in the father's view the child is 'not ill'. In the patrilineal societies of Africa the children 'belong' to the father's descent group and he sanctions all matters relating to their care, welfare and upbringing. Consequently, even when women are not secluded after marriage, as in Lagos, the permission of the father must be given before a child can be brought to the clinic [27]. Similar findings have been reported from East Africa [28, 29].

The geographical mobility of young children is a cultural factor which may affect use of child health services. In many African societies a young child may be sent to a relative, often a grand-parent, when the mother becomes pregnant again. Employed women may also send some or all of their children to grand-parents if they find it difficult to combine child-care and work responsibilities [30]. And yet pre-school children being cared for by grandmothers in our target area in Lagos have extremely low rates of clinic use, presumably because the grandmothers have limited mobility and are disinclined to wait in the clinic for long periods [31].

Increasing numbers of young children in developing countries are in one-parent families, most often being cared for by the mother alone [32]. Not only does the mother have the entire responsibility for family maintenance but the 'under-staffing' of the family makes it harder to find time for clinic visits. Studies in Africa show quite clearly that child health services are used less by family units headed by the mother [21, 31].

Service acceptability

Most studies of service utilisation have examined the issue of acceptability by focussing on the characteristics of the service user or non-user; for example relating maternal education, beliefs, values etc. to utilisation patterns. This approach tends to blame the members of a community for service failures to achieve coverage objectives, citing their irresponsibility, ignorance or distrust for non-use [33]. However individual behaviour is constrained by structural factors. It is suggested here that aspects of service organisation are an important part of the structure of the situation in which an individual decides to use a health service or not. In other words, the way in which a service is organised and operated influences utilisation behaviour. We have noted earlier the negative impact on service use if essential resources, such as staff and drugs are not available or if the service ignores issues of functional or cultural access.

To be fully acceptable the health service must also meet the felt health needs of the community. In the developing world people desire primarily curative care, thus curative care for common conditions must be integrated with the preventive and promotive care which, in the case of children, will do more to improve health status. If preventive and promotive care are offered alone, the service will not be used [7, 11, 14].

Service hours are often incompatible with other demands on the time of women. Government services are invariably organised in the mornings, when the only free time rural women may have is in the afternoons [26, 34]. In the cities, the employed woman will have to take time off from work to attend clinic with her child and the self-employed woman absents herself from her place of trade for a morning, usually the busiest time. If women could be sure of spending no more than one, at most two, hours in the clinic then this schedule of service in the mornings need not be a deterrent. Unfortunately this is not the case. Studies from Africa and South America report time spent in clinics from three to four hours, with waiting time usually comprising the greatest part of this [35–38]. Despite great efforts to streamline care in our own service in Lagos, in order to reduce waiting time, mothers attending for a routine visit spend an average of three hours in the clinic [3].

It is often assumed by those organising child health services that mothers in the developing world have this time to spare [24]. However, it has been pointed out that for both rural and urban women surplus time may be extremely limited, particularly when they are carrying the major economic responsibility for themselves and their children [25, 39–41].

Finally, the reputation of a service and hence its acceptability to a community, is often adversely affected by the perceived attitudes and behaviour of the service staff towards the clients. Numerous reports from developing countries indicate that mothers suffer rudeness, hostility and scolding from service staff [28, 42, 43]. In part, this is a result of the social distance between service providers and service users, who may be of different ethnic groups and who have superior education, income and living standards. Two interesting studies from the USA are relevant here. In one, nurses in a health centre serving a low income area perceived mothers as valuing health care far less than was the actual case [43]. In the other, the health workers studied had very limited and partial information about the actual living conditions and day-to-day difficulties of the poor families in the community served. As such the health workers tended to have stereotyped and perjorative attitudes regarding the health behaviour of the community [45].

In our own service in Lagos, and in most developing countries, the sense of social hierarchy is very strong. This has contributed to the concerted resistance by our service staff to the suggestion that users of the service be brought into the delivery system by incorporating representatives of the community into the monthly clinic meeting. Research elsewhere in Nigeria has illustrated that nurses see patients, or service users, in terms of the extent of their 'control' over them and prefer patients who do not constitute a threat to their authority [46]. Moreover on the part of community members themselves there is often an exaggerated attitude of respect, deference and gratitude towards service staff, which presents obstacles to our efforts to foster self-reliance in health care, for example through the teaching of skills such home-preparation of oral rehydration solution (ORS). It will obviously be a gradual process to develop more egalitarian modes thought on the part of service staff and less dependency on the part of the community [47].

The issue of the acceptability of child health services must include consideration of the numerous alternative forms of care available in a given community. Traditional medicine at present serves the two-thirds of the world's population that is beyond reach of modern medical care. Where modern and traditional care is available people will often tend to use both, sequentially or concurrently depending on preception of problem and/or response to treatment [48–50]. Self-medication probably ranks as the most common form of care for the urban poor [51, 52]. Per capita private expenditure on health care per annum may often exceed quite considerably public spending [13, 20]. As more doctors are trained in developing contries, more personal resources are utilised to purchase medical care from private practitioners. Even a modest degree of relative prosperity may be linked with the purchase of private medical care such that, for example, integrated child health services are scarcely used by the slightly better off [20, 29]. In our target community in Lagos it seems to be an indicator of economic status *not* to use to ICH service but rather a 'private doctor'. Unfortunately, private doctors in most developing countries merely provide ad hoc curative care for children and only very rarely give immunisation or monitor growth and development. Finally, education, as the most important individual characteristic affecting utilisation of services, should be mentioned. It has been demonstrated that the education of women is significantly linked with levels of use of ante-natal services and child-care [53]. Moreover, the education of women in the developing world is linked both to declines in mortality and in fertility [54, 55]. It is obviously important to ascertain the benefits that education confers in terms of increasing the mother's readiness to use child health services and consider how these benefits may be simulated for those women who have not received education.

Promoting contact between community and child health services

The seemingly endless list of barriers, constraints and obstacles to health service use, enumerated above, should not discourage those with responsibilities for delivering child health services to a community. People do desire improved health as shown by the extent to which personal resources are expended on the search for health care. The Primary Health Care approach, with its emphasis on generally available essential health care for common conditions, integrated with prevention and promotive care, use of local personnel and integration with traditional medicine does offer a real prospect for improving the health of the people [5].

Integrating curative, preventive and promotive care breaks down the invidious distinction in child health services between well-child care and curative care, which has had a harmful effect on utilisation of services for far too long. The use of appropriately trained local people at grass-roots level to deliver essential care will bring services within reach of scattered communities. Depending on the local situation a mix of employed personnel and volunteers may be utilised. Where village communities are very small and widely dispersed volunteer health workers (VHWs) can give simple care for the most common conditions and refer cases they cannot deal with [56]. Even in large cities volunteers may be used effectively to refer neighbours and co-tenants for care [2]. It has been suggested that successful users of ORS may volunteer to support others in the community who are trying it for the first time or are uncertain about its use [57].

The 'lay-referral' system has long been recognised by social scientists as influencing the use made of health services. This implies that utilization is highly dependent on the experiences of family and friends [58]. Creating a system of volunteer health workers or referral/support agents in the community helps to increase significantly the extent of the social network which facilitates access to services. Every lay-person, linked with the health system in some form and recognised by it, multiplies the number of community members who receive improved information about the service, is provided with an entry or referral and gain increased confidence in the use of innovations such as ORS or family planning devices.

Reservations have been stated about the use of community volunteers in primary health care. It has, for example, been pointed out that no other welfare sector utilises volunteers [13]. However if health services are to become genuinely more accessible, a large part of the gain must be by utilising the people themselves in the service delivery process.

Facilitating the effectiveness of child health services

The foregoing review of factors affecting service use has indicated that the efficacy of many services is in serious doubt. Where services are poorly equiped and supplied, the immunisation programme, for example, may be of doubtful use having regard to breaks in the cold chain, interrupted supply of vaccines or even expired vaccines in use. Moreover, the technical performance of poorly trained and supervised auxiliaries, functioning in remote areas, may be seriously inadequate. It has been pointed out that primary health care uses simple technology but is extremely complex to manage effectively [59]. Management here is taken to mean the management of human resources (training and supervision of personnel) as well as the material resources of transport, drugs, vaccines, supplies and equipment. As yet the primary health care approach has been successfully applied only in relatively small-scale, tightly controlled projects, usually with outside assistance. To make the extension to the national level requires considerable resources devoted to training and management. These resources would have to be diverted from elsewhere within the health sector, already locked-in to a pattern of provision of urban, curative care. At this time there seem few indications outside the socialist developing countries that this re-allocation of resources for primary health care is being made. Without it, primary health care services are not likely to function effectively on any scale.

Even when efficacy of service functioning is assured services will still lack effectiveness unless there is some effort to focus on priority diseases, to which can be attributed the bulk of the morbidity and mortality, and on high risk groups in the population. Assuming that the service has already selected the care of mothers and pre-school children as its prime focus, high risk groups would then include very young mothers, children cared for by single parents or foster-parents, malnourished or weight-faltering children and any other groups which local conditions suggest are particularly at risk. This kind of focus is also the most efficient use of resources available such that efforts are made to bring about optimum utilisation by those most vulnerable.

In conclusion, the efforts to increase health service utilisation should not focus merely on high coverage of the community with isolated benefits such as immunisation or receipt of ORS packets [60]. Instead what is required is the establishment of high rates of *continuing contact* with child health services, in the form of regular and frequent visits by mothers and children. This is much more difficult and will require that steps be taken to overcome many problems limiting access and acceptability which have been listed above. This in turn will require, above all, a sensitive consideration of the total life situation of mothers and children in the poor areas of the world. However, the establishment of a pattern of regular and frequent visits to child health services and of a relationship of mutual confidence between health worker and client is important enough to warrant considerable efforts to improve access and acceptability. By means of frequent contact the on-going growth and development of the child can be monitored, particularly of children with nutritional and related problems, and the full range of preventive care services provided. Frequent contact also makes it more likely that serious illnesses such as measles, pneumonia and severe diarrhoea will be seen early enough to reduce mortality. Outreach workers, in daily contact with the community, can support mothers in the use of ORS and other innovations. Over time, in partnership with community volunteers and other change agents, real improvements in *health behaviour* may be brought about, providing a sure foundation for technical efforts to improve the health status of children in the developing world.

References

1. Mahler H: Speech at a special convocation of the University of Lagos, 1980.
2. Bamisaiye A: The field health worker: A new cadre of staff for the delivery of family health services. 2nd International Paediatric Conference Nigerian Paediatric Association, Ibadan, Nigeria 1976.
3. Bamisaiye A: Waiting time and its impact on service acceptability and coverage at an MCH clinic in Lagos, Nigeria (in preparation) 1983.
4. Tanahashi T: Health service coverage and its evaluation Bull Wld Hlth Org 56(2):295–303, 1978.
5. WHO/UNICEF: Primary health care. Report of the International Conference on Primary Health Care Alma-Ata USSR. Geneva World Health Organisation, 1978.
6. World Bank: Health sector policy paper. World Bank Washington DC, 1980.
7. Morley D: The child's name is today. Brighton Manton, Westminster, 1982.
8. Federal Ministry of Health Nigeria: The challenge of the basic health services scheme for change. Lagos National Health Planning Division, 1975.
9. Population Reference Bureau: Children in the world. Population Reference Bureau Washington DC, 1979.

10. Progress report. Primary health: a first assessment. People 10(2):6–9, 1983.

11. de Kadt E, Segall M: Health needs and health services in rural Ghana. Soc Sci Med 15A(4):397–518, 1981.

12. Annis S: Physical access and utilization of health services in rural Guatamala. Soc Sci Med 15D(4):515–523, 1981.

13. Golladay F, Liese B: Health problems and policies in the developing countries. World Bank Staff Working Paper. No 412. World Bank, Washington DC, 1980.

14. Cunningham N: The under-fives clinic: what difference does it make? Env Child Hlth J Trop Paed Monograph, pp. 233–333, 1978.

15. Jolly R, King M: The organisation of health services. In: King M (ed) Medical care in developing countries. Nairobi, Oxford University Press, pp. 2:1–2:15, 1966.

16. Fendall NRE: Medical planning and the training of personnel in Kenya. J Trop Med Hyg 68:12, 1965.

17. Kreysler J: Rational development of an 'under-Five Clinic' network. J Trop Paed 16:48–52, 1970.

18. Wray JD: Expanded MCH programmes (editorial). Env Child Health J Trop Paed 20, 1974.

19. Murphy M, Baba TM: Rural dwellers and health care in Northern Nigeria. Soc Sci Med 15 A3(Part 1):265–271, 1981.

20. Lasker J: Choosing among therapies: illness behaviour in the Ivory Coast. Soc Sci Med 15 A(2): 157–1681, 1981.

21. Senanayake IP: Evaluation of a health care system for children under five years of age in Africa. Unpublished PhD thesis, University of London, 1975.

22. Wellman J: The Gbaja Family Health Nurse Project, Lagos, Nigeria, 1967–70. Unpublished PhD thesis, Johns Hopkins University, Baltimore, 1971.

23. Benyoussef A, Wessen AF: Utilisation of health services in developing countries – Tunisia. Soc Sci Med 8:287–304, 1974.

24 Scrimshaw NS: Myths and realities in international health planning. Am J Publ Hlth 64:792–798, 1974.

25. Boserup E: Woman's role in economic development. St Martins Press, New York, 1970.

26. Murthy N: Indian women's need for curative care. In: Blair P (ed) Health needs of the world's poor women. Equity Policy Centre, Washington DC, 1980.

27. Bamisaiye A, Ransome-Kuti O, Ojo May: Health education directed towards the father: new approach within maternal and child health services. 1st International All Africa Conference on Health Education, Lagos, 1981.

28. Bornstein A, Kreysler J: Social factors influencing attendance in Under Fives clinics. Env Child Hlth J Trop Paed 18:150–158, 1972.

29. Bennett FJ, Jellife DB: The health of immigrant babies in an East African town. Trop Geogr Med 17:213–224, 1965.

30. Oyediran MA, Bamisaiye A: A study of the child care arrangements and the health status of pre-school children of employed women in Lagos. Pub Hlth (in press).

31. Bamisaiye A: Selected factors influencing the coverage of an MCH clinic in Lagos. J Trop Paed (in press).

32. Introduction. The condition of women and children's well-being. Assignment Children 49/50, 1980.

33. McKinlay JB: Some approaches and problems in the study of the use of services: an overview. J Hlth Hum Behav 13:115–152, 1972.

34. Ebrahim GJ: Child health in a changing world. Macmillan, London, p 89, 1982.

35. Ashitey GA, Wurapa FK, Belcher DW: Danfa rural health centre: Its patients and services 1970-71. Ghana Med J 11(3):266–273, 1972.

36. Vogel LC: Operational study of the OPD at Government Hospital Kiambu Kenya. E Afr Med J 53(3):168–186, 1976.

37. Keller A, Villareal FS, de Rodriguez AR, Correu S: The impact of organisation of Family

Planning clinics on waiting time. Stud Fam Plan 6(5):134–140, 1975.

38. Zein A: Operational study of the out-patient department at the public health hospital at Gondar Ethiopia. Ethiop Med J 16:45–52, 1978.

39. Popkin BM, Solon SF: Income, time, the working mother and child nutrition. Env child Hlth J Trop Paed 22:156–166, 1976.

40. Longhurst R: Cropping pattern, nutrition and child care in a Nigerian village. Dev Digest 5:86–93, 1981.

41. Okafor SI: Policy and practice: the case of medical facilities in Nigeria. Soc Sci Med 16(22):1971–1977, 1982.

42. Banerji D: Health behaviour of rural populations. Econ Pol Wkly 8:2261–2268, 1973.

43. Stephens AJH: The impact of health care and nutritional education on an urban community in Africa through the Under Five clinics. J Trop Med Hyg 78:97–105, 1975.

44. Brinton DM: Health centre milieu: interaction of nurses and low income families. Nurs Res 21:46–52, 1972.

45. Pratt L: Level of sociological knowledge among health and social workers. J Hlth Hum Behav 10:59–65, 1969.

46. Odebiyi AI, Togonu-Bickersreth V: Nurses perception and preferences for patient types in Nigeria. 10th World Congress of International Sociological Association, Mexico City, 1982.

47. Ransome-Kuti O, Bamisaiye A: The Progressive involvement of the community in planning health care. A plan from Lagos Nigeria. In: Message from Calcutta. Highlights of the 111 International Congress of the World Federation of Public Health Associations, Calcutta, pp. 134–137, 1981.

48. Maclean U: Magical medicine. Penguin Books, Harmandworth, 1971.

49. Kimani VN: The Unsystematic alternative: towards a plural health care among the Kikuyu of central Kenya. Soc Sci Med 15 B(3):333–340, 1981.

50. Chen PY: Traditional and modern medicine in Malysia. Soc Sci Med 15 A(2):127–136, 1981.

51. Gesler WM: Illness and health practitioner use in Calabar Nigeria. Soc Sci Med 13:D23–30, 1979.

52. World Bank: Health. Sector policy report World Bank, Washington DC, 1975.

53. Schaefer EJ, Hughes JR: Socio-economic factors and maternal and child health care. Med Care 14:535–543, 1976.

54. Caldwell JC: Education as a factor in mortality decline: an examination of Nigerian data. Pop Stud 33:395–415, 1979.

55. Caldwell JC: Mass education as a determinant of the timing of fertility decline. Pop Dev Rev 6(2):225–255, 1980.

56. Ofosu-Amaah V: National experience in the use of community health workers. WHO Offset Publication No 71. Geneva World Health Organisation, 1983.

57. Reyes P: Mother's management of child diarrhoea in Lagos Nigeria. Unpublished ScD thesis, John Hopkins University, Baltimore, 1981.

58. Freidson E: Professional Dominance. Aldine, Chicago, 1970.

59. de Sweemer C: Reaching the village: alibi or revolution. People 10(3):3–5, 1983.

60. Walsh JA, Warren KS: Selective primary health care: an interim strategy for disease control in developing countries. N Engl J Med 301:967–974, 1979.

What has medicine in the Western World learned from work in developing countries?

R.E. BROWN

Introduction

Over the years, many individuals have been impressed with the transfer of technology from the developed countries to the lesser developed countries. However, many of these technological improvements have been transferred inappropriately. Nevertheless, in the rush for modernization, a large number of technologic advances have been introduced into developing countries, often causing problems in the use of large amounts of human and financial resources. Unfortunately, some of these transfers have occurred in isolation, without appropriate support services, and without the vital infra-structure that must be present.

More recently, some have been impressed with what the reverse transfer has taught us, that is, what we have learned and adapted from lesser developed countries. There are many examples of unique and on-going benefits that the developed countries have taken from the Third World, over and above the acknowledged 'brain drain'.

This communication will describe changes in process and procedures, modification in roles and training of health providers, changes in therapy and procedures, and finally, changes in awareness.

Changes in process and procedures

Clinics

In many parts of the so-called developed world, Well Baby Clinics have been established. Mothers are encouraged to take their infants to these facilities during the first year of life for check-ups and routine immunizations, as well as for guidance and assessment of growth and development. It became apparent that in places like West Africa, mothers with several children could not afford to invest the time to take a well child only to be examined and checked. There were other children to care for, some of whom were ill when immunizations and physical examinations were scheduled for the well child. It was to accommodate this need that the 'Under Five Clinics' were first developed in Nigeria so that both ill and well children could receive health care. Mothers or guardians could take all of their children at the same time to one location for both curative and preventive services [1].

Although this system appears to be a simple and relatively minor development, in truth it has had significant consequences. Parents could now obtain various health services for all their children at the same time and place. This means more children were being seen for both curative and preventive purposes. In many places, Well Baby Clinics no longer exist; they have been replaced by either Under Five Clinics or Young Child Centers [2].

Records

To closely monitor a young child's growth, particularly in the first 5 years, growth charts were introduced in many parts of the world to record weight-for-age. The plotting of weight-for-age at 1 or 2 month intervals has become an essential ingredient of growth monitoring. Paraprofessional health workers and, in some places, mothers themselves, have been taught to take the weight, plot the weight-for-age correctly, as well as to interpret either an acceptable growth progression or what has been called 'growth faltering' [3]. The routine use of such growth charts has become an essential part of young child care everywhere. The growth chart has also been called 'The Road To Health' chart because a mother or paraprofessional worker can visualize growth progress of a young child under 5 years of age [4].

Along with the routine use of growth charts the introduction of the concept that the mother herself can maintain and retain this record and return with it regularly each month has been a major development. In some places it has been suggested that these charts should be sold to the mother at a nominal fee to ensure safe keeping of the chart. This system has also been employed in the developed countries, usually with unstable populations such as migratory groups [5]. These records, called home-based medical records, contain the weight-for-age curve, a record of immunizations, intercurrent illnesses, as well as a list of medications used routinely for prophylaxis such as antimalarials. Migratory populations, for example the Lapp reindeer herders in Sweden and the migrant farm workers in the United States, have benefitted from the continuity of this record keeping system. With the home-based health record, the parent or guardian joins the health worker in the health maintenance of their children.

Mother infant contact

In many parts of the Third World mothers carry their infants on their backs in a culturally accepted fashion. Recently the developed countries modified this with the use of back-supported carrying frames or the front-supported 'snugglies' in an effort to enhance and increase maternal-infant contact. All these systems free the mother's hands to carry bundles, push a shopping cart, or do other work; more importantly, it makes a very close and continual contact between the mother and her young offspring possible. The psychological and developmental advantages of maternal-infant bonding have been well documented [6]. In fact, in certain developed countries we see a further modification in that the father may get into the act and help carry his young infant.

In an on-going randomized control trial, consisting of 40 mother-infant dyads, significant differences in visual and vocal interactions have been preliminarily documented [7]. Video tapes of a play situation are interpreted by an outside objective observer who found that infants who were held in the 'snugglies' evidenced more eye contact with the mother and were more responsive to the mother than those who were not carried in the 'snugglie'.

Changes in staff, training, and organization

Paraprofessionals

For many years, the developing countries have had limited options in handling their medical needs. Because of insufficient numbers of trained medical workers, health workers other than physicians and nurses have had to deliver medical services. In most countries an indigenous system of health delivery has existed with traditional birth attendants, and traditional practitioners of various kinds (witch doctors, medicine men, brujos, and so forth). In the first world, the development of a paraprofessional health force, organized and trained to deliver many vital health services, is a direct outgrowth of indigenous health systems. In the People's Republic of China, the government issued a directive sanctioning the use of both traditional and/or modern practitioners [8, 9]. Patients could decide which system they preferred or perhaps select a combination of the two. The directive underscored the importance and the validity of alternative health care systems.

Because of the escalating cost of health care, the developed world has been forced to look to alternate styles of medical care already in place in developing countries. The need for the practitioner, as a viable alternative to physicians and nurses, to deliver certain types of health care is gradually being accepted by the orthodox medical community. In addition to being more appropriately trained and demanding a lower level of financial compensation, these health workers are willing to work in rural and other remote areas that are less attractive to doctors and nurses.

Nurse practitioners, for both pediatric and adult patients, are on their way to being accepted as deliverers of various types of health care [5, 10, 11]. Physicians' assistants, community health workers or family health workers represent the next group of paraprofessional health workers who are now delivering care to many needy and underserved populations. The employment of paraprofessional health workers makes a great deal of sense; it creates new jobs; it extends health care to the community; and it is cost effective.

Once paraprofessional health workers are considered a reasonable option in the developed countries, it follows that their training should be more relevant and more appropriate for the types of services they will be delivering. Paraprofessional workers should, if possible, be recruited from their local community and, when appropriate, should be bilingual and/or bicultural. It is easier to train a community person in the necessary technology needed to work effectively in his or her own community, than to take a technically trained individual from outside of the community and acclimate him to the cultural and linguistic needs of the people being served [12]. Since most hospitals can only serve a limited population, those who live within a 5–10 km area, the concept of satellite health posts and neighborhood health centers took root in many developing countries [4]. The design of a comprehensive plan to more adequately meet the needs of peri-urban, suburban, and rural populations can be adopted and incorporated into the health plans of developed countries [11].

It is completely reasonable to develop a tiered system of health delivery, with appropriately trained 'other professionals' at the periphery, to meet the immediate as well as the future programmed health needs of all segments of the population. It is essential to build into the training systems an awareness that referral and transfer of patients up through the tiers is important for efficient management. A progressive system of supervision and evaluation, that is, each level is supervised by the one immediately above it, is invaluable [2]. The logistics of supply management must also be built into such a system. These modifications of health delivery systems are appropriate for both the developed and developing countries because both have 'medically underserved populations'.

Subsidized medical education

It is clear that even in developed countries such as the United States, there are many pockets of medically underserved populations [12, 13]. These groups are found in migrant camps, American Indian reservations, outlying rural areas, as well as in inner city ghettos. The needs of these groups have called for the development of a National Health Corps, which would give financial (governmental) support to health workers, including physicians, nurses, physician's assistants, and nurse practitioners, during their training period. In return, these health workers would be obliged to serve in locations where there were medically underserved populations [2]. This approach has long been necessary in developing countries to ensure that an adequate supply of medical and other graduates would be posted in rural areas considered less desirable from practical, social, and cultural points of view. Since most governments subsidize the high cost of medical and nursing education, it is only fair that graduates compensate their society by working for a prescribed period in areas where it is difficult to recruit health workers.

Changes in therapy and procedures

Triage

In developing countries there often is a shortage of trained personnel in tandem with very heavy patient loads. 'Triage' of military medicine origin has been adopted as the most effective way to handle this quandry. The triage approach, a priority system, identifies patients who need minimal attention, those who require full work-ups, and those whose needs would overburden the system [1, 4, 12].

In most countries in the developed world, planners had the misconception that there were sufficient numbers of graduate physicians and nurses, along with adequate hospitals and other facilities, to diagnose and comprehensively manage all patients. It has become apparent that even in the developed world some system of prioritization and triage is essential. The triage system was adopted first in the emergency rooms and subsequently at various levels of out-patient health facilities [4, 11]. Nurses and other health practitioners, trained to conduct triage, could free physicians for other tasks. This has become part of the new approach which is now incorporated into the standard routine.

Breastfeeding

Based on early documentation from the developing countries, breastfeeding is being promoted as the most acceptable form of infant feeding [3, 12, 14, 15]. In rural areas, almost 100% of the women breastfed. With the advent of artificial infant formula, many of the educated and financially privileged in urban, suburban, and periurban stopped breastfeeding and turned to formula as the modern, technologically and nutritionally advanced alternative [16, 17]. In emulation of their more wealthy neighbors, the poor segment of the population also stopped breastfeeding with disastrous results [18, 19]. Research data in the developed countries leave no doubt that breast milk is not only nutritionally complete but that it also provides maternal antibodies and active cells to protect the infant [18–21]. Formula-fed babies do not receive these antibodies and are therefore at higher risk and are most susceptible to respiratory and gastrointestinal infections rampant in developing countries. Diarrhea, dehydration, and even death can ensue from the inappropriate and unsanitary use of formula [14–16].

A large proportion of educated and financially secure women of the First World are moving away from formula feeding and returning to traditional (on demand) breastfeeding as the most natural, healthy, and psychologically satisfying system of feeding for both mother and child [6, 17, 18]. In most developing countries, regardless of the campaigns against infant formula and government supported efforts to promote breastfeeding, it has been difficult to reintroduce the concept of 'breast is best'. Even in areas lacking clean water, sanitation, or refrigeration, promotion programs and advertising campaigns of infant formula companies have convinced women that it is sophisticated and modern to formula feed [18, 19]. These women are led to believe that their babies will be happier and healthier if they are formula fed even though this is contrary to all recent scientific findings [20, 21].

Relactation

The high maternal mortality rate in the Third World may leave many newborn infants without the availability of a milk supply from his or her natural mother. After this all too common catastrophe, the surviving orphan is customarily given to a female relative to rear and feed [22]. If the woman is healthy and already lactating, providing breast milk for her own infant, there will generally be no difficulty in increasing her milk supply with the additional suckling so that she can successfully provide milk for two infants. With the nonlactating woman, the infant is put to the breast at frequent intervals and a variety of herbal medicines are employed, lactation can usually be initiated. There are many reports from many parts of the world that describe successful lactation in nonlactating, non-postpartum women merely by putting the infant to the breast and allowing him to suckle [23]. Suckling stimulates nerve endings that cause the anterior pituitary gland to produce prolactin, a hormone that acts directly on mammary glands to secrete milk. In the traditional extended family, there are opportunities for relatives or even friends to serve as substitute wet nurses. Health workers should consider the potential for relactation in times of natural or man-made catastrophes, and in times of mass migration or population relocation. In addition, whenever gastroenteritis from contaminated water is associated with interruption of lactation, definite consideration should be given to the reestablishment of lactation for infant feeding even after prolonged periods of time.

In developed countries, for parents who want to breastfeed, the process of relactation may be seriously entertained for low birth weight infants who must remain on premature units for lengthy periods, and for infants who are temporarily taken off the breast during hospitalization for illness or surgery of either mother or infant. Such mothers can be encouraged to relactate, providing of course, that the practitioner is aware of the simplicity of the process so that this can be promoted as a realistic possibility. If the infant is too weak or small to suckle, relactation may be initiated with the expression of breast milk either manually or with the use of a breast pump.

Oral Rehydration Therapy (ORT)

Gastroenteritis is one of the major problems that contribute significantly to high levels of infant and young child morbidity and mortality. Associated with an episode of vomiting and diarrhea, there is generally loss of appetite, a cultural or medical modification of the diet, and the possiblity of significant fluid loss and dehydration. Repeated and prolonged bouts of gastroenteritis present a major problem in the etiology of malnutrition, the immediate concern is treatment of acute dehydration and management of fluid losses.

There was a time when children with severe dehydration were taken to emergency centers for intravenous rehydration. Because of the inaccessability and paucity of such centers in many parts of the world and problems with provision of intravenous fluids, other approaches have been explored. In Bangladesh it was discovered that oral rehydration can provide readily available and appropriate management of acute dehydration. With the addition of glucose, such salt and water solutions have been noted to be readily absorbed through the intestinal wall.

When vomiting and diarrhea are associated with dehydration, oral rehydration therapy (ORT) has been initiated followed by major reduction in mortality rates. Recognition of the signs and symptoms of dehydration have been taught not only to paraprofessional health workers, but can be demonstrated in the villages so that signs can be recognized even by the mother. Some international agencies, governments, and drug companies have put out packets which simply need to be mixed with clean water. If these are not available 'a three finger pinch of salt, a hand grasp of sugar or molasses, and a liter of clean water' are all that are needed to have an excellent oral rehydration fluid [24, 25]. ORT is not only appropriate, but reproducable at the village level and represents both a feasible and an important first line of defense against dehydration. In a 1983 international conference held in Washington, D.C., ORT gained world wide publicity. Health workers from various countries gathered to exchange views on the importance and methods of oral rehydration therapy. This procedure, formulated in less developed countries, has major world wide implications for saving lives and promoting home-based management for dehydration, a serious condition in infants and young children [26].

Geographic pathology

Geographic pathology has recently emerged as an important new field in medicine. The theory of 'balanced polymorphism' was first described by British hematologists working in East Africa where they identified areas with a high gene prevalence rate for sickle cell anemia as being coincident with locations where *Plasmodium Falciparum* malaria was hyperendemic. Subsequently, the geographic distribution of Burkitt's Lymphoma in Africa was found to be similar to areas where mosquitoes were responsible for the transmission of both malaria and certain viral diseases. The correlation which was made implicates viral preconditions in the pathogenesis of malignancies. In infectious diseases as well as in oncology and hematology, scientists continue their investigation of the phenomena of geographic pathology.

Nutrition

We are indebted to the developing world for both the potatoe and corn (maize) as important world wide food staples and our recent awareness of the significance of dietary fiber, an extremely vital basic factor in various disease processes. Nondigestible fiber when present in abundant quantity in the diet tends to reduce intestinal transit time, and is closely associated with low incidence rates of such conditions as hiatal hernia, diverticulosis, appendicitis, colon cancer, and hemorrhoids [27]. Investigation is being pursued that associates the increased ingestion of fiber with a concommitant reduction of coronary heart disease thought to be related to an interference with cholesterol absorption. There is additional interest in the fact that the high cholesterol consumption of East African Masai groups may be counterbalanced by their significant physical activity which results in a low level of serum cholesterol as well as a low incidence of coronary heart disease.

Medical budgeting

In lesser developed countries, associated with the shortage of hospital beds and a lack of trained health personnel, hospital stay has, of necessity, been shortened [1, 4]. Not only have patients not suffered, but it seems that shorter hospital stays following surgical procedures and normal deliveries have a beneficial effect. Certain post-operative complications such as venous thrombosis, intestinal ileus, and problems associated with inactivity and bed rest, can be minimized or avoided by early ambulation. Patients who are ambulated early generally have a shorter period in hospital making it cost effective for the hospital, for medical insurance companies, and for the patient. A procedure introduced out of necessity in developing countries has been incorporated into standard protocols in the developed world because its' benefits have been substantiated [2, 11].

A restricted drug list was initiated in many developing countries by the necessity of limiting the budget for medications [28, 29, 30]. It is inappropriate to have duplication of various forms of the same medication, as well as having combinations of multiple drugs in a single item. From a therapeutic point of view, it is to the patient's benefit to have a more comprehensive diagnostic work-up that yields a specific diagnosis and leads to a more exact course of medical intervention. Whether out of economic concerns and/or improved patient care, the concept of restricting lengthy drug lists should be transferred to the more developed countries.

Changes in awareness

With the training of paraprofessional personnel who have demonstrated a capacity for assuming broader roles in the health care system, a gradual demystification of medicine has been encouraged. An emphasis on health and nutrition education, given the limitations of our information base, has permitted the patient to play an important role in his own care. Certain practitioners have been reluctant to involve the patient in self-care and to relinquish full control, but there are indications of improvement. The development of a community health worker cadre and a community board of directors has involved the community in matters of health care, making it more responsive to the individual's needs. The general population now cares for part of their own health and should assume greater responsibility in this regard.

Practitioners who have worked abroad return to their own countries with a greater appreciation of the importance of cultural and environmental influences on health. Their awareness yields benefits through the recognition of the many factors that directly and indirectly influence health status. A cultural orientation helps clarify the bases for patient compliance or lack of compliance. Traditional therapy has been recognized as playing a major role in disease management, along with Western (or modern) therapy [8, 10].

The tendency to emphasize the esoteric and advanced tertiary care attracts the physician and the medical educator in both developed and developing countries. An awareness is growing of the additional need to emphasize both prevention and routine ambulatory care. It is acknowledged that the majority of any population is not found in medical centers providing tertiary care. Most people are ambulatory and, if not well, may suffer from rather common and often easily preventable conditions. It is both less expensive and more appropriate to emphasize prevention and health education and to provide basic level primary health care. In developing areas health workers may have little option beyond the provision of primary care, preventive measures, and education. Public health workers woold wide agree that preventive efforts deserve more attention, but they are faced with a long delay before benefits are realized from these measures and a recognition that prevention is less exciting an option compared with injections, surgery, and more immediate forms of intervention [2, 11].

Summary

In this chapter there has been presented a potpourri of changes that have been adopted by administrators, trainers, and health workers in the developed countries from documentated experience in the Third World. The reverse transfer from the lesser developed countries must be acknowledged.

The development of Under Five Clinics and the employment of a weight-for-age home based record system have yielded certain benefits. The recruitment, training and employment of paraprofessional health workers of various types has been another positive step in health care delivery systems, as has the use of the triage procedure.

The promotion of breastfeeding for infants in all segments of the population and the universal application of oral rehydration therapy represent positive steps in patient management. The identification of fiber as an important ingredient in normal diets is a simple measure in the area of nutrition and prevention which has universal application.

In conjunction with the employment of paraprofessional health workers, a restricted drug list contributes both to improved patient care as well as having an effect to reduce medical costs.

Finally, physicians and nurses who worked in developing countries, as short term volunteers or with longer commitments, have returned to the developed world with different values, different orientation, and the opportunity to introduce many changes in their professional activities. Health care workers and patients have benefited from these exposures. Some changes are on an individual basis, whereas other modifications have found their way into larger programs and systems. The cross-fertilization process is very interesting, and something of which we all should be aware. It is with deep humility that acknowledgement is given to the many patients and colleagues who have helped in this continuing process. The developed countries must recognize their debt to the Third World.

References

1. Morley D: Paediatric priorities in the developing world. London, Butterworth, 1973.
2. Jonas S (ed): Health care delivery in the United States. New York, Springer, 1977.
3. Jelliffe DB, Jelliffe EFP (eds): Human nutrition. 2: Nutrition and growth. New York, Plenum Press, 1979.
4. King M (ed): Medical care in developing countries. Nairobi, Oxford University Press, 1966.
5. Waife RS, Burkhart MC (eds): The non-physician and family health in Sub-Sahara-Africa.

Boston, The Pathfinder Fund, 1981.

6. DeLorenzo L, DeLorenzo R: Total child care: from birth to age five. Garden City, NY, Doubleday, 1982.
7. Cunningham N, Anisfeld E: Personal communication, 1983.
8. Lee RPL: Chinese and western medical care in China's rural communes. World Health For 3:301, 1982.
9. WHO: The promotion and development of traditional medicine. Technical Report Series 622, Geneva, 1978.
10. Newell KW (ed): Health of the people. WHO, Geneva, 1975.
11. Roemer MI, Roemer RJ: Health care systems and comparative manpower policies. New York, Marcel Dekker, 1981.
12. Brown RE: Starving children, the tyranny of hunger. New York, Springer, 1977.
13. Brown RE: Poverty and health in the United States. Clin Pediat 8:495, 1969.
14. Helsing E, King FS: Breastfeeding in practice. New York, Oxford University Press, 1982.
15. Ghosh S: The feeding and care of infants and young children. New Delhi, Voluntary Health Association of India, 1977.
16. Cameron M, Hofvander Y: Manual on feeding infants and young children. New York, Oxford University Press, 1983.
17. Eiger MS, Olds SW: The complete book of breastfeeding. New York, Bantam Books, 1972.
18. Jelliffe DB, Jelliffe EFP: Human milk in the modern world. London, Oxford University Press, 1978.
19. Mosley WH (ed): Nutrition and human reproduction. New York, Plenum Press, 1978.
20. Cunningham AS: Morbidity in breast fed and artificially fed infants. J Pediat 90:726, 1977.
21. Cunningham AS: Morbidity in breast fed and artificially fed infants II. J Pediat 95:685, 1979.
22. Brown RE: Relactation: an overview. Pediatrics 60:116, 1977.
23. Cohen R: Breastfeeding without pregnancy. Pediatrics 48:996, 1971.
24. Parker RL, Rinehart W, Piotrow PT, Doucette L: Oral rehydration therapy (ORT) for childhood diarrhea population reports. 8 (6), 1980.
25. Rahaman MM, Aziz KMS, Munshi MH, Patwari Y, Rahman M: A diarrhea clinic in rural Bangladesh: influence of distance, age and sex on attendance and diarrheal mortality. Am J Publ Health 72:1124, 1982.
26. Grant JP: The state of the world's children, 1982–83. New York, UNICEF 1982.
27. Burkitt DP: Relationships between disease and their etiological significance. Am J Clin Nutr 30:262, 1977.
28. Gross FH, Inman WHW (eds): Drug monitoring. London, Academic Press, 1977.
29. WHO: The selection of essential drugs. Report of the WHO expert committee, Technical Report Series, No. 615, Geneva, 1977.
30. WHO: The selection of essential drugs. Report of the WHO expert committee, Technical Report Series, No. 641, Geneva, 1979.

Summing up and conclusions

P.G. JANSSENS

From the outset, the symposium on 'Child Health in the Tropics' tackled the number one problem, diarrhoea. It was introduced by an excellent overview of a number of developing countries and Hong-Kong.

In connection with infantile diarrhoea, breastfeeding was scrutinized by Professor Omololu (Ibadan). He reminded us quite rightly that the only one in control of the whole process is the mother. Her role is decisive, she makes the decision between breast and bottle, she decides about a rhytmn on demand or in accordance with some timing. She also decides about the length of breastfeeding and the start of weaning.

A follow-up study in the Bakau community (the Gambia) by Dr. Rowland provided useful complementary information about weaning. He was able to ascertain that the age of weaning is not as critical as the weaning itself. It may be induced at an early stage without exaggerated risks. The advertisements about commercial foods may give risk to weaning at a much earlier stage than the traditional one. Anyway, weaning will produce at its onset a drop in growth performance, start intestinal and other infections and malnutrition. This trend is, however, neither consistently nor necessarily severe. Furthermore an early onset of weaning is not incompatible with prolonged breastfeeding. Inexperienced young mothers have on the whole a good judgment about the moment to start the weaning. Breastfeeding as such does not prevent diarrhoeal disease.

Ir. W. Klaver (Wageningen) gave a well-illustrated documentation about proportions of staple foods and complementary foods, visualized in a table of double mixes, that allow the quick formulation of multiple mixes without having to resort to detailed food composition tables. Oil is added to the mixes in order to correct the energy gap without compromising the level of utilizable protein.

Dr. L. Sinisterra discussed the basic problems of the socially disrupted organization of the mixed population of tropical America, and more especially of Colombia. The contrast between the socio-economic state of the top and the other strata is appalling: this should be recognized as the key to the problem. The situation is, moreover, deteriorating due to the increasing urbanization, which ends up in a 'ruralization of the cities'. The nutritional situation requires a serious and adapted solution: second zone citizens are undersized, have muscles of lower quality and are less bright. Improvement of nutrition on the contrary decreases the number of diarrhoea and fever episodes. Incorpar, which is adapted to the needs and traditions of Indians, had to be adapted to the other groups.

The improvement of laboratory techniques made it possible to identify the etiology in 80% of the diarrhoeas, whereas this percentage referred previously to the unknowns. Salmonella, shigella, campylobacter, yersinia staphylococcus, enterotoxic and enteropathogenic E coli, rotavirus etc. are the main offenders, sometimes even in association. Convulsions and meningitis may be produced by several of these organisms.

Those are the facts, but what is their real meaning? It is obvious that they are not the major cause of diarrhoea in children, but are epiphenomenon on the basic disturbances facing infants living in unsanitary surroundings. Lack of drinking water, inadequate sanitation, excessive crowding, low personal hygiene, malnutrition, low degree of education of the parents – a situation comparable to the one prevailing in the slum areas of New York in 1900, as Professor Feris (Santo Domingo) reminded us.

This relation was clearly demonstrated by Professor Yeung (Hong Kong). In his country the improvement of the standards of living and education has indeed changed the whole picture for the better.

A major break through in the treatment of diarrhoeal diseases has been oral rehydration, combined with continuing breast or other feeding, notwithstanding the diarrhoea. Dr. Abdul Molla (Dacca) pleaded aptly for the replacement of glucose by rice powder in the ORS and produced some solid facts about the thus induced purging rates and lowered volume, which support his efficient adaptation of rehydration and maintenance of hydration.

A consensus came forward about the capital role of the mother in the implementation of ORS. She should prepare the solution. This direct participation in the fight against diarrhoea will become a major factor in her trust and in the motivation of other mothers, as was underlined by Professor Okeahialam (Enugu). The salt content of the available water may be a problem. It has also been emphasized that, however important the role of well trained community workers might be, the mother is the pre-eminent primary health care worker. Moreover some resistance against ORS must be overcome, even in some doctors. Dr. Kahn (Lahore) and Dr. Suharyono (Djakarta) drew attention to many of those points.

All agree that effective early ORS administration and early refeeding are of paramount importance to break the vicious circle and Professor Feris (Santo Domingo) underlined that spoon administration of ORS is to be preferred over bottle administration in order to avoid dangerous practices. The 'ROSE system' rehydration, orally too, simultaneous education recommended by Dr. Suhanyono has been generally approved.

Mrs. Ayesha Molla (Dacca) provided an excellent survey of practical feeding during diarrhoea. She also presented interesting data on all kinds of correlations between malabsorption and nutrient losses.

For this 'most serious disease in infancy' and threat for lower class children, vaccination programmes, even against the major organisms, are no substitutes for better sanitation.

The role of drugs was incidentally involved without practical conclusions.

The second day made a good start with two complementary presentations about assessing nutritional and health status, as seen from the National Institute of Nutrition (Indian Council of Medical Research) and as lived at the village level. Dr. Mathur (Hyderabad) presented an impressive study about the scientific methodology of evaluation. How to collect data, how to quantify major health problems, how to handle anthropometric indications, how to implement an assessment, how to change attitudes and motivate those concerned.

Professor Morley (London) reminded us, in his own unadulterated lively style, of the cycle of undernutrition and the importance of energy density. This became the occasion to emphasize the need for good and easy measurements by the use of simple easily-understandable charts, of the usefulness of simple gadgets and short cuts on the road to health. The 'arm circumference growth chart' was for some amongst us a newcomer.

On the previous day Professor Voravarn Tanphaichitr (Bangkok) had captivated the audience with her experience about the bodily growth in thalassaemia. A good example of the high quality of research at the faculty of medicine, Mahidol University.

Professor Vichai Tanphaichitr treated us with an equally brilliant exposé on the epdemiology and clinical assessment of vitamin deficiencies in Thai children. Its survey of the Infantile Beriberi will become a classic. The description of suggestive signs and diagnostic clues, including laboratory assessment through erythrocyte transketolase activity (ETKA) and other such techniques, was fascinating. He also stressed that beriberi will follow an inadequate intake of thiamine, but also increases thiamine requirements. He discussed further riboflavine and vitamin A deficiencies, so important and dangerous for infants and children in many developing countries.

Dr. D. Brasseur and Dr. Ph. Goyens provided the symposium with some of the results of the Brussels study in depth of P.E.M. in the Kion. It was an excellent opportunity for discussing the interest and obscurities of lactose malabsorption and the atrophy of the jejunal mucosa, persisting after recovery. Some trace elements (zinc, copper, selenium), which interfere with the physiopathology, have been analyzed also by reliable metallo enzymetic methods. However, therapeutic selective trials were without influence on the mortality or on the healing process. The interpretation and practical value of these data still remain obscure.

The possible sources of the high percentage of L.B.W. in the developing countries, and especially in Africa, have been scrutinized by Professor Tafari (Addis Ababa). He analyzed both the foetal and maternal factors. He put emphasis on the precedence of energy over protein, the effect of zinc deficiency on the outcome of pregnancy, the role of perinatal infection, the importance of chorioamniotitis and maternal hypovolemia.

Professor Olowe (Lagos) could highlight with understandable satisfaction that the L.B.W. Nigerian infants have on the whole a better chance of survival and grow better than elsewhere. Therefore the Nigerian child is not endowed genetically to be smaller. Good living standards will improve the prevailing situation. Dr. Boersma (Curaçao) devoted much work and research to the perinatal growth in the tropics.

Dr. Canosa (Valencia) reported his recent experience in Bangladesh as a WHO consultant, where he studied the urban and rural situation on 65 precoded variables in high and low income groups. He provided thus a wealth of information on age of marriage, miscarriages, stillbirth, low birth weight, risk factors etc.

The organization of neonatal intensive care in Bombay, presented by Dr. Daga, was rich in useful information and data. Dr. Daga showed that efficient help can be given without the western high costs practiced by emphasizing breastfeeding, providing thermo regulation, prevention of infection, effective use of maternity wards and still saving nurse hours. In this setting septecaemia and umbilical sepsis remain killers, but diarrhoeal episodes can be reduced markedly.

Dr. Alisjahbana (Bandung) and Dr. Martodipuro (Surabaya) introduced us to situations regarding Indonesian newborns. It is difficult to get good data on poor reporting. This was an incentive for Dr. Alisjahbana to develop a methodology of survey based on interviews by traditional birth attendants. The determinants of intro-uterine and postnatal growth in rural areas are undoubtedly age, parity, birth interval, all of which are factors associated with L.B.W. Dr. Martodipuro is using under guidance and supervision a 'pregnancy monitoring chart' which serves to raise the awareness of the mother, improves the antenatal and selects the high risks. The education process of the mother and attendants can be improved by simulation games, an excellent methodology to improve consciousness.

The correlation of the monitoring chart and the observed facts are good; the indicators are manageable and scientifically sound. Financial contribution comes from the village head and not from governmental salaries.

The Indonesian symphony was achieved by Professor Kusin (Amsterdam), who presented so lively and convincingly the nutritional aspects of the mother-infant dyad in Madura. Having underlined that L.B.W. is not the same problem all over the world, she emphasized further that this is also true for Indonesia. In Madura the situation is typical for a developing country: L.B.W. and P.E.M. in infants and a poor nutritional state of the mothers, not less during pregnancy. This situation can be improved by the administration of enriched food during the last 90 days of pregnancy. The condition of the newborn will benefit from a slowly progressive supplementary 99 kcal (banana) from the first month on. All this follows monthly home visits and antenatal clinic, ensured by locally trained and supervised ancillary personnel, to weigh, measure, monitor growth, and convince and educate. This programme is successful because of its continuity, generating indispensable participation and confidence. This illuminating example will certainly bear fruit outside of Madura.

I kept for the dessert the important and substantial communication of Professor Hendrickse (Liverpool). He focussed the interest of an attentive audience on the mycotoxins much neglected by the medical profession.

Nevertheless 'ochatoxins' of Aspergillus and Penicillium may produce nephropathy beyond the Balkans. 'Zearalones' of fusarium, in cereals, beer and sour porridge, show oestrogenic effects in pigs, why not in gyneacomastia of man.

'Trichothecenes' are known to produce toxic aleutia, as happened previously in the Sovjet Union. But of course, blue and green Aflatoxins and Aflatoxicol with the many metabolic effects of this dynamic complex got, for good reason, the main attention. The reason being that 'the more malnutrition, the more susceptibility to Aflatoxin', which is present in so many households (up to 80%) and meals (46% in Sudan); these deleterious potentials are moreover enhanced by malnutrition. The multifactoral origin of malnutrition versus marasmus is in need of better understanding. Aflatoxin may be associated with it.

'Child Health in the Tropics' has been more than the Sixth Nutricia – Cow & Gate Symposium, it has been a highly successful encounter. It brought together, on an excellent programme covering the main problems of the newborn and their mothers, a group of educators and practitioners active in this field selected by a Nigerian/Belgian association of quality.

The unabated attention of the audience and the lively discussions produced evidence of a good choice of items and speakers. All of us are waiting for the proceedings. They will offer a more thorough knowledge of the invaluable facts and data presented at this symposium. It will stimulate our future activities in our respective fields and also our thinking and our approach of the 'Child Health in the Tropics'.

Index of subjects